DISTANCE
RUNNING

Robert M. Lyden

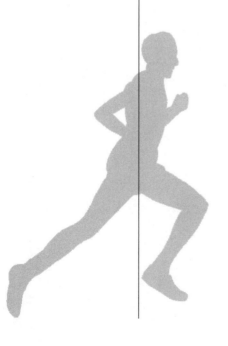

Published privately in the United States of America

Printed by Sheridan Books, Inc., Ann Arbor, Michigan

ISBN: 0-9724144-0-1

Library of Congress Catalog Card Number: 2003093464

Book layout, cover design: Paul Lewis

Cover photo: The author running at Cannon Beach, Oregon, 1999. Photo by Shellie Lyden.

Published by The Running Book, LLC

For information, contact: therunningbook@yahoo.com

DEDICATION

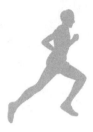

*T*o my wife Shellie, our son Kieran,
and my parents for their love.

ACKNOWLEDGMENTS

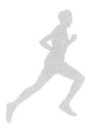

I wish to thank the following persons and institutions for their assistance or contributions to this work: Per-Olaf Åstrand at the Karolinska Institute, Franz Berghold at the University of Salzburg, the late Bill Bowerman, Russell Burrows of New York, Forbes Carlile of Sydney, Australia, Karen Carpenter at Sports Illustrated, Peter Cavanagh at Penn State University, Nancy Cerutty of Portsea, Australia, Scott Cheshier and Corbis Photo Archives, David L. Costill of Muncie, Indiana, Edward F. Coyle at the University of Texas at Austin, George Dales of Kalamazoo, Michigan, Jack Daniels at Cortland State University, Erin Davis at Butler University, Bill Dellinger of Eugene, Oregon, Herb Elliott of Perth, Australia, Jim Ferstle of St. Paul, Minnesota, William H. Freeman at Campbell University, Edwin S. Fox and Jon Hendershott at Track & Field News, E.C. Frederick of Brentwood, New Hampshire, Rustem Igor Gamow at the University of Colorado, Roy Griak at the University of Minnesota, Joe Henderson of Eugene, Oregon, George Herringshaw and sporting-heroes.net of Leicester, England, Chick Hislop at Weber State University, Nobuya Hashizume of Plymouth, Minnesota, John Idstrom of Santa Cruz, California, Tom Ivers of Washougal, Washington, Peter Janssen of Deurne, Netherlands, Karl Keska of Wolverhampton, England, Damien Koch of Fort Collins, Colorado, B. Kummer at Sportverlag, Berlin, Chester Kyle of Weed, California, Arthur Lydiard of Auckland, New Zealand, Sarah Maddock at Penguin UK / Pelham Books, Milan Mader of Lakeville, Minnesota, John McKenzie of Fort Worth, Texas, Carolyn McMahon and AP / Wide World Photos, George Mitchell and USA TODAY Photo Archives, Melanie Moenig and Keystone Photos of Germany, Kenny Moore of Kailua, Hawaii, Klaus-Jürgen Müller and Heribert Simons at the University of Freiburg, Germany, Eric Newsholme at Oxford University and John Wiley & Sons Limited, Dr. Tim Noakes at the Sports Science Institute of Cape Town, South Africa and Retesha Thadison at Human Kinetics, Scott Pengelly of Eugene, Oregon, Steve Plasencia at the University of Minnesota, John Pottage of Mount Eliza, Victoria, Australia, Loan Osborne at Princeton University Press, Victah Sailer and Photorun of Smithstown, New York, Mike Salmon and the Amateur Foundation of Los Angeles, Ron Sass of White Bear Lake, Minnesota, Kristine Schueler and Allan Steinfeld at the New York Road Runners Club, Bob Sevene, of Boston, Massachusetts, Frank Shorter of Boulder, Colorado, Martyn Shorten of Portland, Oregon, Emil Siekkinen and Tomas Lindberg of Stockholm, Sweden, Graem Sims of Sydney, Australia, Bob Stewart of Shoreview, Minnesota, Susan Storch and the University of Oregon Archives—The Knight Library, Anthony Sullivan and Getty Images, Leo Tarantino at Duomo Photography, Edith Unold of Oetwil, Switzerland, Dr. Marc Wiessbluth at Northwestern University School of Medicine, and special thanks to George Dales and John Pottage for editing an early draft of the manuscript, and to Paul Lewis of Monterey, California for his contributions to the book layout and cover design.

CONTENTS

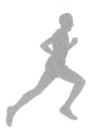

This is the first really original work on distance training in several decades. Most recent books on this subject primarily focus on the physiology of training, and associated training schedules—essentially "man-as-machine." These treatments give us no real philosophical underpinnings for sport, for training, and for their relation to life as a whole. They are one-dimensional theories dealing with multi-dimensional human beings. This book is a return to the "whole person" approach to training—once popular in the era of the great coaches like Bill Bowerman of the United States, Percy Cerutty of Australia, and Arthur Lydiard of New Zealand—where athletes are treated as more than just the sum of abstract physiological constructs, where heart and attitude and desire are as important, and perhaps more so, as measurable physical capacities. For every great champion, there are a hundred or thousand others with the same physiological traits, yet who fail to reach the same level.

This work is divided into four parts: (1) The Foundation and Principles of Training, (2) Strength, Flexibility and Injury Prevention, (3) Special Considerations for Distance Runners, and (4) Appendices, including the Training Schedules. The first part introduces a comprehensive model that reveals the structure, nature, and substance of the training process. In particular, Chapter 1 on Cycles of Acquisition and Training, provides elegant graphics by which the process of athletic development can be clearly visualized and understood. Chapters 2 through 6 address in consecutive order the Base, Hill, Sharpening, Peak, and Post-Season Recovery Periods, following their normal sequence during an athletic season. By the end of part one, you will have an excellent understanding of athletic training and be able to plan and illustrate entire seasons, and multiple years of athletic development.

The next two parts of the book, Strength, Flexibility and Injury Prevention, and Special Considerations for Distance Runners are devoted to often-overlooked essentials. Chapter 7 on Stretching, Flexibility and Movement, teaches a novel form of stretching especially suitable for distance runners, which draws upon particular teachings of *T'ai Chi* and *Yoga*. Certain aspects of the mind-body relationship are also discussed in relation to athletic performance. Chapter 8 expounds the importance of Strength Training for achieving success in distance running. This chapter also provides fitness guidelines for strength training and detailed weight training progressions. Chapter 9 reflects on Injuries and Athletic Shoes, examines numerous common running injuries and indicates possible

conformational, biomechanical, environmental and training errors that contribute to injury. It also examines the historical development of athletic footwear, and problems sometimes associated with specific footwear designs and constructions. The insights provided in this chapter may help you ask the right questions and make more informed choices when purchasing running shoes.

Part three, Special Considerations for Distance Runners, includes five chapters on specific factors affecting running performance, and concludes with two detailed chapters on the Steeplechase and Marathon. Chapter 10 reveals the dramatic effects of Shoe Weight and Mechanical Efficiency upon athletic performance. Chapter 11 on Iron Deficiency Anemia, provides vital information, guidelines, and certain precautions that can be discussed with a medical doctor. Chapter 12 considers the effects of Heat and Humidity upon athletic performance, and teaches how to prepare and successfully compete in these conditions. Chapter 13 on Altitude Training, explores various acclimatization scenarios associated with competition, and also the possible benefits of training at altitude for athletic performance at sea level. Chapter 14 examines the considerable influence of Aerodynamic Drag and Drafting upon athletic performance in the middle-distance and distance events. Chapter 15 addresses the highly specialized training required for The Steeplechase. Chapter 16 discusses training and competition in The Marathon, and raises worthwhile questions concerning participation in this popular event.

The Appendices offer detailed training schedules for runners competing at 800, 1,500, 3,000, 5,000 and 10,000 meters, as well as the marathon. This detailed illustration of how to apply the model and teachings provided in the first part is invaluable. The appendices also include sample schedules for bridging the gap between national championships and major international competitions, such as the World Championships or Olympic Games. These schedules will prove helpful to coaches and athletes facing these challenges for the first time, since relatively few athletes have numerous opportunities to compete in these international events.

The Glossary precisely defines the meaning of various terms used in this text. An extensive Bibliography has been included that should be useful to those who desire to pursue the subject further, and an Index has also been provided for easy reference.

This book is a welcome addition to the running canon. No serious coach or runner should be without it.

—William H. Freeman

Author, *Peak When It Counts.*,
Co-Author with Bill Bowerman,
High Performance Training for Track and Field,
Co-Author with Bill Dellinger,
The Competitive Runner's Training Book

PREFACE

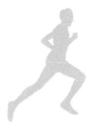

This book originated with the expressed need of coaches and athletes who were searching for understanding and success in distance running. Both are faced with the challenge of acquiring the knowledge and wisdom of a lifetime—while still in their youth. Accordingly, this work is intended to provide you with the benefit of what other sucessful coaches and athletes have learned in their efforts to excel in distance running.

Within this text you will find a comprehensive model of athletic development that integrates discussion of relevant exercise physiology with detailed training programs for specific events. After finishing this book, you will be able to review your training diary and understand what happened, and also why it happened. You will better understand the implications of what you are doing at the present time, and be able to plan your training so as to peak and deliver your personal best performance at the right time and place. Moreover, the principles found in this text can be applied to many other physical activities and sports.

Early drafts of this work have circulated amongst coaches and athletes. As a result, it has been affectionately christened "The Cookbook." Enjoy the recipes, but also strive to transcend them as you master the art. Upon attaining enlightenment, Zen students sometimes ceremoniously burn a copy of the sutras as an outward sign of mastery and liberation. Perhaps, you might instead make a gift of this book to someone else in need.

—Robert M. Lyden
Portland, Oregon 2003

PART I

FOUNDATION AND PRINCIPLES OF TRAINING

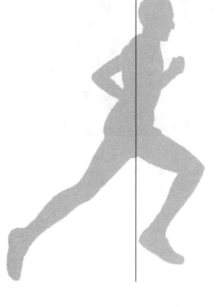

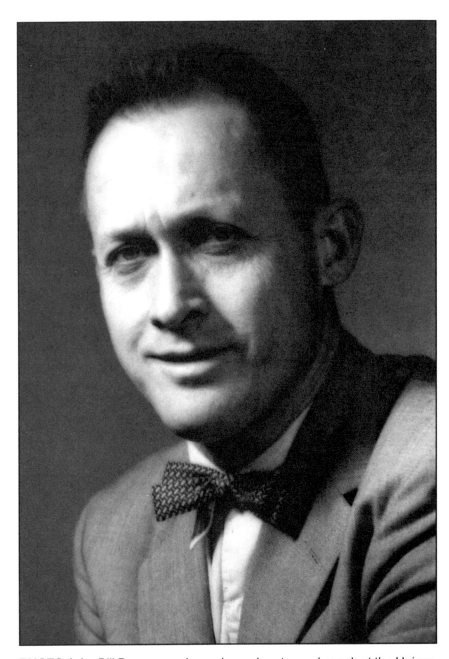

PHOTO 1.1—Bill Bowerman, legendary educator and coach at the University of Oregon, and co-founder of Nike, Inc. Photo by B.L. Freemesser, published by the Oregon Alumni Association, Old Oregon, February-March, 1960. Photo reproduced by permission.

CHAPTER 1

CYCLES OF ACQUISITION AND TRAINING PERIODIZATION

This chapter provides essential information concerning the structure and principles that govern athletic training. While challenging, it provides answers to the most fundamental questions associated with athletic training and development. The model is simple, yet comprehensive, and numerous figures are provided to help you grasp the key concepts. Once a few important relationships are understood, the mystery sometimes associated with training for distance running will be dispelled. As a result, coaches and athletes can plan their training and racing schedules with confidence and enjoy success.

Training Loads and Adaptation

The aim of athletic training is to bring about positive physical and mental adaptations to enable higher levels of performance. A *training load* is an appropriate stimulus, dosed so as to determine a progression effect in the training activity, (Pedemonte, 1982). Of course, we normally refer to training loads as workouts. The components of a training load or workout being:

- Quantity
  - Volume
  - Duration
- Quality
  - Intensity
  - Frequency
  - Density

Adaptation is the first law of survival, and a progression of suitable workouts can enhance athletic performance. However, work for the sake of work is not the answer. You must train intelligently in order to realize improvement. In this regard, planning workouts and performing them are two different things. Here lies the difference between an external training load and an internal training load. In simple terms, an external load is a workout written on a piece of paper. The internal load is the degree of effort the workout imposes on an athlete. For example, let's say two individuals are given the identical external training load of running a five-minute mile. However, one individual is a four-minute miler and the second a five-minute miler. Accordingly, the internal load placed on the first will be nothing compared to that placed on the second. The relationship between an external and an internal training load can be illustrated using the following interval training session including: 4 (5 x 200 meters at 30 seconds) with a 100 meters jog recovery (jr) on the series (S), 200 meters jr on the series break (SB) or set, as shown in Figure 1.1.

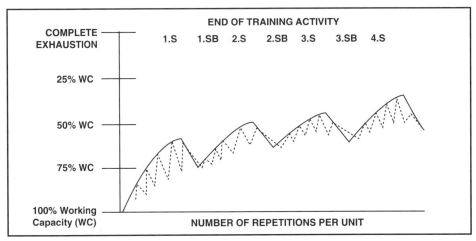

FIGURE 1.1—From Schmolinsky, 1978

As the workout progresses, maintaining the 200 meters series in the pace of 30 seconds requires greater effort. At the same time, maintaining the limited duration of the recovery period also becomes more difficult as the workout progresses. Given that an athlete enters the recovery period in a progressively higher state of fatigue as the workout continues, the recovery becomes progressively inadequate or too short, as compared to the earlier periods. As a result of the increasing internal load, the original recovery period is, in effect, being compressed during the workout. This can condition the athlete to physically and mentally put forth greater effort, and thus maintain the pace during an actual competition. Understanding the relationship between external and internal training loads can help an athlete shape the physical and mental conditioning taking place during training.

Coaches and athletes need to respect and focus upon the internal training load, that is, what is actually happening in a workout, as opposed to what they might have planned on a piece of paper. Do not attempt a planned workout if your body is telling you that it is not ready, or has had enough for the day. The body does not lie, but a piece of paper may do so. Trust, listen and attend to what your body tells you. Have a specific goal for each workout, and keep the workouts simple. Beware of losing touch with reality when planning workouts, as abstract ideas can have an intellectual or emotional appeal when you put pencil to paper. So long as you accomplish the desired physical and mental tasks, simple is best.

The Effect of Training Effort on Improvement

Emil Zatopek, the Olympic Champion at 5,000 meters, 10,000 meters, and the marathon in the 1952 Olympic Games, once drew an analogy between the human body's response to a workout and the reaction of a spring. If you push the "spring" down a bit with a light training load, it will rebound in a relatively short time to a higher level than before. If you push the spring down with a heavier training load, it will take longer to recover and will rebound to an even higher level. However, be careful not to push too hard or too often, because you can damage the spring! (Spear, 1982).

This rebounding of the "spring" and an athlete's fitness to a higher level is commonly known as super-compensation. Accordingly, supercompensation is a cyclical phenomenon. When you undertake a training effort, your body becomes tired and your performance capability temporarily decreases. However, after a period of recovery, your body bounces back more fit than before. It is important to understand the practical effect that different training loads, or workout training efforts, have upon the rate of recovery and the amount of supercompensation. The essential unity of optimal loading and recovery constitutes the building block for all athletic development. The basic supercompensation model is shown in Figure 1.2.

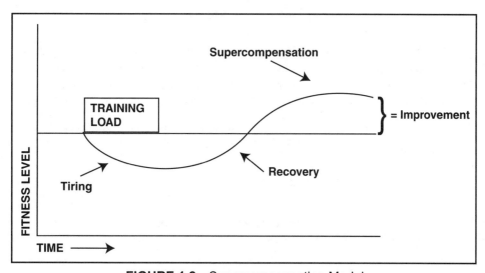

FIGURE 1.2—Supercompensation Model

This model represents only one possible training scenario. In reality, one of three different things can happen depending upon the magnitude of the training load in a given workout. The training load can either be:

1. *Too easy*—A training load that requires little effort provides for some supercompensation and improvement, but not a great deal as shown in Figure 1.3. This is commonly known as under-training. When under-training, athletes can conduct a workout without fear of hurting themselves, and the net result will still be positive.

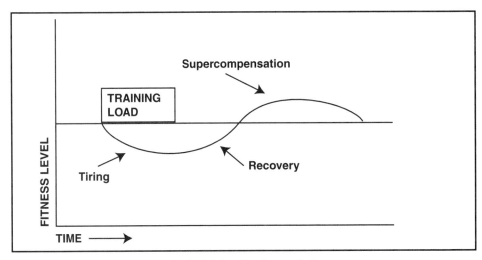

FIGURE 1.3—Under-training

2. *Too hard*—A training load that is too difficult can actually set an athlete backwards and result in a loss of fitness, as shown in Figure 1.4. This is commonly known as overtraining. Recognize that athletes can injure not only their muscles and tendons, but also their metabolism.

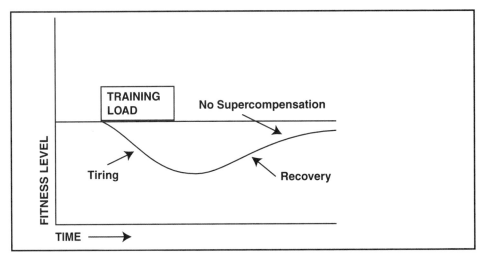

FIGURE 1.4—Over-training

3. *Just right*—A training load that solicits an optimal effort which provides substantial supercompensation and improvement, as shown in Figure 1.5.

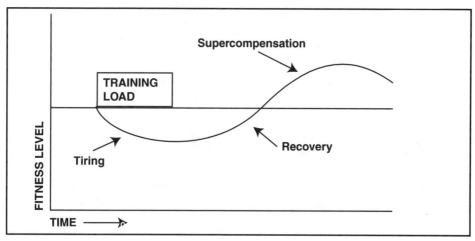

FIGURE 1.5—Optimal training

Figure 1.6 shows the alternate effects of under-training, optimal training, and overtraining on the rate of recovery and supercompensation. Figure 1.7 also shows the effects of various training efforts on the rate of recovery and supercompensation.

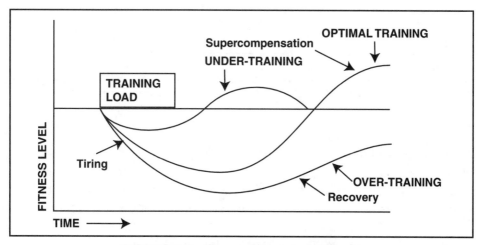

FIGURE 1.6—Three different resultants

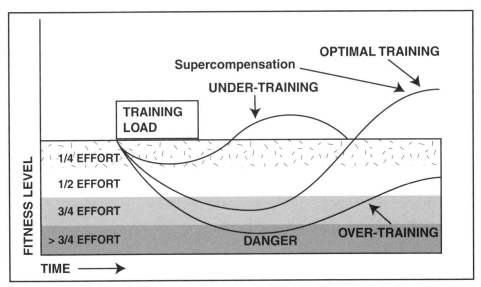

FIGURE 1.7—Three different resultants with effort levels

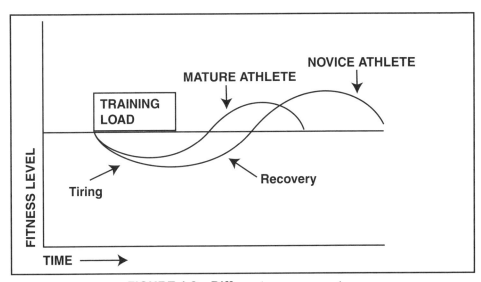

FIGURE 1.8—Different recovery rates

As shown in Figure 1.8, mature athletes recover faster from a given training load than their younger counterparts, but mature athletes do not as a rule enjoy as much resulting supercompensation, or convertibility from supercompensation to improved performances. Moreover, the suitability of any exercise for competitive training should be defined exclusively by how useful it is for developing performance in any given competitive event (Harre, 1982).

In light of the above, under-training is always better than overtraining. Under-training provides for some potential improvement, but overtraining actually destroys athletic fitness. When in doubt, risk under-training rather than overtraining. As a rule, whenever coaches or athletes find themselves asking whether they should call it a day, *the mere posing of the question provides the answer.*

The Effect of Training Frequency on Improvement

Another important variable effects supercompensation and improvement: the training frequency as it relates to the summation of the supercompensatory effects. Here again, one of three things can happen, depending on whether succeeding training loads or workouts are properly timed:

1. *Too far apart*
2. *Too close*
3. *Just Right*

The proper time for an athlete to apply the next training load is while he or she is still at the peak of the supercompensation resulting from the preceding training load. In simple terms, an athlete first pushes down the spring, then allows it to rebound. The idea is to catch the spring while it is at the highest point of rebound and then to repeat the process. Consider what happens in the three scenarios indicated above.

Too far apart—If too much time slips by, the enhancement of ability is lost, and the athlete has to repeat the work all over again. From the standpoint of training frequency, the athlete is under-training. Figure 1.9 shows this by representing an athlete's fitness level on the left axis over time. There is no difference between the initial and final position on this axis, so no enduring adaptation or improvement in the athlete's performance potential has taken place.

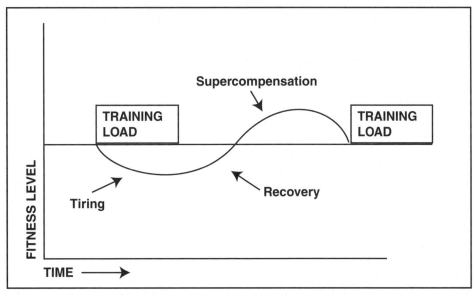

FIGURE 1.9—Training frequency too low.

Too Close—If succeeding workouts are placed too close together the result will be cumulative overloading and overtraining. In the abstract, the succeeding training load could be well within the athlete's capabilities, but in actual practice, coming too soon after the preceding training load, it will impose an overload while the athlete is insufficiently recovered. If a runner does not wait long enough for the resulting supercompensation to arrive, the process can be undermined and the athlete will then go backwards, as shown in Figure 1.10.

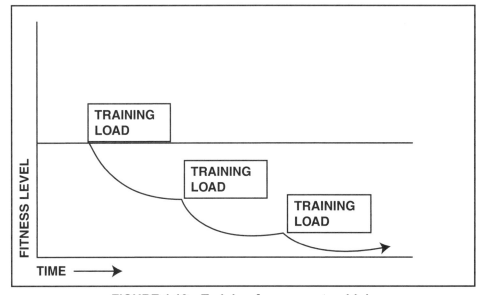

FIGURE 1.10—Training frequency too high.

In this case, from the standpoint of the frequency of training loads, an athlete is overtraining. The athlete will become more and more fatigued and the probability of illness or injury greatly increases. Over-training can result in the following symptoms commonly associated with overstress:

• Insomnia
• Illness
• Injury
• Anxiety
• Loss of appetite
• A higher resting pulse rate

Just Right—Given optimal training frequency, the timing or spacing of the training loads will be just right. As shown in Figure 1.11, the succeeding training load should be placed at the crest of the resulting rebound and wave of supercompensation. The difference between the initial and final position as indicated on the fitness level (left) axis indicates the amount of change or positive adaptation. This change corresponds to an improvement in the athlete's level of fitness and performance potential:

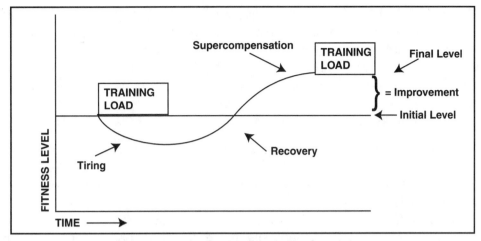

FIGURE 1.11—Optimal training frequency

Keep in mind that the training load tolerances and powers of recovery of individual athletes will vary. More mature athletes have greater training load tolerance and powers of recovery. Thus, relative to young athletes they require more frequent or heavier training loads in order to realize optimal improvement. In sum, the rebound of the spring results in improvement. The trick is to know what is a suitable training load and effort, and how long to wait in order to recover and catch the spring at the crest of the resulting rebound.

What constitutes 1/4-effort, 1/2-effort, and 3/4-effort workouts for mature and relatively fit athletes? And what is the length of the recovery period normally required afterwards? Table 1.1 correlates subjective effort with physiological response parameters (Adapted from Freeman, 1989).

EFFORT	INTENSITY	HEART RATE	% VO$_2$ MAX
FULL	MAXIMUM	190+	100+
3/4	SUB-MAXIMUM	180-190	90-100
	HIGH	160-180	70-90
1/2	MEDIUM	150-160	60-70
1/4	LIGHT	130-150	50-60
	LOW	110-130	30-50

TABLE 1.1—Example of an elite athlete. The maximum heart rate and response characteristics will vary greatly between different individuals.

In the training of mature and relatively fit distance runners, coaches often advocate the so-called hard-day/easy-day rule. However, this rule cannot be used in every circumstance. As shown in Table 1.1, training loads corresponding to 1/4-effort, 1/2-effort, 3/4-effort, and full-effort each require a different recovery period for an athlete to rebound, supercompensate, and then be ready for another quality training load. Given the various training loads commonly assumed by distance runners, the corresponding recovery periods are approximately:

- 24 hours, or 1 day following a 1/4-effort training load, or low intensity workout
- 36 to 48 hours, or 2 days following a 1/2-effort training load, or medium intensity workout
- 48 to 72 hours, or 3 days following a 3/4-effort training load, that is, a high or sub-maximal intensity workout—generally two such training efforts should be kept 3 to 4 days apart
- 72 to 96 hours, or 3 to 4 days minimum following a full effort, but as discussed below, most workouts should not exceed 3/4-effort

These parameters generally dictate the required training frequency between succeeding training loads or workouts for distance runners. Optimal training is a lot like playing music. If you play the right notes with proper rests, you have a melody, otherwise you have nothing but useless noise. Again, recognize that the more gifted, fit, or mature athlete possesses a faster rate of recovery from any given training load than a less gifted or fit individual. The former will rebound earlier and be ready for the next demanding workout while the latter is still tired and inadequately recovered. Therefore, the workouts must be individualized. Otherwise, the combination of quantity (volume and duration) and quality (intensity, frequency and density) could be ideal for one athlete, but counterproductive and perhaps even destructive to another. How do you accomplish this in practice? Let's say a coach is planning to have a boy's high school cross-country team conduct the following interval workout during the sharpening period: 4 (4 x 200 meters) at 32 seconds with a 100 meters jog recovery during the series, and 200 meters jog recovery at the set or series break. This workout could be fine for mature athletes who possess state championship potential, but the following changes could be made to individualize the routine for other team members:

- The quantity (volume and duration) could be reduced to perhaps just two sets for the freshmen, and three for the sophomores and less talented or less fit juniors and seniors
- The intensity could be reduced from 32 seconds to 34 or 36 seconds
- The density could be decreased by providing a 200 meters jog recovery during the series, and 400 meters at the set, or series break

In this way, athletes of all levels of ability can conduct the same type of workout on the same day, and the entire team can maintain the same training frequency. Normally, this is the best course of action when athletes having different levels of ability are following the same competitive schedule. An unfortunate situation can occur when workouts are constructed and directed towards only the most talented or mature athletes, and the rest are left to chase the leaders. As a result, the younger athletes overtrain, and soon experience residual or chronic fatigue problems. If and when they survive the process, the practical effect is to sharpen them faster than the mature athletes—that is, to give them more, when they actually require less! The younger athletes will then peak at a lower level of performance than they otherwise would, and relatively early in the season. Most of these athletes will then be on a downhill slope by the time of the championship competitions.

A training load having excessive magnitude can cause injury or exhaustion. As a result, athletes could be highly susceptible to illness and incapable of resuming demanding training for days or even weeks. Accordingly, the dose of training that will produce a supercompensatory effect has a practical limit: Optimal training loads do not normally exceed 3/4-effort. Optimal training does not correspond to maximal effort. However, a 3/4-effort for an elite runner generally corresponds to a heart rate between 160 and 190 beats per minute (bpm). This level of effort is no "walk in the park" by layman's standards.

All things being equal, the greater the training load, the longer the requisite period of recovery—and within certain limitations, the greater will be the supercompensatory effect. But remember, nothing in the various figures and tables found herein determine an athlete's response. It takes much to build, but little to destroy. *A single workout can end an athletic season or career.* Moreover, the price of freedom of the will is a degree of indeterminance in human affairs, and so we face the machinations of chance. The coach and athlete should attempt to reduce, if not completely eliminate the influence of chance or so-called luck on the course of events. In short, those who aim for success strive for certainty. A large part of what passes for luck stems from a positive attitude and a habit of doing all those so-called extra "little" things. They are not extra, nor are they little, because by the end of a season they add up a mountain high!

MICRO-CYCLES: THE WEEKLY VIEW OF ATHLETIC TRAINING

In the course of the preceding discussion and illustration of supercompensatory effects, load-wave phenomena have been introduced. The graphs depict so-called short load-waves corresponding to what are commonly called micro-cycles—the interfacing of day-to-day training, or weekly view of athletic development. We can now address the indissoluble unity of the cycles (loading, recovery, supercompensation, higher loading) and the interfacing of succeeding supercompensatory effects that are characteristic of micro-cycles.

Again, improvement results from a correct alternation of loading and recovery. As shown in Figure 1.12, suitable workouts of varying effort are conducted successively, following appropriate recovery periods. The difference between the initial and final position on the vertical axis indicates the amount of improvement, and the slope of the line drawn between any two given points indicates the rate of change with respect to improvement.

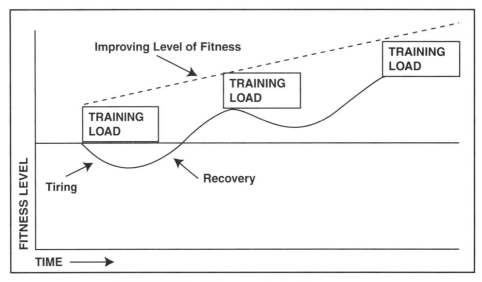

FIGURE 1.12—Micro-cycle loading waves

It is now possible to depict the complex and delicate relationship between optimal loading and recovery required for significant athletic development. In contrast, Figure 1.13 shows a complex series of hypothetical effects that can result from poorly administering the various indicated training loads and recovery periods.

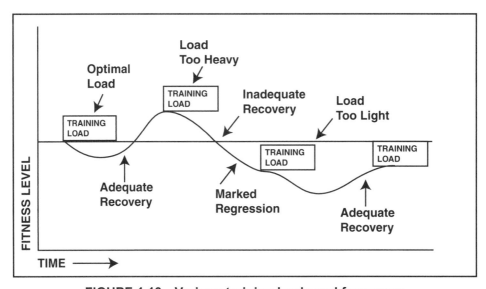

FIGURE 1.13—Various training loads and frequency

In mathematics and physics, a vector represents direction and magnitude. Here, an individual vector arrow can be used to represent the result of each individual supercompensatory cycle by showing the magnitude of gain or loss, and also the direction over any given time period. Moreover, the slope of each vector indicates the rate of change for any given interval of time. Further, adding a given string of individual vectors tip-to-tail determines the final product of an extended series, thus deriving the larger resultant vector. The individual and resultant vectors can sometimes be used to illustrate the momentum developed by a series of training efforts. Again, the larger resultant vector sums the entire group of individual events, and its slope represents the rate of change over the entire series, as shown in Figures 1.14 and 1.15.

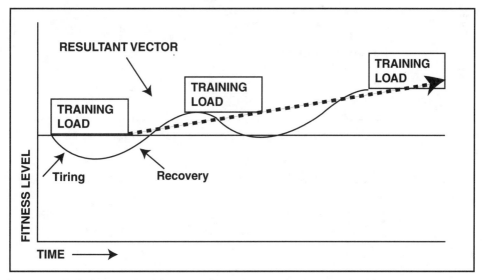

FIGURE 1.14—Vector = direction and magnitude of change

An ideal unity of loading and recovery fosters optimal athletic development, because the athlete successively assumes optimal training loads after appropriate recovery periods. The difference between the initial and final position on the left axis indicates the amount of change and positive adaptation. If the training loads suit an individual's athletic development, this change directly corresponds to improvement in the runner's performance potential.

As shown in Figure 1.15, the resultant vector indicates the end result of a series of non-optimal training events. The difference between the initial and final position represents the change in performance potential. The slope [slope = change in y (vertical) over change in x (horizontal)] of this resultant vector indicates the rate of change in performance potential.

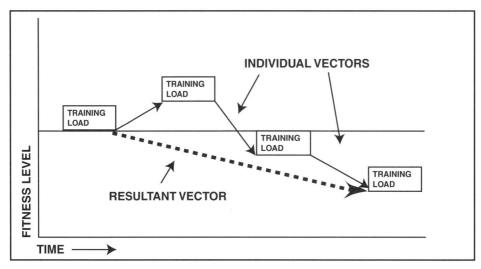

FIGURE 1.15—Individual and resultant vectors

Coaches or athletes would do well to take their training schedule or diary and to diagram the various training loads and recovery periods. Seeing is believing. Due to the importance of our visual sense, this exercise can provide clarity and understanding. Figure 1.16 shows an example of a micro-cycle for possible use during an athletic season:

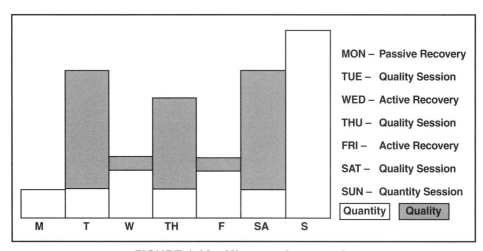

FIGURE 1.16—Micro-cycle example

When using this weekly model or training schedule during the base period, a 3/4-effort anaerobic threshold session would be conducted on Tuesday, a 1/2-effort fartlek session on Thursday, and a 3/4-effort evenly paced steady state on Saturday. During subsequent hill and sharpening periods, days of heavier training loads would again be placed on Tuesday and Saturday. This consistency results in better acquisition and a faster rate of athletic development. The content of the passive and active recovery sessions undertaken on Monday, Wednesday, and Friday are essentially unchanging. Whenever possible, throughout the base, hill, and sharpening periods, retain a 1/2-effort fartlek session on Thursday, and an easy long run on Sunday.

Obviously, associating specific days of the week with particular training tasks is quite arbitrary, serving only as an illustration. It is the pattern and balance of the training that is important. The special needs and requirements associated with delivering optimal performance renders the nature of the activities undertaken during the peak period a special case. Once within the peak period, an athlete is largely sustained by the momentum gathered during the preceding athletic season. However, from the standpoint of enabling optimal performance, this momentum will run its course in just a few weeks.

It is now possible to consider medium load-waves, or meso-cycles—the interfacing of micro-cycles, or weeks of training, to create what could be called the monthly view of athletic development. Following this, long load-waves, or macro-cycles, associated with entire competitive seasons, and finally mega-cycles, which correspond to multiple years of training, can be addressed. However, the micro-cycle is the most critical in its immediate effect upon an athlete. It is the basic building block or *sine qua non* upon which the larger cycles and periodization of training depend.

MESO-CYCLES: THE MONTHLY VIEW OF ATHLETIC TRAINING

The coach and athlete should now be able to visualize and diagram the day-to-day training program and plan several weeks of training. However, the preceding information is insufficient for the purpose of successfully planning an entire athletic season. Consider the following:

Question: Even if you manage to conduct workouts with optimal effort and training frequency, can you continue to train indefinitely and realize improvement?

Answer: No. It is not possible. Even if you provide training loads with appropriate effort, as determined by the quantity (volume, duration) and quality (intensity, density and frequency), it is simply not possible to train strenuously for an indefinite period of time and continue to realize improvement. The primary problem involves the onset of residual fatigue.

The Role of Variation in Preventing Fatigue

The brief recovery periods taken between individual workouts deal effectively with the phenomenon of acute fatigue. Specifically, you work hard and get tired, but over a period of a few hours or days, you recover. However, if you continuously train over many days or weeks, your body may be unable to keep up with the much larger demands placed upon it. As a result, your body can become depleted of essential mineral salts and nutrients. For example, when athletes deplete their calcium, potassium, magnesium, or phosphorus, they can experience lingering muscular fatigue and become susceptible to stress fractures. When runners deplete their iron, they risk a bout with anemia. The solution may be as simple as eating well, avoiding things associated with depletion—such as hard training efforts, sun tanning, saunas, and diuretics—and resting your way back into shape.

Many other biochemical processes can also be compromised and result in the onset of residual fatigue. If, over a long time an athlete ignores the warning signs of residual fatigue and does not attended to them, a more serious condition can result, known as chronic fatigue, or the so-called "burned-out" syndrome. To use the analogy of a factory, it is not then a matter of being out of the materials required for production, rather, there has actually been some damage done to the factory itself. In particular, the body's ability to make and use essential hormones associated with the endocrine system, and to maintain the delicate balance between anabolic and catabolic processes can be adversely affected.

Any number of processes in the body can go awry when residual fatigue progresses to the point of causing a state of chronic fatigue. Once this happens, the coach or athlete has opened a Pandora's Box of troubles. Chronic fatigue syndrome can result in serious physical and mental breakdown, and can be potentially life threatening. An essential part of the solution includes the cessation of hard work and competition, and going out to pasture for a while. Professional medical help should be sought to properly diagnose and treat the condition. This could include both an endocrinologist and a clinical psychologist. However, beware of seeking medical assistance for a quick fix, such as medication, only to continue upon the path of overtraining and possible self-destruction. This may bring a period of apparent "recovery," but afterwards, an athlete can become even more seriously affected, and possibly addicted to the medication. When the body habitually gets something for nothing, the "factory" normally responsible for manufacturing that something within the body often curtails its production and shuts down, perhaps never to start up or function as well again. Unfortunately, many take the pharmaceutical approach to solving chronic fatigue problems. In the short term, this method is easier and less costly than teaching an athlete how to train properly or change their mental outlook and behavior. And when the problem lies with faulty athletic training, few doctors or psychologists have the knowledge to assist in this area. When your body suffers a breakdown, it is telling you that you have violated a natural law. Ultimately, athletes need to educate themselves and take responsibility for their own physical and mental health.

The Role of Variation in Preventing Habituation

Variation not only serves to dodge the onset of residual or chronic fatigue, but also prevents habituation. Over time, the human body grows accustomed to any given type of training load or workout. As the athlete's body habituates to the would-be training stimulus, physical and mental stagnation is the most likely result. In this case, there is a direct relationship between an athlete's physical state and mental state. In time, as the athlete habituates to a workout, the magnitude of positive adaptation will decline, if not cease altogether. What once provided a suitable physical and mental stimulus now comes to resemble a state of equilibrium. On the mental side, this produces a decline in the athlete's interest and motivation. The athlete becomes bored with the dull routine and loses enthusiasm.

Workouts must vary from day to day and week to week. Moreover, the potential enhancement of fitness created by the individual training sessions needs to be stabilized and consolidated. Variation and recovery are necessary, not only with respect to the day-to-day composition of training, but also with respect to larger blocks of work consisting of several days or weeks. Accordingly, if athletes want to continue improving, they must periodically take a worthwhile break. To allow the body to recover, they should take a respite from hard training lasting between seven and 14 days. So, after a period of continuous training lasting days or weeks, the training loads should be eased in order to avoid the onset of residual fatigue and habituation. This also permits the proper stabilization and consolidation of performance potential created by previous hard work. Thereafter, athletes will be able to resume training until they once again require a subsequent worthwhile break. In this regard, training is a lot like climbing a ladder, or laying bricks. If athletes try to take too many rungs too quickly, they will miss one and take a fall. Alternately, if they lay too many bricks before the mortar has had a chance to set properly, then the entire structure could tumble down, and the athletes would have to start over again.

Often, runners fear to back off and take a worthwhile break, because they think someone else is out there training hard and getting ahead. They need to be reminded that a worthwhile break forms an integral part of the larger process of acquisition and improvement, and that the activities of others have nothing to do with their own athletic development and fitness. An old Zen story tells about a student being impatient and disappointed upon hearing that it would take five to ten years to attain mastery of a certain martial art. He asked his master what would happen if he tried twice as hard. The master replied that it would then take him twice as long to reach his destination.

The importance of introducing variation with respect to consecutive weeks of training, thereby creating blocks of training, will now be addressed. Here it is necessary to address medium load-waves or meso-cycles, which correspond to the monthly view of athletic training and development.

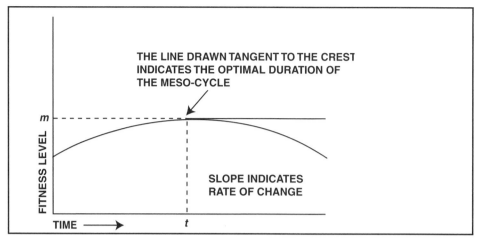

FIGURE 1.17—Training regression

Meso-Cycle Structure and Duration

Again, after days or weeks of demanding training, the rate of acquisition and performance potential of the athletes will eventually crest. With the onset of residual fatigue, if runners continue with demanding training they can actually suffer a regression in fitness and go backwards. As shown in Figure 1.17, maximum fitness (m), being achieved at time (t), with a subsequent decline in fitness, indicates that the duration of the meso-cycle ought not to exceed t days.

Question: How long can athletes train before they need an easy worthwhile break?

Answer: It all depends upon the degree to which they tax their metabolism. Weight lifters can sometimes train for five to six weeks without requiring a worthwhile break. At the beginning of the base period, distance runners can normally undertake three to four weeks of training before requiring a worthwhile break, but as the quality of the training loads increase during the course of the athletic season, they will need to cut back to 21-day, 14-day, and ultimately, 7-to-10-day meso-cycles.

However, a middle-aged athlete who resumes training after a long lay-off could require a worthwhile break after the first week of training. If you are unfit and attempting to train for the first time, you might even require a break after just a few days. It could take a while for you to become fit enough to put two weeks of continuous training together. Even mature athletes might require a worthwhile break after a week of training if they increase their training loads too aggressively. For example, athletes who suddenly increase their mileage from 80 to over 100 miles per week may require a worthwhile break the following week. It could take several weeks or even months for these athletes to be capable of sustaining 100 mile per week.

Question: How do you know when to take a worthwhile break?

Answer: After a 3/4-effort workout, it is not abnormal to be fatigued and recovering for two or even three days, but this fatigue should not linger for much longer. Any time athletes expect to be recovered but find themselves still fatigued, and two similar days follow, they could be suffering from the effects of residual fatigue. At that point, athletes could actually be going backwards in their training. One or more of the following symptoms can warn of this impending condition: insomnia, illness, injury, anxiety, loss of appetite, and a higher resting pulse rate. As a normal training practice, athletes do not want to run themselves into a state of residual fatigue. Athletes should plan and conduct their training so that they take a worthwhile break before they encounter signs of overtraining or other difficulties. An experienced coach or athlete will be able to predict with great accuracy how long the athlete can train before a worthwhile break is needed. If you do not intelligently plan a worthwhile break, then the body will force you to do so at a time that could prove especially disadvantageous. If you do not control the process, then it will control you—and more often than not, to the detriment of your athletic goals.

In brief, the greater the training loads and stress on the metabolism, the more frequently athletes require a worthwhile break. Thus, as an athletic season progresses (and with it, the quality of the work being conducted), the meso-cycles shorten in duration and increase in frequency. Figure 1.18 shows the optimal time for introducing a worthwhile break given the training loads being conducted during the various training periods.

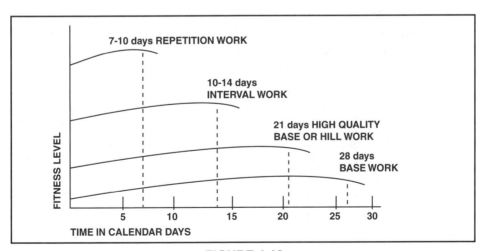

FIGURE 1.18

Generally, 21 to 28 days of base work, or 21 days of hill work, or seven to 10 days of sharpening work can be undertaken before athletes need a worthwhile break. Remember, a maximum of two 3/4-effort workouts and one 1/2-effort workout can be conducted during a typical week. So working backwards, runners can conduct a maximum of two or three 3/4-effort interval or repetition workouts over seven to 10 days, perhaps six 3/4-effort hill workouts over 21 days, and between six and eight 3/4-effort anaerobic threshold and steady state workouts over a period of 21 to 28 days. If runners attempt to exceed any one of these prudent limits—they will often run straight into trouble.

When runners attempt to squeeze in "just one more" demanding workout, and encounter substantial residual fatigue, then the price to pay can easily be a 10-to-14-day recovery period. So trying to get one workout "ahead" can easily put an athlete one or two weeks behind. And if an athlete thereby becomes injured or ill, the price to pay can easily be the desired outcome of the current athletic season. As we have seen with the micro-cycle or weekly view of athletic training, it is better to under-train than over-train. With the meso-cycle or monthly view of athletic training, this is doubly important. If and when athletes make a mistake with a larger training cycle, they pay a greater price.

Meso-Cycle Structure and the Consolidation and Stabilization of Fitness

Habituation to training can be avoided by introducing well-timed worthwhile breaks. Also, by shifting from general to more specific training tasks, variation can be introduced within the larger meso-cycle. In truth, it is necessary to shift the emphasis of the training program to specific tasks such as the conduct of time trials or competitions, since these cannot be performed to good effect when suppressed by previous hard work. Every coach and athlete needs to appreciate this simple, but profound truth: hard training suppresses performance. It is impossible for athletes to conduct a time trial or compete to good effect when insufficiently recovered from demanding training. If and when they make such an attempt, they cannot deliver optimal performances, and their true level of fitness could be difficult to discern. More importantly, when demanding training suppresses the quality of the time trials or competitions, stabilization and consolidation of the potential improvement created by the training efforts will be thwarted.

The task of stabilizing and consolidating the potential created by previous hard work is accomplished by taking a worthwhile break lasting between seven and 14 days, and then conducting a time trial or competition at the end of the worthwhile break. At that point in time, the actual performance level of the athletes will then rebound and reflect their true performance potential. Thus, athletes should not race in practice, nor practice in races. They should not "train through" races and make a muddle of the acquisition process. That would be counterproductive to obtaining the physical and mental fitness required for superior athletic performance.

Again, a direct relationship exists between the worthwhile break and realizing improvement. Athletes train for a length of time in order to raise their performance potential, but it is only potential because they have not actually performed at this new level. When fatigued from demanding workouts, they will not be able to demonstrate their performance potential. Accordingly, the worthwhile break must be introduced. The end of the worthwhile break then concludes with a time trial or competition, which serves to stabilize and consolidate the potential enhancement of performance created by previous acquisitive training efforts. Performance potential can then be realized as actual performance. The time trial or competition also provides a concrete reference point with respect to the athletes' level of fitness. The information it provides can then be used to reevaluate the training plan for the next training meso-cycle.

Meso-Cycle Structure and Load Leaping

By adapting the height, size, and shape of a block of training, the magnitude of training loads assumed over time can be represented as a percentage of maximum working capacity. As shown in Figure 1.19, athletes can progress from lower to higher training loads consistent with the model of Matveyew. Alternatively, they can begin with higher training loads and then back off consistent with the model of Vorobyew. More complex models will be provided later in this chapter.

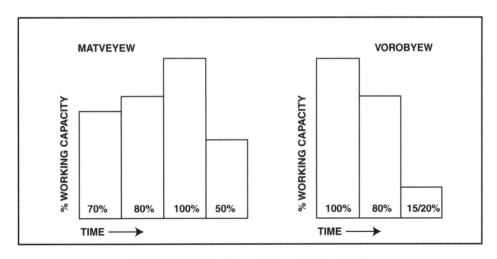

FIGURE 1.19—From Schmolinsky, 1978

Figure 1.20 illustrates the effect of a series of weekly training loads on potential and actual performance levels. Here, the bar columns, indicating the magnitude of the training loads and the percentage of working capacity assumed by the athletes, properly support the solid blue line representing their performance potential. The broken red line, indicating the actual performance level, reflects the degree that hard work suppresses their performance potential. The symbol X indicates a time-trial or competition at the end of the worthwhile break to consolidate acquisitive training efforts and check on athletic development. At this point, the performance potential and actual performance of the athletes are both approximately at the same level, and these lines should intersect. Alternating a series of blocks of hard training with required worthwhile breaks within a meso-cycle is commonly called load-leaping.

Provided here are abstract 14 and 21-day acquisitive meso-cycles corresponding to work conducted during the base, hill, or sharpening period.

14-DAY MESO-CYCLE	21-DAY MESO-CYCLE
1 Passive Recovery	**1** Passive Recovery
2 3/4-Effort, Quality Session	**2** 3/4-Effort, Quality Session
3 Active Recovery	**3** Active Recovery
4 1/2-Effort, Quality Session	**4** 1/2-Effort, Quality Session
5 Active Recovery	**5** Active Recovery
6 3/4-Effort, Quality Session	**6** 3/4-Effort, Quality Session
7 Active Recovery	**7** Easy-effort, Long Run
8 Easy-effort, Long Run	**8** Passive Recovery
9 Passive Recovery	**9** 3/4-Effort, Quality Session
10 3/4-Effort, Time Trial	**10** Active Recovery
11 Active Recovery	**11** 1/2-effort, Quantity Session
12 Easy Recovery	**12** Active Recovery
13 Day Before Race Routine	**13** 3/4-Effort, Quality Session
14 Race	**14** Active Recovery
	15 Easy-effort, Long Run
	16 Passive Recovery
	17 3/4-Effort, Time Trial
	18 Active Recovery
	19 Easy Recovery
	20 Day Before Race Routine
	21 Race

Meso-Cycle Structure and Duration of the Training Periods

Based on the preceding discussion, it will now be possible to address the meso-cycle structure and also the duration of the base, hill, sharpening, peak, and post-season recovery periods in an athletic season. Ultimately, the number of competitive athletic seasons assumed during the calendar year, and the length of the hill, sharpening, peak, and post-season recovery periods defines the duration

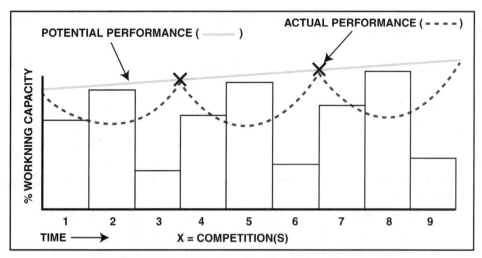

FIGURE 1.20—Actual and potential performance

of the base period. Mature athletes should normally undertake two athletic seasons and at least two weeks of post-season recovery, but young athletes should normally undertake a post-season recovery period of at least one month. During the early part of the base period athletes will be attempting to increase their training volume. Normally, the quality of the work is low, and so they will have no difficulty with training for three to four weeks before taking a worthwhile break. However, as athletes undertake high quality base work they will require a break after only two to three weeks of hard training. As shown in Figure 1.21, a meso-cycle structure of progressive loading over succeeding weeks is usually ideal during the base period.

The hill period is often reduced to a training emphasis during the cross-country season. However, middle distance runners often conduct more highly structured hill repetition work in preparation for the outdoor track and field season. In this regard, the hill period could include two to three weeks of progressive work, followed by a worthwhile break, thus determining a hill period of three to four weeks. Alternately, a five-to-six-week hill period could be broken up into two meso-cycles—each including two workweeks followed by a worthwhile break, as shown in Figure 1.22.

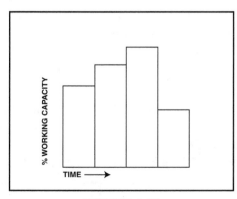

FIGURE 1.21

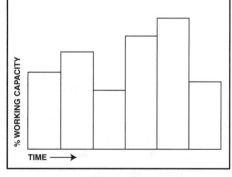

FIGURE 1.22

Again, always conclude a given training period with a worthwhile break that ends with a time-trial, or performance. This practice will:

- Consolidate and stabilize previous work
- Serve as a check upon athletic development
- Permit athletes to enter a new training period fully refreshed

The sharpening period incorporates especially demanding interval and repetition training. Also, athletes normally begin to compete more frequently during the sharpening period. Unfortunately, many high school and college athletes might then find themselves competing far too often. Given the effects of anaerobic work on the metabolism, the sharpening period is the most stressful. Normally, the length of the sharpening period is limited to three to four weeks. In order to realize optimal results, female distance runners and young male athletes (who enjoy less aerobic ability than mature male athletes) often only require three weeks of sharpening work. Mature athletes intending to compete in 10-to-12-kilometer cross-country races sometimes also enjoy optimal results with only three weeks of sharpening work. However, mature male and female athletes normally achieve optimal results with a sharpening period of four weeks. Arthur Lydiard arrived at this realization by years of experimentation, and the best evidence from exercise physiologists and other coaches also support the discovery: The human body does not require more than approximately four weeks of sharpening work. When athletes exceed that duration, they often waste valuable time and energy, and the results prove counterproductive to a successful outcome.

During the sharpening period, athletes should not attempt four weeks of intensive training without taking a worthwhile break. Accordingly, the sharpening period is divided into two meso-cycles. A worthwhile break should be introduced approximately seven to 10 days into the sharpening period after completing the early progression of quality interval work. The first worthwhile break normally extends seven to 10 days, and then concludes with a competition in the main race event. After completing the early interval work and taking a worthwhile break to freshen up, athletes should be already coming into a respectable level of competitive fitness. This is the best time, and normally should be the only time, that athletes compete in their main race event during the sharpening period. Because the later repetition workouts can be tailored to eliminate any areas of weakness, it is important to obtain a clear picture regarding the athletes' fitness and performance in the main race event. In addition, given the rebound of energy that accompanies the worthwhile break, athletes will be better able to conduct the repetition workouts during the second seven-to-10-day meso-cycle of the sharpening period.

A meso-cycle model characterized by progressively increased loading best corresponds to the pattern of response and training requirements for athletes during the early part of the sharpening period. Accordingly, the training load can and should be increased over the first seven to 10 days of the sharpening period prior to taking the worthwhile break. However, during the second sharpening period, a meso-cycle model characterized by declining loading best corresponds to the pattern of response and training requirements for athletes during the more stressful repetition workouts. The worthwhile break that follows the second seven-to-10-day meso-cycle then simultaneously comprises the beginning of the peak period, and in particular, the nine-to-10-day ascent (or so-called taper) to the plateau of peak performance which will then last approximately two to three weeks. This meso-cycle model of acquisition for the sharpening period is illustrated in Figure 1.23.

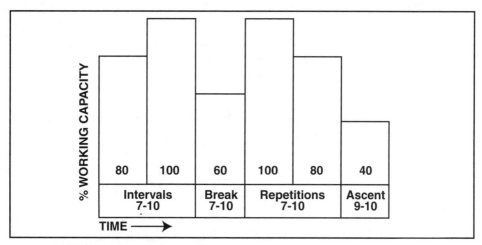

FIGURE 1.23—Meso-cycle structure of the sharpening period

Once the peak period begins, athletes normally do not undertake demanding acquisitive training efforts. For the most part, athletes essentially time trial, race and recover. However, three distinct types of peak periods should be discussed. A short peak period normally begins with a nine-to-10-day worthwhile break that simultaneously comprises the ascent or taper to a plateau of peak performance that will then last two to three weeks. Relatively few athletes desire to maintain race fitness beyond the normal two-to-three-week duration of the plateau of peak performance associated with a short peak period. However, sometimes important championship or qualifying competitions are more widely separated.

The plateau of peak performance can be extended beyond two to three weeks by reintroducing a delicate prescription of regenerative or stabilizing work, but this requires a relatively high level of sophistication. This more complex type of peak period is known as an extended peak period. For example, collegiate conference championships sometimes precede the national championships by several weeks. Accordingly, some maintenance or stabilizing training efforts can then be done to bridge the gap and extend the plateau of peak performance. In this case, athletes could perform one or more select workouts previously conducted during the athletic season. However, the effort of these workouts should be reduced relative to those conducted previously.

Occasionally, qualifying meets come one or more months prior to a major championship. For example, high school athletes might peak for their state cross-country championships, but then compete one or more weeks later in regional championships, and then again one or more weeks later in the national championship. Athletes face this same situation if they compete in the USATF National Championships in mid-June or July, and then compete in the World Championships or Olympic Games in August or September. Often, athletes qualifying for international competition in the USATF National Championships, later fail to perform well in major international competitions in August or September. If and when athletes dash off to race in Europe immediately after the USATF National Championship, they could lose substantial fitness before the World Championships or Olympic Games. Therefore, they need to conduct a multiple peak period. In this regard, they would undertake at least one acquisitive or regenerative meso-cycle (including base and strength work), then conduct sufficient sharpening work to bring them back into a competitive level of fitness prior to re-ascending to the second plateau of peak performance for the World Championships or Olympic Games.

A post-season recovery period should be taken after the peak period. Mature athletes should normally take at least two weeks of post-season recovery. Since demanding training tends to suppress maturation, young athletes should take at least four weeks of post-season recovery. If necessary, more post-season recovery should be taken by the athletes to clear up any possible injuries and restore their enthusiasm.

MACRO-CYCLES: PLANNING THE ATHLETIC SEASON

Three phases of training activity characterize athletic development. How do these three phases relate to the training undertaken by runners during an athletic season?

Acquisition corresponds to the preparatory phase in which athletes conduct general and specific conditioning work in order to improve their athletic performance potential. This phase includes the workweeks conducted during the base, hill, and sharpening periods. An acquisitive training load, micro-cycle, or meso-cycle is intended to actively raise the performance potential of athletes and often includes ground-breaking or novel workouts.

Consolidation corresponds to the competitive phase in which athletes stabilize and realize their performance potential via actual performance. This phase includes the worthwhile breaks taken during the athletic season, but primarily corresponds to the peak period. A stabilizing training load, micro-cycle, or meso-cycle is designed to maintain and consolidate fitness. Accordingly, selected workouts previously conducted during the athletic season can be repeated with some decrease in the training effort. In contrast, a regenerative training load, micro-cycle, or meso-cycle is designed to more substantially rebuild certain aspects of fitness. It normally includes a brief recap of activity assumed during one or more distinct training periods (such as the base, hill, sharpening, or peak periods), and the work will be conducted in like-sequence. Stabilizing or regenerative work is sometimes performed during the peak period in order to extend its duration.

Decline corresponds to the transitional phase—required to prevent habituation to the training and the onset of residual or chronic fatigue. It also permits delayed transformation and thus allows improvement of performance potential between two successive athletic seasons. The decline or transitional phase is associated with the post-season recovery period. Figure 1.24 shows a prudent modulation of quantity, quality, and performance over the various training periods.

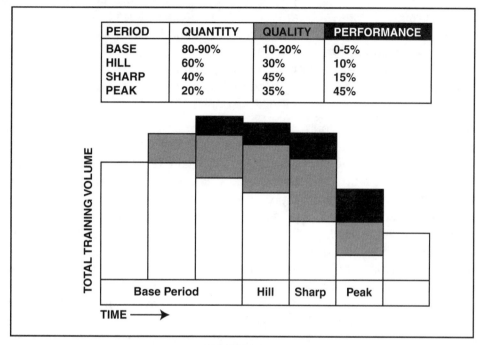

PERIOD	QUANTITY	QUALITY	PERFORMANCE
BASE	80-90%	10-20%	0-5%
HILL	60%	30%	10%
SHARP	40%	45%	15%
PEAK	20%	35%	45%

FIGURE 1.24

Macro-Cycles: Planning the Structure of the Athletic Season

Based on this framework, you can now construct a detailed plan for an entire athletic season. To make the plan, begin with a tentative competitive schedule and a large desk calendar. Then prepare to work backwards! Cut and tape the calendar months together into a continuous scroll encompassing the entire athletic season. It will help if you denote the major peak competition of the season with a zero, and then number the calendar backwards in the manner of a countdown. After you establish the first athletic competition to fall within the projected two-to-three-week plateau of peak performance:

- Count back 9 to 10 days to establish the beginning of the peak period, thus allowing for the worthwhile break constituting the ascent, or so-called "taper" leading to the plateau of peak performance
- Count back approximately 28 days or 4 weeks from that point to define the beginning of the sharpening period
- Count back approximately 4 to 6 weeks, depending on which of the meso-cycle models has been adopted, to define the beginning of the hill period
- Anything previous would then constitute the base period

Once the general structure, length, and placement of the training periods has been determined, they can be color-coded on the calendar with a highlighter. Then, working backwards from the peak period, select three to four competitions (each separated by at least 10 to 21 days) as possible targets for performance in the main race event. These contests should become more competitive as the season progresses. Preferably, any other competitions during the season should be over-distance or under-distance relative to the main race event. The selection regarding over-distance versus under-distance competitions should be determined by what will best balance the individual athlete's fitness, given the composition of the larger training program. Generally, runners should compete more frequently in their weaker off-distance event.

Again, athletes should only compete in the main race event at the end of an acquisitive training meso-cycle, after taking a seven-to-14-day worthwhile break. Normally, runners are best prepared for the main race event by assuming a preceding time-trial or under-distance race. With mature athletes in a high level of fitness, best results are generally obtained with the conduct of a time trial or under-distance race three to four days before the main event, within a worthwhile break lasting seven to 10 days. For high school or collegiate athletes, best results are normally provided by a time trial or race four to five days before the main event, within a worthwhile break lasting nine to 10 days. However, this latter scenario could also benefit mature athletes when substantial travel enters the equation. A time trial or competition between 300 to 600 meters is generally advisable for specialists at 800 meters; 600 to 1,200 meters for specialists at 1,500 meters; 1,000 to 1,500 meters for specialists at 3,000 meters; 1,500 to 2,000 meters for specialists at 5,000 meters; and 2,000 to 3,000 meters for specialists at 10,000 meters.

The training and racing schedule should be created to facilitate the best competitive results during the peak period. Do not simply take the same old conference schedule that has been handed down year after year as if it were the Ten Commandments, and then plan the current athletic season so as to neatly fit into the mold. If you do, the results will likely be the same as with every other coach or athlete who has used it. Think outside the prevailing box, or conventional un-wisdom. Apply your knowledge, experience and creativity when planning a training schedule for the athletic season. Remember, the duration of the meso-cycles should decrease and their frequency should increase as the quality of the training improves during the season.

This procedure will determine both the number and structure of the meso-cycles within the macro-cycle, or athletic season. You might then number and indicate the structure of the meso-cycles along the edge of the calendar. Now you can plan the workouts for each day of the athletic season! Obviously, circumstances may lead you to modify the schedule, but you will literally be able to see (and thus, better judge) the effect of any adjustment on the balance of the season's training. And sometimes an athletic season does happen to unfold according to plan without making a significant change. The planning process may take the better part of one or more evenings for an experienced coach or athlete. Creating a plan for an athletic season is much like solving a difficult jigsaw puzzle.

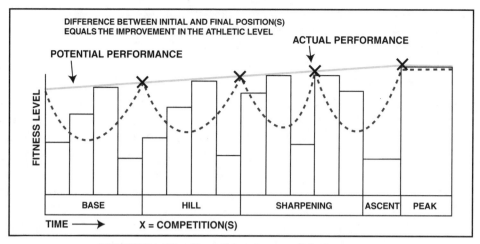

FIGURE 1.25—Macro-cycle, or athletic season

Completing the seasonal plan is well worth the time and effort. Coaches will be able to use the final product to educate athletes, and intelligently answer questions concerning what they are doing, and why. The tyrannical "do this" and "do that" coaching style can be abandoned, and instead, the style of an educator can be adopted. Coaches might even hold a class and teach the subject of athletic training during the first few days of organized team practice. Athletes can then "learn by doing," and actually plan their individual training schedules for the athletic season. The two-way communication afforded by a mature coach-athlete relationship will enhance the quality of the decision-making process, and thus, competitive results. An additional reward will be the confidence and enthusiasm generated amongst the athletes. A direct causal connection exists between enlightenment, self-directed physical and mental activity, and excellence. The sooner athletes acquire the knowledge, experience and confidence required to plan their own training and assume responsibility for their athletic destiny, the better will be the results both on and off the field (Cerutty, 1964, 1967, and Harre, 1982).

Figure 1.25 illustrates a macro-cycle model that integrates the various training periods and meso-cycles. The left axis indicates the athlete's level of fitness, and the bar graphs (indicating percent working capacity) represent the workload assumed by the athlete. The difference between the initial fitness level and the highest fitness level indicates the amount of improvement in the athlete's potential and actual performance level over the athletic season. The slope of the blue line of performance potential indicates the rate of change in improvement over the athletic season. The dashed arcuate line of actual performance illustrates both the suppression of performance potential by hard work, and the subsequent dramatic rebound by the end of each worthwhile break. The X symbols indicate primary competitions, and should be placed at the end of the worthwhile breaks, when the potential performance and actual performance levels become equated, and their lines intersect.

Figure 1.26 shows a macro-cycle including a multiple peak-period for bridging the gap between the USATF National Track and Field Championship and a major international competition.

Date Pace and Goal Pace

How do you properly progress the date pace, goal pace and finishing speed during the macro-cycle or athletic season? At the beginning of the sharpening period the athlete should conduct quality work at goal pace for the main race event. Goal pace corresponds to the pace of the desired goal performance in the main race event during the peak period. Date pace work is normally conducted once a week during the base and hill periods to enable a gradual progression of physiological and biomechanical function, and to establish a sound foundation for later work at goal pace during the sharpening period (Dellinger, 1973). Normally date pace work should be incrementally reduced in quality from goal pace by 1 second per 400 meters in each meso-cycle preceding the sharpening period. Date pace work can also maintain or improve an athlete's running economy, and thereby facilitate high quality base and hill work. Finishing speed work is intended to advance or improve an athlete's closing speed over the last 400 meters of a race. The desired maximum closing speed over 100 or 200 meters constitutes goal finishing speed. This work is normally conducted as a brief series of controlled accelerations or repetitions no longer than 400 meters, and the athlete then takes full recovery periods. Finishing speed work can be progressed by .5 seconds / 200 meters in each meso-cycle leading up to the plateau of peak performance, thus enabling goal finishing speed and optimal performance to be achieved during the peak period.

Figure 1.27 shows an abstract prescription and progression of date pace, goal pace and goal finishing speed for an athletic season. It indicates the various training periods, as well as the structure of the meso-cycles and larger macro-cycle. The duration of the workweek and worthwhile break segments, and also the ascent and peak, are shown in days. The athlete's potential and actual performance levels are also indicated at any given point in time. Figure 1.27 has also been modified and left blank for use as a worksheet by coaches and athletes, and appears as Figure 4.3 in Chapter 4. The abbreviations main race event (MRE), over-distance event (ODE), and under-distance event (UDE) also appear, and their significance will be addressed.

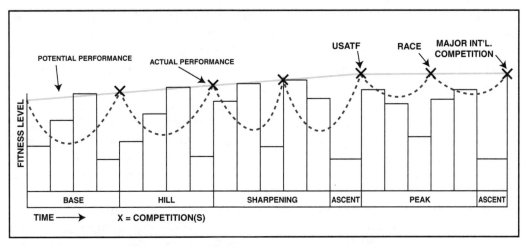

FIGURE 1.26—Extended athletic season for senior U.S. athletes

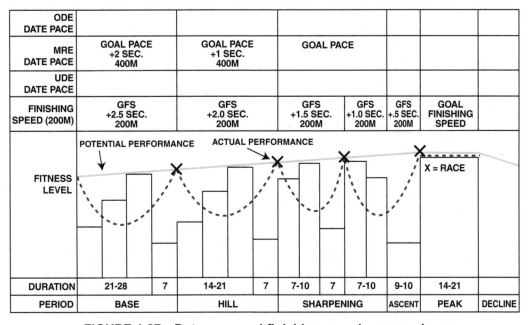

ODE DATE PACE								
MRE DATE PACE	GOAL PACE +2 SEC. 400M		GOAL PACE +1 SEC. 400M		GOAL PACE			
UDE DATE PACE								
FINISHING SPEED (200M)	GFS +2.5 SEC. 200M		GFS +2.0 SEC. 200M		GFS +1.5 SEC. 200M	GFS +1.0 SEC. 200M	GFS +.5 SEC. 200M	GOAL FINISHING SPEED
FITNESS LEVEL								X = RACE
DURATION	21-28	7	14-21	7	7-10	7	7-10	9-10	14-21
PERIOD	BASE		HILL		SHARPENING		ASCENT	PEAK	DECLINE

FIGURE 1.27—Date pace and finishing speed progressions

Figure 1.28 illustrates an athletic season model for a 1,500 meters performance of 3:42, corresponding roughly to a 4-minute mile. It indicates date pace, goal pace and also the potential and actual performance levels in the main race event (MRE), over-distance event (ODE) and under-distance event (UDE). Athletes will normally conduct several meso-cycles of base work, and only the last meso-cycle corresponding to the base period is shown in Figure 1.28. The illustrated base period meso-cycle could include approximately 21 days of demanding training in which the training load is gradually increased, then a worthwhile break lasting seven to 10 days. It would thus contain a maximum total duration of less than four weeks. A time trial or competition should be conducted at the end of the first worthwhile break, marking the conclusion of the base period and beginning of the hill period. Normally, an athlete with the potential to run a time of 3:42 in the 1,500 meters main race event (MRE) during the peak period will have an actual performance level of 3:54 at this time. The equivalent performance in the 800 meters under-distance event (UDE) is then approximately 1:54, and in the 5,000 meters over-distance event (ODE), about 14:18. These performances can be expected if an athlete elects to compete in an over-distance or under-distance event at this time. The over-distance performance is normally much easier to attain, since not enough sharpening work will have then been conducted to permit an equivalent performance over 800 meters (For determining equivalent performances, see Tables 4.8 and 4.9 in Chapter 4, and also, Daniels and Gilbert, 1979, and Daniels, 1998). The date pace work conducted for the main race event during the first meso-cycle would be 62 seconds/400 meters and a performance corresponding to that pace would be delivered at the end of this meso-cycle. Figure 1.28 also indicates the quality of date pace work corresponding to the over-distance and under-distance events, and also the athlete's finishing speed progression.

The next meso-cycle consists of 14 to 21 days of hill work followed by a worthwhile break lasting seven to 10 days, thus has a total duration of three to four weeks. The progression of date pace and finishing speed is also indicated. At the end of the hill period, the athlete should be capable of delivering a 3:50 performance in the 1,500 meters. The equivalent under-distance performance in the 800 meters is then approximately 1:52, and the equivalent over-distance performance in the 5,000 meters is about 14:05.

Again, the duration of the sharpening period should be limited to approximately four weeks or 28 days. The sharpening work is too demanding to be conducted in one continuous block of ever-increasing training loads. Instead, it should be divided into two meso-cycles. The first seven-to-10-day meso-cycle should have gradually increasing training loads, including interval training, and should be

ODE: 5,000M **DATE PACE** **FITNESS LEVEL**	68 14:18		67 14:05		66 13:51				13:37
MRE: 1,500M **DATE PACE** **FITNESS LEVEL**	62 3:54		61 3:50		60 3:46				3:42
UDE: 800M **DATE PACE** **FITNESS LEVEL**	56 1:54		55 1:52		54 1:50				1:48
FINISHING SPEED (200M)	25.0		24.5		24.0	23.5	23.0		

FITNESS LEVEL	POTENTIAL PERFORMANCE / ACTUAL PERFORMANCE — 3:54, 3:50, 3:46, 3:42 (X = RACE)								
DURATION	21-28	7	14-21	7	7-10	7	7-10	9-10	14-21
PERIOD	BASE		HILL		SHARPENING			ASCENT	PEAK / DECLINE

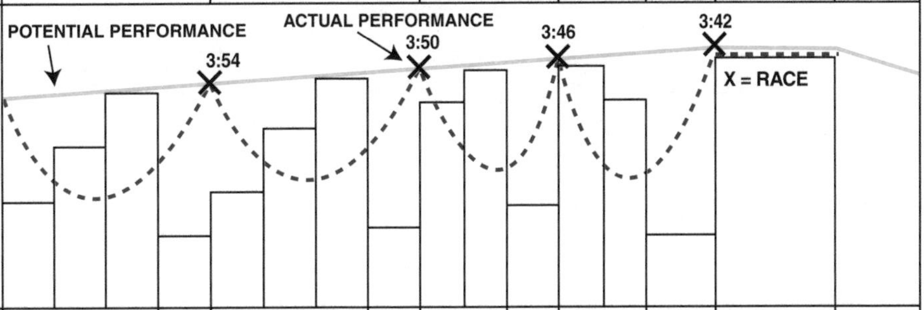

FIGURE 1.28—Schedule for a 1,500 meters performance of 3:42

followed by a worthwhile break of seven to 10 days. At the end of this worthwhile break, the athlete should be capable of delivering a 1,500 meters performance of 3:46. The equivalent under-distance performance in the 800 meters is then approximately 1:50, and the equivalent over-distance performance in the 5,000 meters is about 13:51. The second seven-to-10-day sharpening period meso-cycle then follows, and is characterized by repetition training and a decline in training loads. Afterwards, the next worthwhile break lasts between seven to 14 days, but nine to 10 days normally provides the best results. This worthwhile break permits the ascent to the plateau of peak performance, thus it can be viewed as part of the sharpening period or the beginning of the peak period. In this text, it will be treated as part of the peak period. Once upon the plateau of peak performance, the athlete will be able to deliver a 1,500-meter performance of 3:42 (roughly corresponding to a four-minute mile) in the targeted champion-ship competition. The equivalent under-distance performance in the 800 meters is then 1:48, and the equivalent over-distance performance in the 5,000 meters is 13:37. This figure also shows the final progression of finishing speed work.

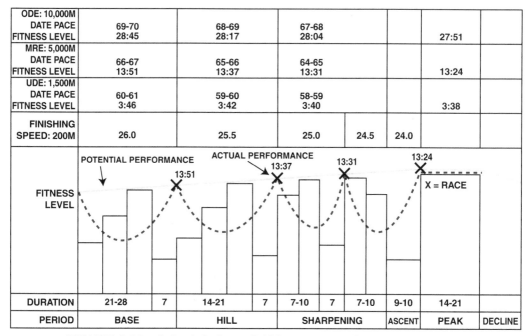

ODE: 10,000M DATE PACE FITNESS LEVEL	69-70 28:45	68-69 28:17	67-68 28:04				27:51	
MRE: 5,000M DATE PACE FITNESS LEVEL	66-67 13:51	65-66 13:37	64-65 13:31				13:24	
UDE: 1,500M DATE PACE FITNESS LEVEL	60-61 3:46	59-60 3:42	58-59 3:40				3:38	
FINISHING SPEED: 200M	26.0	25.5	25.0	24.5	24.0			
DURATION	21-28	7	14-21	7	7-10	7	7-10	9-10	14-21	
PERIOD	BASE		HILL		SHARPENING		ASCENT	PEAK	DECLINE

FIGURE 1.29—Schedule for a 5,000 meters performance of 13:24

Figure 1.29 illustrates a similar model of an athletic season for an athlete who would deliver a 5,000-meter performance of 13:24. Abstract finishing speed progressions for world class women and men in various events are shown in Table 1.2, and Table 1.3, respectively.

TRAINING PERIOD	800 METERS	1,500 METERS	3,000 METERS	5,000 METERS	10,000 METERS
BASE	26.0 5x150	27.0 5x200	28.0 5x200	29.0 5x200	30.0 5x200
HILL	25.5 5x100	26.5 5x150	27.5 5x200	28.5 5x200	29.5 5x200
SHARPENING PART 1	25.0 4x100	26.0 4x150	27.0 4x200	28.0 4x200	29.0 4x200
SHARPENING PART 2	24.5 4x60	25.5 4x100	26.5 4x150	27.5 4x200	28.5 4x200
ASCENT	24.0 3x60	25.0 3x100	26.0 3x150	27.0 3x200	28.0 3x200

TABLE 1.2—Finishing speed progression for world class women by event

TRAINING PERIOD	800 METERS	1,500 METERS	3,000 METERS	5,000 METERS	10,000 METERS
BASE	23.0 5x150	24.0 5x200	25.0 5x200	26.0 5x200	27.0 5x200
HILL	22.5 5x100	23.5 5x150	24.5 5x200	25.5 5x200	26.5 5x200
SHARPENING PART 1	22.0 4x100	23.0 4x150	24.0 4x200	25.0 4x200	26.0 4x200
SHARPENING PART 2	21.5 4x60	22.5 4x100	23.5 4x150	24.5 4x200	25.5 4x200
ASCENT	21.0 3x60	22.0 3x100	23.0 3x150	24.0 3x200	25.0 3x200

TABLE 1.3—Finishing speed progression for world class men by event

Figures 4.6 and 4.7 in Chapter 4 provide date pace and finishing speed progressions for performances of 4:38 and 4:00 in the 1,500 meters, corresponding to the athletic levels of high school girls and boys who would qualify for their state championships. In addition, Tables 4.2 and 4.4 provide finishing speed progressions for national caliber high school athletes.

MEGA-CYCLES: MULTIPLE YEAR DEVELOPMENT AND PEAKING SCENARIOS

How can multiple macro-cycles or athletic seasons be illustrated? What can be seen and understood by doing so? By illustrating a progression of macro-cycles or athletic seasons, a multi-year model of athletic development can be created. This is essential for properly planning how to develop and peak for a major competitive event held periodically, such as the Olympic Games.

Athletes normally complete an athletic season at a higher athletic level relative to the preceding season. This can be expected provided that runners train properly and athletic development takes place. The training and development that occurs during the course of an athletic season can be classified by one of three phases:

1. *Acquisition* corresponds to the preparatory phase, and includes the base, hill, and sharpening periods
2. *Consolidation* corresponds to the competitive phase, and in particular, the peak period
3. *Decline* corresponds to the transition phase, and is associated with the post-season recovery period

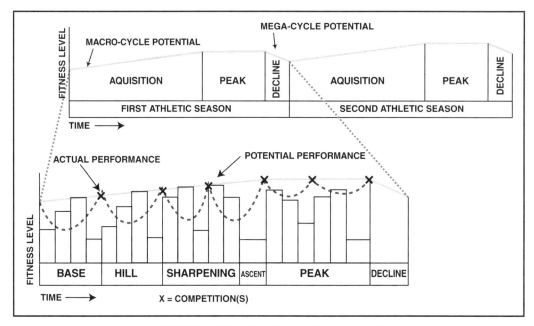

FIGURE 1.30—The Mega-Cycle model

In Figure 1.30, the yellow line supported by the crest of the larger macro-cycles or athletic seasons represents mega-cycle potential. This line indicates the direction and momentum of athletic development over a series of macro-cycles, or athletic seasons. The prefix "mega" has been used because it agrees with established vocabulary, and indicates thousands of training days, thus is true to scale. The slope of the ascending yellow line representing mega-cycle potential indicates the rate of change for the mega-cycle over months or years of training. Moreover, the projection of this line into the future represents potential future development, but also the prudent limits of acquisitive training and load tolerance over the next macro-cycle.

Acquisitive training efforts always suppress performance. For this reason athletes never see all of the development effected by the training within a given season. This is known as delayed transformation, and it is responsible for the continued improvement of performance potential realized during the decline or transition phase of training when athletes undertake post-season recovery (Harre, 1982). The continued positive slope of the yellow line representing mega-cycle performance potential during the post-season recovery period illustrates this phenomenon.

When runners attempt a too rapid Herculean acquisition effort within a given athletic season, they fail to reap the full benefit of improved performance during that particular season. The demanding acquisitive training efforts suppress athletic performance in much the same way as rapid physical maturation and

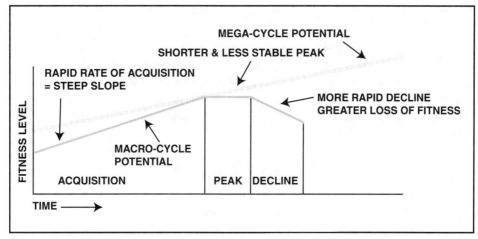

FIGURE 1.31

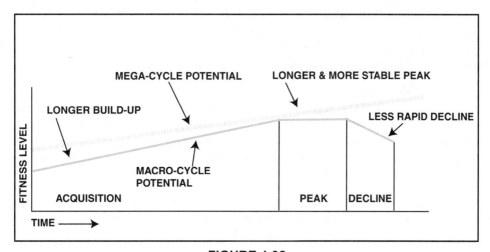

FIGURE 1.32

growth. This can be explained and graphically represented using the mega-cycle model. Remember, if athletes make an aggressive training effort during a macro-cycle, the slope of the blue line representing performance potential will be steep. This creates a wide gap between the yellow line representing mega-cycle—and the blue line representing macro-cycle performance potential. It also results in greater area between these two lines during all three stages of athletic development. This gap and area is proportional to the degree to which performance potential will be suppressed within that particular macro-cycle. Moreover, as shown in Figures 1.31 and 1.32, a rapid rate of acquisition normally results in a shorter, and less stable peak period, and also a longer period of decline relative to a longer and less aggressive training build-up.

Again, if athletes are aggressive with acquisitive training efforts over a given macro-cycle or athletic season, the blue line representing macro-cycle performance potential will be steep, thus reflecting rapid acquisition. The magnitude of the training loads will then necessitate more frequent meso-cycles, that is, if residual and chronic fatigue are to be avoided. Nevertheless, even with frequent meso-cycles, the heavy training loads inherently have a sharpening effect, thus accelerate the rate of reaching peak fitness, and shorten the effective duration of the athletic season. As a result, the athletes could peak too early and be on a downhill slope by the championship competition. Figure 1.33 illustrates this phenomenon by reproducing Figures 1.31 and 1.32 in a simplified form on the same set of axes.

Figure 1.33 also illustrates how a relatively long period of decline brought on by too aggressive a training program can also suppress future potential. As a result, there is a greater variance at the beginning of the next athletic season, as shown between the blue line representing macro-cycle potential, and the yellow line representing the mega-cycle potential. A longer, more stable build-up results in less suppression of performance potential and a longer, more stable peak. All things being equal, it also results in a shorter period of decline and less suppression of actual performance levels during the next athletic season.

Athletes who engage in Herculean acquisition efforts might perform quite well in an Olympic year, but perhaps then be outstanding a year later. The presence of preliminary heats and the focus upon competitive outcomes accounts, in part, for the quality of the performances delivered in the course of an Olympic Games. However, delayed transformation is one of the reasons why a surge of world records often takes place during non-Olympic years.

As shown in Figure 1.34, when the aim of the athletic season is to refine the product of previous acquisition with minimal suppression of athletic performance, the blue line indicating macro-cycle performance potential should have nearly the same slope as the yellow line representing mega-cycle performance potential. In this regard, a relatively long and gradual build-up during an athletic season is best.

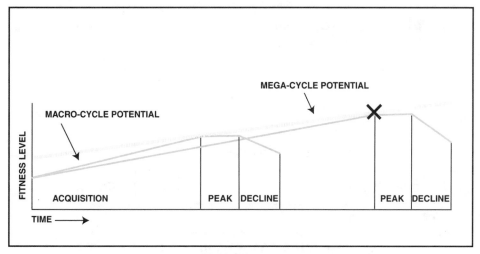

FIGURE 1.33

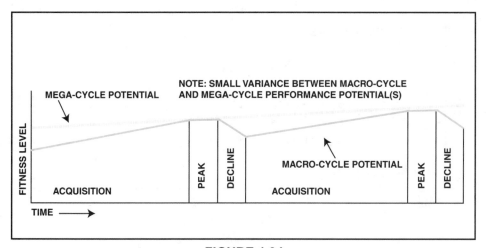

FIGURE 1.34

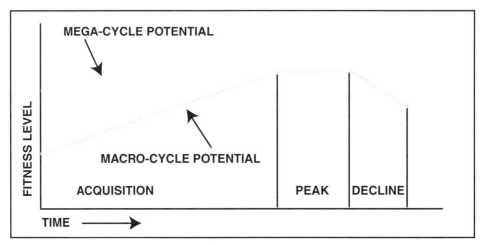

FIGURE 1.35—Young athlete

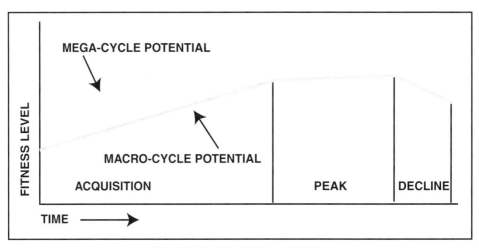

FIGURE 1.36—Mature athlete

As a result of many years of training, the mature athlete's peak period will lengthen. It also will be more stable, and support more frequent and higher quality performances. The required post-season recovery period will also normally be shorter. With a mature athlete, the slope of the peak performance plateau does not rapidly level off perpendicular to the left axis, but can continue to maintain a positive slope, thus reflecting their higher performance potential. In the case of mature athletes, the period of decline corresponding to post-season recovery will also have a less sudden drop-off and negative slope. Figures 1.35 and 1.36 represent this.

The better an athlete's preparation, the easier it will be to achieve a high athletic level during the peak period. Moreover, it will be easier to maintain athletic fitness and conduct an extended or multiple-peak period. Again, a multiple-peak period is required whenever athletes must peak in mid-June or July for the Olympic trials, and then again for the Olympic Games in late August or September.

Multiple Annual Athletic Seasons

The presence of two macro-cycles or athletic seasons within a calendar year will be identified as a bi-annual or two-season configuration, and three macro-cycles as a tri-annual or three-season configuration. Recognize that the amount of improvement in athletic fitness that is possible to achieve over a calendar year will normally be greater in a bi-annual configuration. Accordingly, the slope of the yellow mega-cycle line (representing performance potential) is steeper, and attains a higher value than in a tri-annual configuration. As shown in Figures 1.37 and 1.38, this happens simply because the bi-annual structure devotes more time to acquisition, whereas the tri-annual configuration sacrifices preparation for short-term competitive outcomes.

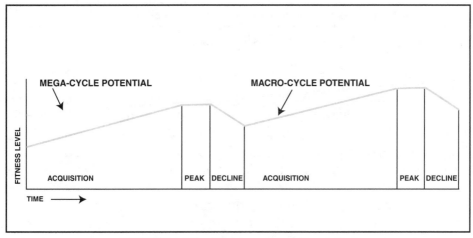

FIGURE 1.37—Bi-annual configuration

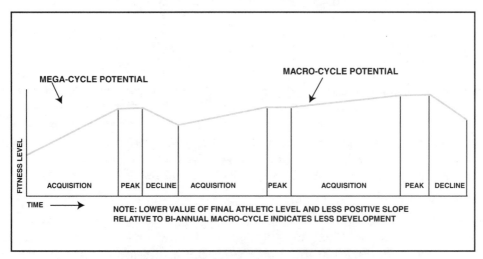

FIGURE 1.38—Tri-annual configuration

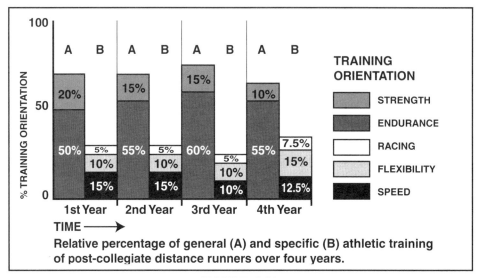

Relative percentage of general (A) and specific (B) athletic training of post-collegiate distance runners over four years.

FIGURE 1.39

In the United States, it would be commendable for the NCAA to address the year-round competition that collegiate distance runners contend with in cross-country, indoor, and outdoor track and field. No other group of collegiate athletes has a year-round competitive schedule. Developmentally, it does not make sense for distance runners to have three competitive seasons. This situation not only hurts their athletic development, but also their academic performance. The fact that distance runners tend to be fine students only serves to disguise the adverse impact of year-round athletic competition upon their academics. Institutions of higher learning have a responsibility to teach progressive educational practices and to demonstrate by example. For this reason, middle distance and distance runners should be limited to participation in only two of these three possible athletic seasons each year.

Peaking for the World Championships or Olympic Games

How can athletes optimize performance in the last year of a four-year developmental cycle? This is an important question for the collegiate coach, and also for post-collegiate athletes who aspire to competition in the Olympic Games. It is necessary to create sufficient vocabulary to describe scenarios for developing and peaking at the end of two, three, or four-year mega-cycles. A two-year developmental and peaking scenario will be referred to as biennial, and three or four year scenarios as triennial, and quadrennial mega-cycles, respectively.

In order to develop and peak in a quadrennial mega-cycle, athletes should progress the quantity and quality of acquisition efforts to optimal levels through the third year. This includes the progression of individual sharpening workouts that would be undertaken in the fourth year. But in the fourth year the training loads should level off, and in some cases, the volume and duration should actually be decreased. Further, athletes should work on their relative areas of weakness in order to balance their abilities in the over-distance versus under-

1st year	2nd year
3,000 meters	3,000 meters
1,500 meters	1,500 meters
3,000 meters	3,000 meters
5,000 meters	5,000 meters
5,000 meters USATF Prelims	10,000 meters USATF Final
5,000 meters USATF Final	3,000 meters Europe
3,000 meters Europe	5,000 meters Europe
5,000 meters Europe	10,000 meters Europe

3rd year	4th year
3,000 meters	3,000 meters
1,500 meters	1,500 meters
3,000 meters	5,000 meters
5,000 meters USATF Prelims	10,000 meters USATF Prelims
5,000 meters USATF Final	10,000 meters USATF Final
3,000 meters	3,000 meters
10,000 meters W.C. Prelims	10,000 meters Olympic Prelims
10,000 meters W.C. Final	10,000 meters Olympic Final

TABLE 1.4—Racing Schedule

distance events prior to the athletic season corresponding to the Olympic Games. For example, if athletes are weak on the 1,500 meters side of the 5,000 meters event, they should work to correct that deficiency. Athletes should then train towards their natural strength during the athletic season of the Olympic competition. In the fourth year, the quality of the sharpening workouts should be enhanced by placing greater emphasis upon race practice, that is, the ability to execute surges, breakaways and the finishing kick. In some cases, athletes should use competition to a greater degree, as a method of sharpening and advancing their athletic level. In sum, the aim should be to refine and polish the fruit of previous acquisitive work by placing greater emphasis on quality, technique and actual performance, as illustrated in Figure 1.39. Table 1.4 shows a progression regarding the number and type of competitions assumed by a U.S. distance runner who would move up from 5,000 meters to 10,000 meters over a four-year period in preparation for the Olympic Games.

Plan Ahead and Qualify Early

Athletes should normally obtain the qualifying time needed for the following year's major international competition, such as the World Championships or Olympic Games, during the preceding year's track and field season, after the stipulated qualifying date. They should not wait until they have qualified in their national championships (which are often tactical affairs conducted in poor weather conditions), and then suddenly realize that they also need to meet the international qualifying standard. If athletes put themselves in this situation, they could easily lose control of their athletic destiny. For example, in order to make an attempt to obtain the standard, athletes might have to travel overseas and compete at an inopportune time. If and when the attempt succeeds—they may then have compromised optimal preparation for the major international competition. Athletes need to think ahead and intelligently plan their athletic careers with the big picture in mind.

This chapter merely describes and illustrates some of the laws of nature that relate to distance running. Coaches and athletes need to master this subject in order to effectively plan training schedules, but they must also prudently modify workouts in the light of circumstances. Planning a training schedule for a high school or collegiate team for an entire season can easily take one or two days, and an additional hour of preparation each day in order to individualize the workouts. Those who deny the merit of planning—pay the penalty. They fail to deliver their best performance at the right time and place.

When you look beyond the superficial differences in the vocabulary and training habits of successful coaches and athletes—you discover how much they actually have in common. For example, Bill Bowerman corresponded and visited with the accomplished coaches of his day, including Arthur Lydiard and Gosta Holmer. This exchange of information contributed to the development of the "Oregon system." While it is true that "many roads lead to Rome," they are all paved with the same stone.

In conclusion, coaches and athletes should appreciate the degree to which the nature and substance of athletic training is over-determined. There are reasons within reasons for what must be done, and they must all be consistent and harmonious with the desired end. The question of whether a particular workout is efficacious can only be answered by considering everything that has preceded and all that will follow in the training program. And here there must be unity and coherence. Everything enters the picture, everything matters, and everything is interrelated.

> *If you do not look at things on a large scale it will be difficult for you to master strategy.*
>
> —Miyamoto Musashi

References

Bowerman, William J., *Coaching Track & Field*, William H. Freeman, Editor, Boston, Massachusetts: Houghton Mifflin Co., 1974.

Bompa, Tudor O., *Theory and Methodology of Training*, 3rd Edition, Dubuque, Iowa: Kendall/Hunt Publishing Company, 1994.

Daniels, Jack, and Jimmy Gilbert, *Oxygen Power*, Tempe, Arizona: Published Privately, 1979.

Dellinger, Bill, "A Runner's Philosophy", *Track & Field Quarterly Review*, Volume 79, Number 3, 1979, pages 13-16.

Dellinger, Bill, "University of Oregon Distance Training," *Track & Field Quarterly Review*, Volume 73, Number 3, 1973, pages 146-153.

Dellinger, Bill, and Georges Beres, *Winning Running*, Chicago, Illinois: Contemporary Books, 1987.

Dick, F.W., *Training Theory*, London: British Amateur Athletic Board, 1984.

Freeman, William H., *Peak When It Counts,* Mountain View, California: Track & Field News Press, 1989.

Harre, Dietrich, Editor, *Principles of Sport Training*, Berlin: Sportverlag, 1982, page 48.

Kim, Hee-Jin, *Dogen Kigen: Mystical Realist*, Translated by Victor Harris, Tuscon, Arizona: University of Arizona Press, 1987, page 152.

Lydiard, Arthur, and Garth Gilmour, *Run To The Top*, Auckland, New Zealand: Minerva, Ltd., 1962.

Matveyev, L., *Fundamentals of Sports Training*, Moscow: Progress Publishers, 1981.

Musashi, Miyamoto, *A Book Of Five Rings*, Translated by Victor Harris, New York: The Overlook Press, 1982, page 48.

Pedemonte, Jimmy, "Updated Acquisitions About Training Periodization," *NSCA Journal*, October-November, 1982.

Schmolinsky, Gerhardt, Editor, *Track & Field*, Berlin: Sportverlag, 1978.

Spear, Michael, "Emil Zatopek gives Modern-Day Runners the Truth Behind the Myth," *Runner's World Annual*, 1982.

Suzuki, Daisetz, *Zen and Japanese Culture*, Princeton, New Jersey: Bollinger Foundation, Inc., Princeton University Press, 1973.

Tschiene, Peter, "The Further Development of Training Theory," *Science Periodical on Research and Technology in Sport*, Volume 8, Number 4, 1988.

Yakolev, N.N., *Sports Biochemistry*, Leipzig: DHFK, 1967.

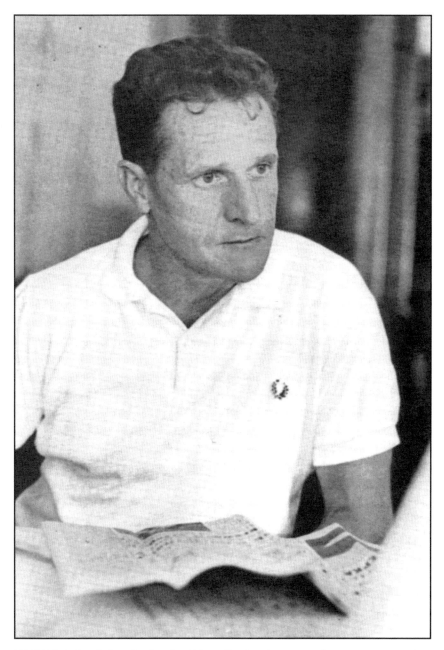

PHOTO 2.1—Arthur Lydiard of New Zealand captured at a press conference in 1964. From the title page of Arthur Lydiard and Garth Gilmour, *Run to the Top*, Auckland: Minerva, Ltd., 1967. Photo courtesy of Arthur Lydiard.

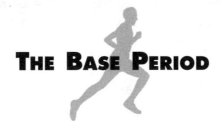

CHAPTER 2

THE BASE PERIOD

The base period is the first and longest of the five training periods of the athletic season, and its primary aim is to enhance aerobic ability. Improvements in aerobic ability result from adaptation to chronic training loads, thus take place over many months and years of training. Distance runners do not reach the peak of their development until well into their late twenties or thirties, and also must be willing to devote something on the order of ten years to achieve optimal results. A brief look at the relevant exercise physiology will demonstrate why the development of aerobic ability is so important for distance runners.

Exercise Physiology

The human body has three energy systems available for use in athletic performance:

- ATP-PC
- ATP-Lactic Acid
- ATP-Aerobic

Two of these energy systems are anaerobic, that is, they operate in the absence of oxygen, while one is aerobic, functioning in the presence of oxygen. Of the two anaerobic systems, the ATP-PC (Adenosine Triphosphate-Phospho-creatine) energy system dominates in explosive efforts up through 45 seconds, whereas the ATP-Lactic Acid system predominates in exhaustive efforts ranging from 45 seconds to three minutes. The aerobic pathway predominates beyond the temporal range of the ATP-Lactic Acid system, and is used almost exclusively in the marathon event. Table 2.1 provides an estimate regarding the predominant energy system used in various events.

The ATP-PC system provides a large power capacity, but is exhausted in 45 seconds duration. Its half-life—that is, the time required for it to reconstitute 50% of its capacity—is 20 seconds, 75% in 45 seconds, and 100% within 3 minutes duration (Kraemer, Fleck, 1982). Note that continuous slow jogging or running will postpone, if not completely thwart recovery of the ATP-PC system. Continuing intense efforts of relatively short duration, using a running-jog recovery, will then primarily stress the ATP-Lactic Acid energy system. Keep in mind which aspect of fitness the athlete is attempting to condition. If an athlete sets out to enhance their ATP-Lactic system, but walks or stands around between repetitions, then actually the ATP-PC system is recovering. For example, if an athlete runs reps of 200 meters at high speed with a relatively long walk recovery, then most of the training

Event	% Aerobic	% Anaerobic
400	15	85
800	35	65
1,500	60	40
3,000	85	15
5,000	90	10
10,000	95	5
Marathon	99	1

TABLE 2.1—Adapted from Sparks & Bjorklund, 1984

	Percentage of Fibers	
Athlete	Slow Twitch	Fast Twitch
Sprinter	24	76
Middle Distance	62	38
Marathon Runner	79	21
Cross-Country Skier	80	20
Untrained	53	47

TABLE 2.2—From Costill, Daniels, and Evans, et. al., 1976

session will utilize the ATP-PC system, whereas the use of a continuous jog recovery would stress the ATP-Lactic Acid energy system.

The third energy system is the aerobic pathway, also known as the Krebs Cycle, and it serves as the primary energy source for race events lasting over three minutes. Compared with the aerobic pathway, the anaerobic systems are extremely inefficient in their energy production. The ATP-PC system essentially constitutes a one-time-only source of energy in the early seconds of a race. In contrast, the ATP-Lactic system can be engaged whenever the athlete exceeds the capacity of the aerobic pathway to provide requisite energy. However, the ATP-Lactic Acid system produces a net of only two ATP's from available energy stores compared to 38 ATP's by the aerobic pathway, thus it is relatively inefficient on the order of 19:1!

That is one of the reasons why, once an athlete substantially begins to use the ATP-Lactic Acid system, energy reserves are quickly exhausted and metabolic by-products bring activity to a rapid halt. A recent study indicates that the metabolites phosphate and magnesium are responsible for muscle fatigue—not lactic acid (Posterino, Dutka, and Lamb, 2001). In addition, both anaerobic systems are limited to using carbohydrates as energy substrates, whereas the aerobic pathway can draw upon fatty acids and proteins. Female middle distance runners should not attempt to reduce weight by undertaking a non-carbohydrate diet and then engage in training or racing efforts that place demands on the ATP-

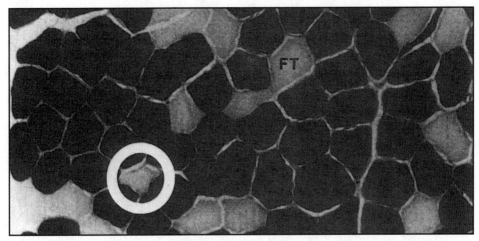

Photo 2.2—A microscopic view of Frank Shorter's leg muscle fiber type. The black fibers represent the slow twitch (type I) type, whereas the unstained cells are the fast twitch (FT, type II) fiber. Shorter's muscle was 80 percent slow twitch. From David L. Costill, *Inside Running*, Carmel, Indiana: The Cooper Press, LLP, 1986, page 5. Photo courtesy of David L. Costill.

Lactic Acid system, because they will become exhausted. The possession of superior aerobic ability also serves to enhance the efficiency of the anaerobic energy systems, because all the systems inhabit and utilize the same structure, and to some degree, the same arsenals. Further, the anaerobic systems depend upon the aerobic pathway for their recovery, so the athlete's aerobic ability serves as the limiting factor governing performance in distance running.

Many believe that an athlete's natural aerobic ability can be enhanced 25 to 35% over years of training. In response to chronic training loads, more capillaries will form, that is, their number as measured per square millimeter can increase 40% in a highly conditioned athlete, relative to a sedate individual (Åstrand and Rodahl, 1986). The mitochondria (the powerhouses of the cell) also greatly increase in number. The heart's stroke volume becomes larger, and it will then be able to pump more blood.

Further, we are all born with different ratios of one of two types of muscle fibers: slow twitch Type I muscle fibers (associated with endurance and aerobic ability), and fast twitch Type II muscle fibers (largely associated with explosive speed, power, and anaerobic ability). In addition, there are three different kinds of Type II muscle fibers: Type IIa is closely associated with the ATP-Lactic Acid system, Type IIb with the ATP-PC system, and Type IIc exhibits the ability to cross-train and assume many characteristics of the slow twitch Type I muscle fiber. Accordingly, specificity of training can, to some degree, influence the enzyme characteristics of various muscle fiber types so as to optimize performance in a given competitive event. Table 2.2 indicates the percentage of various muscle fiber types possessed by individuals competing in the different running events. Photo 2.2 shows a microscopic photograph of the leg muscle fiber type of Frank Shorter, the 1972 Olympic Gold Medalist in the marathon event.

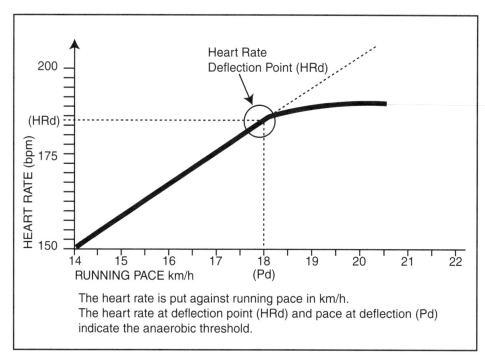

FIGURE 2.1—In well-trained athletes the heart rate (HR) in beats per minute (bpm) at the deflection point (HRd) is five to 20 (average 10.6) beats per minute lower than maximal heart rate. In untrained persons, the heart rate at the deflection point is 20 to 27 beats per minute lower than maximum heart rate (Adapted from Janssen, 1987).

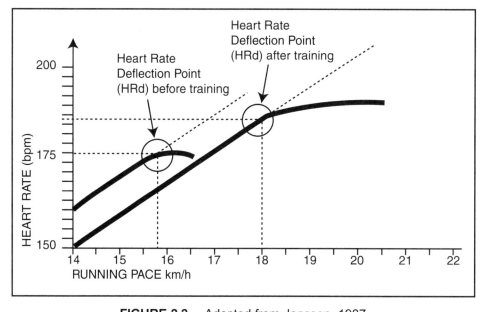

FIGURE 2.2 —Adapted from Janssen, 1987

Aerobic Training Theory

Again, an individual's aerobic ability is the primary limiting physiological factor in distance running performance. Once energy demands exceed the capacity of the aerobic pathway, exhaustion sets in geometrically. This exercise threshold is sometimes called the aerobic-anaerobic passing zone, or simply the anaerobic threshold. The heart rate of an athlete normally responds in a linear manner to increasing running speeds, that is, up to the point of the anaerobic threshold. Beyond this point, the heart rate will deviate from a linear progression and drop off, as shown in Figure 2.1.

As shown in Figure 2.2, with training and improved fitness, an athlete will be able to maintain a higher pulse rate and working level, and conversely, will be able to perform sub-maximal training loads at a lower heart rate than previously. Figure 2.3 shows one possible relationship between an elite runner's anaerobic threshold, running pace, and lactate production.

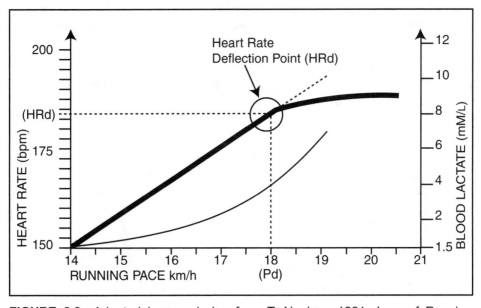

FIGURE 2.3—Adapted by permission from T. Noakes, 1991, *Lore of Running*, 3rd Ed., Champaign, IL: Human Kinetics, page 95.

The anaerobic threshold generally corresponds to a blood lactate level of approximately 4mM/liter. However, as fitness improves, the athlete will be able to run at higher continuous speeds with lower levels of lactate production, and will then cross the 4mM/liter anaerobic threshold when moving at higher speeds than before, as shown in Figure 2.4. Different training efforts can be associated with specific ranges of exhibited heart rate and lactate production, as shown in Figure 2.5. More specifically, Figure 2.6 shows the relationship between training effort, intensity, heart rate, blood lactate accumulation, and training activity.

See again Table 1.1, which provides a general guideline for relatively fit young athletes concerning the relationship between training effort, exercise heart rate, and VO$_2$ maximum. Our bodies can utilize fatty acids (primarily intra-muscular triglycerides), carbohydrates, or proteins as energy sources during exercise. Given low intensity exercise, runners use a high relative percentage of fatty acids as an energy source. However, the fatty acid metabolism is relatively slow and it cannot meet sudden high-intensity energy demands. In contrast, carbohydrates can satisfy relatively sudden high-intensity energy demands, but the human body can only store enough carbohydrates for about 90 minutes of high-intensity aerobic effort. When athletes function anaerobically, using the ATP-lactic acid energy system, they can exhaust the available carbohydrate stores in less than two minutes.

The brain can only use carbohydrates as an energy source, so when glycogen or carbohydrate stores are extremely low, an individual's mental concentration can be impaired. When high school or college students study intensively for final

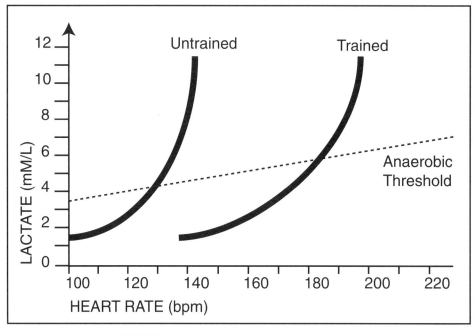

FIGURE 2.4—Adapted from Janssen, 1987

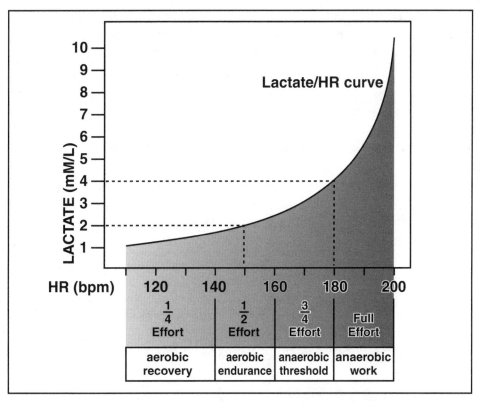

FIGURE 2.5—Adapted From Janssen, 1987

$\frac{1}{4}$ EFFORT	$\frac{1}{2}$ EFFORT
• Low Intensity Effort • Heart Rate 100 - 140 bpm • Lactate 1 - 1.5 mM/L • Passive Recovery • Easy Recovery • Active Recovery • Long Run, as Extensive Endurance Work	• Moderate Intensity Effort • Heart Rate 140 - 160 bpm • Lactate 1.5 - 2 mM/L • Active Recovery • Extensive Fartlek • Long Run, as Intensive Endurance Work (e.g., preparation for marathon)
$\frac{3}{4}$ EFFORT	FULL EFFORT
• High and Submaximum Intensity Effort • Heart Rate 160 - 180 bpm • Lactate 2 - 4 mM/L • Steady State Runs • Anaerobic Threshold Steady State Runs • Intensive Fartlek • Extensive Intervals • Extensive Repetitions • Early Date Pace Work • Early Finishing Speed Work	• Maximum Intensity Effort • Heart Rate 180 - 200 bpm • Lactate 4+ mM/L • Races • Time Trials • Intensive Intervals • Intensive Repetitions • Later Date Pace Work • Later Finishing Speed Work

FIGURE 2.6

exams, the depletion of carbohydrate stores is similar to what occurs during a 3/4-effort workout. Accordingly, it is prudent to adjust the training program during "finals week" and encourage athletes to consume sufficient carbohydrates.

Normally, proteins are not greatly used as an energy source during exercise. If and when this does happen, as it can during the marathon, an athlete's legs will be slow to recover. And it generally takes at least seven to 14 days for an athlete to recover from competition in the 10,000 meters. Sometimes the presence of bad breath can indicate that an athlete has consumed muscle tissue protein during hard exercise.

In distance running, an important adaptation concerns the enhanced ability to use fatty acids as an energy source, thus sparing the more limited carbohydrate stores. A fitter athlete can use fatty acids as an energy source to a greater degree during a race, thus preserving a greater portion of available carbohydrate stores for executing surges, breakaways, and the finishing kick. Figure 2.7 illustrates this adaptation with respect to fatty acid utilization.

Of course, the enemy of adaptation and enhancement of an individual's aerobic ability is father time. Maximum heart rate decreases with age. To make an approximation, take the maximum heart rate of 220 bpm, and then subtract the individual's age in order to predict their maximum heart rate, as shown in Figure 2.8.

Steady-state Distance Runs

What is the most efficient way to improve our aerobic ability? Performing quality work near the anaerobic threshold enables high training loads to be sustained for a relatively long duration. The state of equilibrium achieved near the anaerobic threshold is commonly known as an individual's steady state. Highly conditioned athletes will commonly perform at 86 to 88% of their VO_2 maximum for one hour, or approximately ten miles, while running at their steady-state pace (Daniels, 1999). So when athletes perform a steady-state run are they actually functioning below, within, or above the anaerobic threshold? The answer can be any of the above, depending on the individual and the particular circumstances. Athletes tend to intuitively optimize their performance in the steady-state run based on their limiting physiological factors on a given day. Some days the limiting factor could be that they had too little for lunch, and are low on carbohydrates. However, it is probably more accurate to say that an athlete performs at the "proton threshold," that is, at the limit of the body's ability to remove and buffer the acidity associated with blood lactate. Once the blood pH drops below 7.0, the enzyme functions and biochemistry required for continued exercise are quickly rendered inoperable (Newsholme, 1983). This variable ability to remove or buffer the protons associated with lactic acid production accounts, in part, for why some individuals can sustain higher blood lactate levels than others during a steady-state training session. Stroke volume, mitochondria and capillary density, and muscular strength are a few of the variables that affect the clearance of blood lactate. Since an athlete's improvement will be determined by the performance of

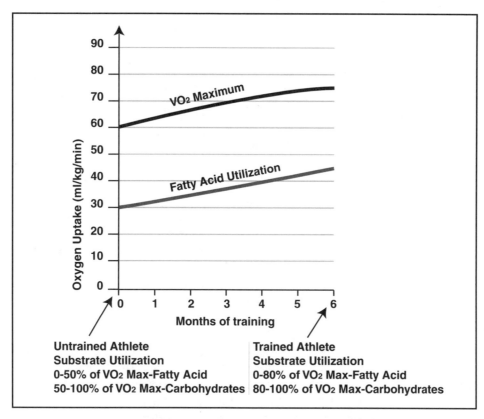

FIGURE 2.7—Adapted from Janssen, 1987

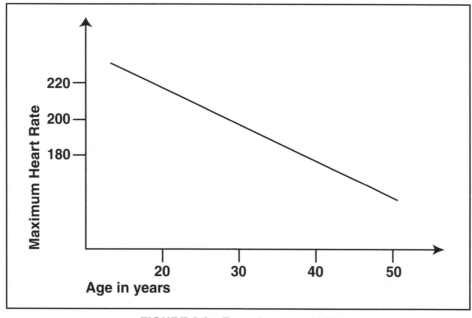

FIGURE 2.8—From Janssen, 1987

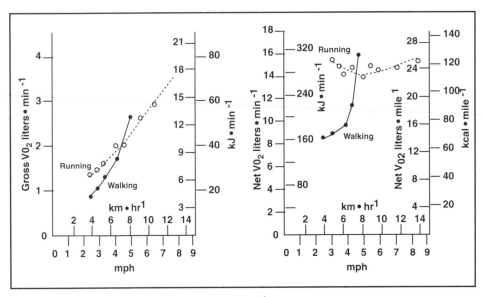

FIGURE 2.9—From Åstrand, 1986

optimal training loads and training frequency, the athlete should run at paces as close to the steady-state as possible, and nearly as often as permitted by adequate recovery. In practice, this translates into two workouts at 3/4-effort, and one at 1/2-effort each week. Given the nature of the anaerobic threshold, the steady-state run can be sustained longer when conducted at a relatively even pace. From the standpoint of available energy reserves, running an even pace at 3/4-effort does not pose a problem, since the slight difference in total energy consumption while functioning aerobically at five, six, or seven minutes/mile pace is not a significant limiting factor. Practically speaking, athletes can run for almost as long at five, as at seven minutes/mile, provided they do so aerobically, as shown in Figure 2.9.

In simple terms, this is the theory behind steady-state training of an athlete's aerobic ability. A steady-state run comprises a relatively long and evenly paced effort: the athlete running near the edge, but not quite crossing the "proton threshold," or then falling rapidly into a state of complete exhaustion. For the exceptionally fit athlete, the 3/4-effort steady-state training session is generally characterized by a heart rate between 165 to 185 beats per minute (bpm), as the athlete functions at roughly 86 to 88% of their VO_2 maximum, and often within 95 to 97% of their maximal heart rate (Janssen, 1987, Coyle, 1995, Daniels, 1998). However, recognize that older, untrained, or relatively unfit individuals perform at much lower physiological values when exercising at 3/4-effort.

To make significant and rapid gains, considerable pressure must be placed on the cardiovascular system. In the late 1970's, Arthur Lydiard shocked many would-be disciples during a visit to Minneapolis by personally demonstrating how the steady-state run should be conducted. Picture a man in his 60's running ten miles at 6:30 minutes/mile pace and lecturing most of the way! The popular

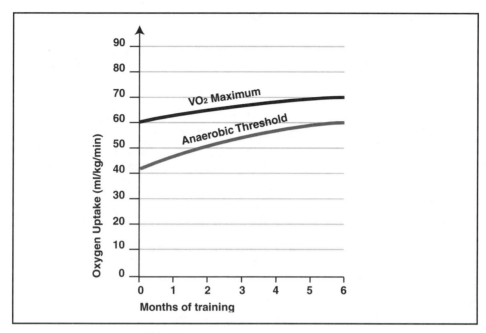

FIGURE 2.10—Adapted from Janssen, 1987

notions of Lydiard as a long slow distance advocate were quickly dispelled. There are different approaches to athletic training. Some are more suited, and some are less suited for a given athlete. But there is no easy way. There was something else about steady-state training that eluded many of Lydiard's listeners. Steady-state training of aerobic ability is necessary, but if used exclusively, it has certain liabilities. It is neither self-sufficient nor the most efficient means of enhancing aerobic ability. What actually happened during those steady-state runs over the testing New Zealand terrain?

Anaerobic Threshold Steady-State

Three variables are highly correlated with running performance: maximum oxygen uptake (or VO_2 maximum), anaerobic threshold (the point below VO_2 maximum associated with the heart-rate deflection point and pronounced blood lactate accumulation), and running economy (how much of an athlete's aerobic ability is actually translated into useful biomechanical work). Evenly paced steady-state runs are actually being conducted near and slightly below the anaerobic threshold, and not an individual's VO_2 maximum. Healthy athletes, who are not yet conditioned, typically encounter the anaerobic threshold at about 70% of their VO_2 maximum. However, given proper training, an evenly paced 3/4-effort steady-state can be run for an hour, covering approximately ten miles, and their anaerobic threshold elevated to approximately 86 to 88% of VO_2 maximum. In practice, athletes will have raised their functional aerobic ability by 16 to 18%. This results in the delayed onset of anaerobic metabolism, and in greatly improved performances, as shown in Figure 2.10.

How can the anaerobic threshold be raised?

> To develop the A.T., the pace must be faster than the highest steady-state pace, but yet not so fast as to push the body into deep anaerobic lactic acid metabolism. In effect, the body carries on a conversation with itself saying "I want to be aerobic and if I can raise my A.T. slightly so as to still metabolize aerobically, I will have made a positive adaptation to stress. So to raise my A.T. all I need to do is raise the triggering mechanism to a higher percentage because I have the maximum VO_2 capacity to handle the workload (John McKenzie, Unpublished Manuscript).

To define an individual's steady-state pace and provide a format for anaerobic threshold training, take the pace that a young athlete can run for ten kilometers (or alternately, ten miles for mature athletes), and use it as a guideline. Relative to the quantity that could be undertaken in an evenly paced effort over that distance, an athlete should subtract 20% for the anaerobic threshold training session. So if an individual can run 10 miles in an evenly paced steady-state, then plan on covering roughly 8 miles in the anaerobic threshold workout. This is an allowance for the inefficiency of the uneven surging efforts undertaken in the anaerobic threshold training session relative to the evenly paced steady-state. Young athletes should then introduce surges 20 to 30 seconds faster than steady-state pace, lasting anywhere between 10 seconds and three minutes, whereas elite athletes can progress to conducting faster segments lasting up to five to 10 minutes. The athletes recover by slowing back down from this faster segment, and then running at their steady-state pace again. However, if one had to pick a single "magic" distance or duration to conduct, it would be 1,000 meters, or approximately between 2:30 to 3:30 minutes duration.

In the abstract, it is not possible to accurately predict or prescribe target heart rate response characteristics for different athletes. For example, an extremely fit elite athlete might run the faster segments with a heart rate over 180 bpm, but the slower segments still above 175 bpm. However, a young untrained athlete or a relatively fit 40-year-old might run the faster segments near 160 bpm and the slower at 150 bpm. Pay close attention to the effort, and if you wish, record the heart rate. But do not prescribe training efforts in terms of heart rate unless it is for an individual athlete whose fitness and characteristic heart rate responses are well known. There is simply too much variability from person to person due to differences in age, sex, athletic level, and training background. Because of this, coaches and athletes should not get too hung up on technology. Technology can be useful, but it is no substitute for judgment and experience. In truth, experienced athletes know what a 3/4-effort is, and also when their pulse rate has recovered to 120 beats per minute. And experienced coaches know a full-effort, 3/4-effort, or 1/2-effort workout when they see it. Moreover, top level coaches and athletes also know what is required in athletic training, and when. Technology such as heart rate monitors and oxygen uptake analyzers can be helpful.

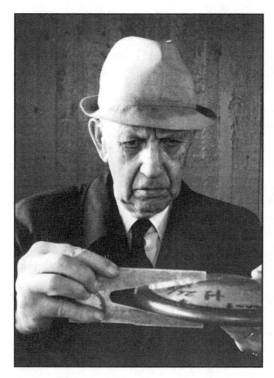

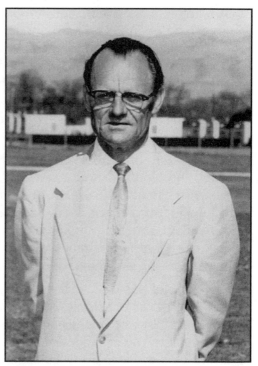

Photo 2.3—Swedish Coach Gosta Holmer, the creator of Fartlek training, who influenced World Record Holders Gunder Haegg and Arne Andersson. Photo courtesy of Emil Siekkinen, Sweden.

Photo 2.4—Coach Mihaly Igloi, who coached Hungarian World Record holders Istvan Rozsavolgyi and Sandor Iharos during the 1950's. Photo courtesy of Mike Salmon, Amateur Athletic Foundation of Los Angeles.

However, if the fundamental decisions upon which the athletic training is based are faulty, then all runners will have at the end of the athletic season is a lot of fancy data to document their mistakes.

Coaches and distance runners are sometimes overly meticulous when it comes to measurement and recording of detail. Psychologically, this can be a way of exorcising fear, blame, or perhaps bolstering one's confidence. As a result, athletes sometimes become unduly gratified by recording their daily training. Sometimes this comes from the need to prove themselves to themselves, and can be a sign of weakness, rather than strength. For every successful athlete with a detailed diary and various gadgets, at least a dozen other unsuccessful athletes have the same. This doesn't mean you should throw all record keeping and science away, but do not attach too much to it.

> *No one ever won the olive wreath with an impressive training diary.*
>
> —Marty Liquori

A reporter once questioned Arthur Lydiard while Peter Snell was running a workout in an open field. The reporter asked Lydiard how far Snell was running. His answer: "I don't know." Next, the reporter asked how fast Snell was running. Lydiard's answer: "I don't know." The reporter then asked how many repetitions Snell was doing. Again, his answer: "I don't know." At that point, Lydiard explained to the reporter that what really mattered was whether Snell was accomplishing the desired training effect with the appropriate effort.

The same principle holds true in the performance of an anaerobic threshold training session. In order to enhance the quality of the training session, runners can vary the length of the faster segments, and alternate shorter and longer surges throughout the session. It is most effective to begin with shorter and slightly faster surges and work into the longer segments, and then return and finish by conducting shorter surges. The anaerobic threshold workout should be tailored to an individual's main race event, with consideration being given to the distance, number, and intensity of the surges.

This form of training has been around for decades under various names and guises. The practice of fartlek or "speed play" on nature trails, as practiced by Gosta Holmer and the Scandinavians, was a form of anaerobic threshold training. Emil Zatopek ran so-called interval workouts, covering upwards of 10 to 15 miles, stressing various distances while constantly changing the tempo. Some of the so-called intervals were run in the pace of 70 to 80 plus seconds, thus the structure of the interval format as it appeared in the abstract tended to disguise what was actually being accomplished (Kožík, 1954). Mihaly Igloi, a trained Hungarian military observer, spent a winter watching Zatopek's training through binoculars and meticulously recorded the details (Mader, 1979). Igloi then coached the next wave of World Record holders in distance running. Certainly, the training of Percy Cerutty's athletes in the sand dunes surrounding Portsea, Australia, included considerable training of the anaerobic threshold. Many have also misconceived what Lydiard actually accomplished during steady-state runs. Given the hilly New Zealand terrain, many steady-state efforts were, in reality, anaerobic threshold workouts, as opposed to evenly paced steady-state efforts conducted on the flat.

Accordingly, runners can conduct an unstructured anaerobic threshold work-out by simply running a steady-state over a demanding course. Athletes will surge with greater effort on the hills and briefly cross the anaerobic threshold, but then recover on the downhill sections or while running as close to the anaerobic threshold as possible. Mentally, this unstructured approach is less exhausting, and can actually be exhilarating when performed in beautiful natural surround-ings. However, merely training the anaerobic threshold is not the most productive way to elevate an individual's aerobic ability.

Anaerobic threshold and evenly paced steady-state training are both neces-sary and are actually complimentary. Neither one is fully sufficient as the most efficient means of improving aerobic ability. The most efficient way of doing this during the base period is to alternate the training efforts. On one hand, the evenly paced steady-state too much resembles simple equilibrium. For the body, equilibrium is bliss, but change and variation results in greater improvement. In the evenly paced steady-state runs, athletes face the constant danger of stagnating by forming neuromuscular stereotypes that will ultimately hinder the acquisition of fitness. They can easily fall into a groove and run at nearly the same pace in the steady-state runs week after week because it has become the dominant habit. Moreover, athletes who only run at an even effort will not be physically or mentally conditioned for executing surges or breakaways in competition. We train to race after all! However, the anaerobic threshold training sessions also have certain liabilities. If athletes only conduct anaerobic threshold work, they might not be physically or mentally conditioned for competitions in which no respite or easing of the pace is provided. Constant change and variation also presents the danger of not adequately stabilizing and consolidating newly gained performance potential. A runner's enhanced aerobic ability would be realized and practically demonstrated by sustaining a faster even pace during a steady-state run. Remember, the pace of the evenly paced steady-state over a given duration is the practical measure of the anaerobic threshold, and indirectly, of the individual's maximum oxygen uptake. The anaerobic threshold training session is like taking a step up on a ladder into empty space: the potential for climbing higher is there, but to fully consolidate that new potential the athlete needs to connect with the next rung on the ladder, in the form of an evenly paced steady-state.

Let's say an individual's steady-state pace over 10 miles is 6:00 minutes/mile, and the athlete conducts an eight mile anaerobic threshold session averaging under 6:20 minutes/mile while alternating surges of 30 seconds and a minute duration at a pace of 5:40 minutes/mile. Suppose that four days later the runner has recovered so that his or her aerobic ability is in a temporary state of enhancement. Now let's suppose the athlete's steady-state pace over 10 miles has potentially improved to 5:55 minutes/mile. If this individual were to conduct another anaerobic threshold session this new potential might not be fully consolidated. The athlete has the potential to run 5:55 minute miles for 10 miles (the concrete and practical measure of the individual's aerobic ability), but the runner's body has never done it! It remains only potential. In a sense, the athlete's performance capability is floating on air. Better to run an evenly paced steady-state at 5:55 minutes/mile so as to assimilate and consolidate this new level of ability. The athlete would then proceed from this building block or rung on the ladder to conduct another anaerobic threshold session, and so repeat the process. Accordingly, the anaerobic threshold and evenly paced steady-state training sessions are complimentary, and both necessary to the most efficient acquisition of aerobic ability. When conducted at 3/4-effort and separated by approximately three to four days, they constitute the two primary quality training efforts undertaken on a weekly basis during the base period.

Many Factors Contribute to an Athlete's Aerobic Ability

The formula for calculating VO_2 maximum is shown below (Fox and Mathews, 1981):

$$MAX\ VO_2 = (SV \times HR) \times (av\ O_2\ difference)$$

SV = Stroke Volume

HR = Heart Rate

Cardiac Output = $(SV \times HR)$

However, the contributing factors to an athlete's demonstrable aerobic ability are many, and their interrelationships are infinitely more complex than this simple formula would seem to suggest. Edward F. Coyle, Director of the Human Performance Laboratory at the University of Texas at Austin, has attempted to define some of these interrelationships and measure how they correlate with athletic performance. As shown in Figure 2.11, many factors can influence an individual's anaerobic threshold and performance capability.

- Muscle capillary density increases as a result of chronic training loads. The long run on the weekend, and the steady-state and anaerobic threshold running efforts, all stimulate the creation of greater capillary density. Capillary density can enhance performance by providing a greater supply of oxygen, but also by more rapidly clearing and neutralizing the by-products of work associated with lactic acid production.

- If an athlete lacks muscular strength, then running can solicit relatively forceful muscular contractions and result in the occlusion of blood flow in muscle tissue. This would neutralize the practical effects of increased capillarization. Accordingly, Chapter 8 discusses the importance of strength training for middle distance and distance runners.

- Maximal heart rate and stroke volume can also influence aerobic ability. As the heart enlarges, the morning pulse will frequently slow to less than 50 bpm, a condition known as bradycardia. The imposition of a sudden venous preload upon the heart (as when briefly recovering from high-intensity exercises) can enhance stroke volume. For this reason 10 x 100 meters accelerations should be conducted with a short and fast 50 meters jog recovery several times each week during an athlete's warm-up or warm-down. This can be accomplished by running diagonals on the infield of a track and field facility or soccer field.

- Aerobic enzyme activity is largely defined by an individual's genetically determined muscle fiber composition, but can also be influenced by the type of training being conducted and its volume. Proper diet and sound training practices can greatly benefit the central nervous and endocrine systems, and positively influence aerobic enzyme activity.

- Taking naps and getting adequate sleep can have dramatic effects upon athletic development and performance. Like infants or young children,

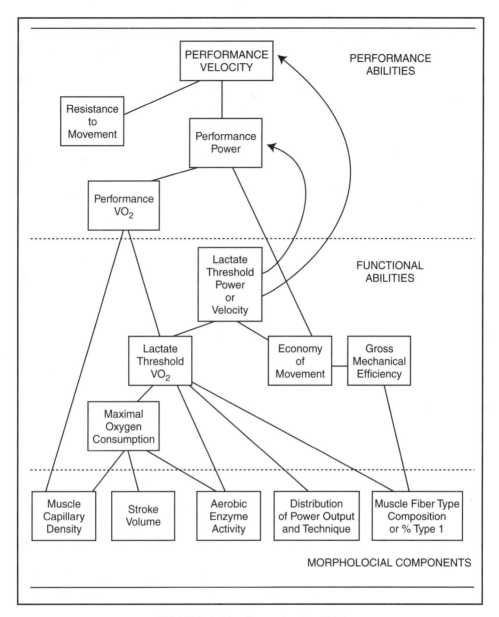

FIGURE 2.11—From Coyle, 1995

developing athletes are also in the mode of acquisition and physical transformation. Young children should take naps in the morning and afternoon, and get to bed at an early hour (Weissbluth, 1987, 1995). Taking even a 20-minute nap several times a day will lower cortisol levels and thereby stimulate anabolic, as opposed to catabolic metabolism. Marc Weissbluth, M.D., Director of the Sleep Disorder Center at Children's Memorial Hospital, Chicago, recalls that Bob Mathias, the 1948 and 1952 Olympic Decathlon Champion, was able to take naps between his events. Herb Elliott, the 1960 Olympic Champion at 1,500 meters, was also able to nap prior to a major contest.

There is a fundamental aspect of athletic training that needs to be understood: The human body is the handiwork of the ages. We are hunter-gatherers, and yes, predators—the twentieth century has certainly proved it (Maile and Selzer, 1975, Goodall, 1990). The human body knows nothing of "athletic training." When we call upon it to exercise at the intensity athletic training demands, it is genetically programmed to presume that the situation is a case of fight or flight, or alternately, a potentially life-threatening quest for sustenance.

When a leopard makes a kill, it will drag the carcass up a tree, then gorge itself and sleep. However, when the leopard misses, it must stay in the hunt until it succeeds, and its metabolism then continues to function in an energy efficient starvation mode, or catabolism. The same thing holds true for athletes out hunting fitness by way of training sessions. If athletes do not drink and eat soon afterwards, and then take a nap or sleep, their metabolisms will remain parsimonious and unduly catabolic. That translates into meager acquisition and transformation of functional ability, thus little or no improvement in athletic performance.

In order to transform its performance potential, the human body needs a few simple cues to tell it that it's an environmentally safe time to spend energy in a relatively uneconomical manner. After all, the process of acquisition and adaptation is something of a luxury, because in nature, a mistake can result in certain death. And the primary cues that the human body pays heed to are exercise, drink, food, and sleep. Athletes do not need to take anabolic steroids or various hormones in order to be successful, rather, they need to train intelligently, and eat and sleep well.

- Running economy is much more significant to performance in the distance events than commonly appreciated. In aerobic exercise, an athlete's running economy directly influences their oxygen demand. All things being equal, as the intensity of aerobic exercise increases, a less economical runner will encounter the anaerobic threshold sooner than another who is more efficient. This is partly why each week, during the base and hill periods, athletes should conduct a 1/2-effort short interval session at date pace that includes reps having a distance between 100 to 400 meters. It is also one reason why athletes should do some barefoot running on grass or a sandy beach whenever possible. The effect of a runner's distribution of power output is discussed in greater detail in Chapter 16. Briefly, athletes who demonstrate a greater range of motion, and more subtle variations and improvisations in their running technique, can effectively distribute the work load over greater muscle mass. Therefore, specific muscle groups and individual muscle fibers do not have to work as hard and will not produce high levels of blood lactate as early during exercise or performance. Many do not recognize and appreciate this aspect of running economy.

- Nutrition can greatly influence a runner's aerobic ability and anaerobic threshold. Athletes and coaches should read and consider Percy

Cerutty's views on diet, and also the similar conclusions of James Autio (Cerutty, 1961 and 1964, Autio, 2000). See also the brief discussion on pre-race diet in Chapter 16.

An entire book could be written on the subject of nutrition, but that lies beyond the scope of this treatment. Accordingly, only a few things will be discussed here. An individual athlete's food intolerances or allergies must be avoided. For example, many are intolerant to lactose (found in milk products), and others to wheat. If you are intolerant and don't know it, then your ability to assimilate nutrition can be compromised, and your immune system may be severely stressed. This will not promote good health or athletic development.

After a demanding workout, athletes should quickly restore their blood pH to a slightly base condition, since this can greatly impact their recovery rate and subsequent performance. A blended citrus fruit juice such as pineapple-grapefruit works well for this purpose. The relatively simple sugars in this juice will also help to restore normal blood sugar levels. Cantaloupe, peaches, watermelon, bananas, mandarin oranges, and almost any form of bread, can also be used. Moreover, taking not only carbohydrates, but also small amounts of protein and fat can enhance recovery. Yogurt can provide about the right amounts, and is easily assimilated. When traveling in foreign countries, a trusted brand of yogurt can also help restore the right bacteria, and provide quick relief from digestive problems that can cause dehydration and severely affect athletic performance. Obviously, an athlete needs adequate stores of carbohydrates for optimal performance. Accordingly, in order to perform at optimal levels, an athlete requires foods with a moderate or high glycemic index in meals preceding a hard workout or competition.

After decades of continual use, the soils in which our food is grown have become nutritionally depleted. For this reason, and because athletes require more than non-athletes, they should take vitamin and mineral supplements.

Obviously, athletes should stay away from all manner of drugs. Alcohol adversely affects performance potential for at least several days thereafter, and is seldom a good idea. Greasy foods or excitotoxins, which create false appetites or tastes similar to MSG, should also be avoided. Note that MSG can be listed as an ingredient under many other names, such as "natural flavors." The caffeine present in coffee is another drug that can impair an athlete when its consumption becomes an addictive habit.

Diet includes what we eat, drink and breathe, but it can also include substances that permeate our skin. In terms of air quality, avoid smog, smoke, paint, new cars and recently laid carpeting. That new car smell is comprised of volatiles, most of which are toxic, and do not enhance performance. Beware of exposure to petroleum products, other harsh chemicals and toxins, and new clothes that have not yet been washed. They can include chemicals that penetrate the skin. Absorption of such chemicals through the skin can sometimes render an athlete anemic. Most people recognize that they can become sick by breathing or eating something harmful, but many are not aware of the skin being a permeable membrane. Playing or swimming in a clean lake or ocean that is rich in minerals can facilitate recovery from demanding exercise and promote health, since the skin is actually a more porous membrane than commonly imagined, and water is the most remarkable solvent in the world. The use of mineral springs to aid or restore health also has merit. The skin can then serve as a selectively permeable membrane, enabling the body to pull from the water what it needs—and simultaneously eliminate what it does not. Accordingly, by taking a dip in the ocean after running in the sand dunes, the athletes who trained with Australian coach Percy Cerutty enjoyed an ideal environment and training practice. Often, runners who fear their athletic season ruined due to excessive training, racing, or travel can quickly recover and deliver their personal records by getting proper nutrition, rest, and taking several dips in a refreshing lake or ocean.

- An athlete's vital capacity, (i.e., the maximum volume of air they can inhale while breathing) and breathing technique can directly affect their aerobic ability and performance. After all, running has a lot to do with breathing. To inhale, the pressure on the lung cavity must be relieved to create a vacuum. It requires muscular effort to take the pressure off of the lung cavity so that the atmospheric pressure (14.69 pounds per square inch and 760 mm of mercury) can do its handiwork and refill the lungs with needed oxygen. How many athletes today conduct breathing exercises? How many coaches even think they should? The intercostal muscles and diaphragm can benefit from strengthening and stretching, particularly after a demanding running workout. An athlete can accomplish this by conducting pull-ups, push-ups, jumping jacks, the bench press, or by hanging vertically from an overhead bar. Lying flat on your back on a firm floor, and sleeping on a firm futon are also beneficial. Again, an athlete should consider Percy Cerutty's writings on the subject of breathing (Cerutty, 1964, and 1967). He observed that many athletes insufficiently fill their lungs while breathing during strenuous exercise. Cerutty also taught and understood tidal, or so-called Zen breathing, and the physical, mental, and "spiritual" implications of correct practice. An in-depth treatment on the subject of breathing can be found in the works of Karlfried Graf Dürckheim (Dürckheim, 1986, and 1988).

- Concerning an athlete's demonstrated aerobic ability and anaerobic threshold, one should also consider the human body as an electrical phenomenon. Ultimately, all the chemical processes in the body are electrical in nature, with muscular contractions being an obvious case in point. The earth has a charge. So does the atmosphere. Man has a charge or electrical potential. And the human body contains different electrical potentials and gradients, some of which generally correspond to the meridians known in acupuncture or acupressure. Hard work necessarily changes some of those potentials, and an individual's recovery and acquisition of fitness is dependent upon their restoration (Becker, 1987).

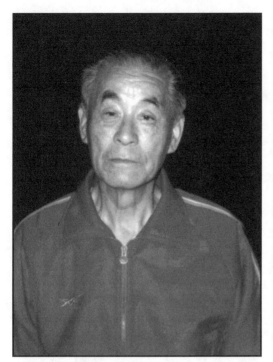

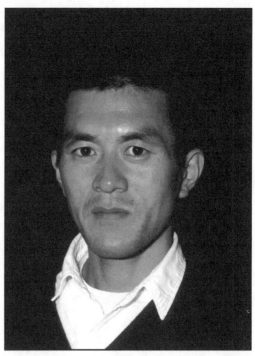

Photo 2.5—Master Kiyoshi Nakamura, coach of Japanese distance runner Toshihiko Seko. Photo courtesy of Nobuya Hashizume.

Photo 2.6—Toshihiko Seko, Boston, Massachusetts, 1987. Photo from Victah Sailer/ Photorun.

Accordingly, walking or running barefoot on grass or a sandy beach influences the electrical potentials within the body and speeds recovery. Swimming may be even better in this regard, although runners can do without the chlorine found in indoor pools. However, swimming or splashing about in a lake or the ocean surf can greatly accelerate recovery. Massage therapy can also be effective, for the same reason. Athletes in the United States often run in electrically non-conductive footwear, and upon hard asphalt surfaces. That is not natural, and what is not natural is generally not good. Perhaps, this bioelectrical phenomenon can be measured and scientifically proven, but only with great difficulty (given the number of variables and the subjective nature of human perception). However, when you see the same positive reaction from a large number of athletes to certain stimuli over a number of years, the question concerning just how or why becomes something of a moot point. All the science in the world cannot tell us as much about the effects of a given training variable upon an individual as one simple question: "How do you feel?"

An individual's mental state can greatly influence the anaerobic threshold. Physical tension resulting from anxiety, and the associated biochemical changes it induces in the body, can dramatically reduce an athlete's exhibited aerobic ability. Make sure you have the mental game in hand. Otherwise, the fittest athlete in the world will not be able to demonstrate it on the appointed day and hour.

PHOTOS 2.7 — Toshihiko Seko running the Boston Marathon, 1987
photos from Victah Sailer/Photorun

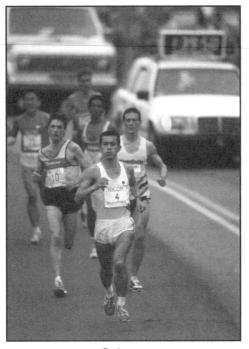

Going…

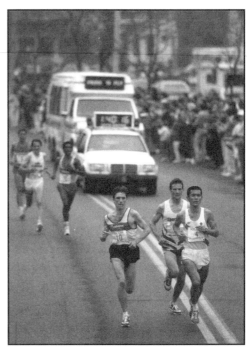

Going…

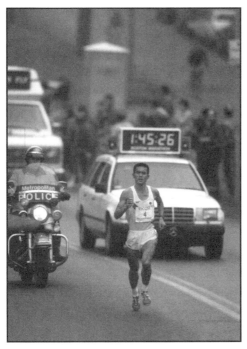

Gone!

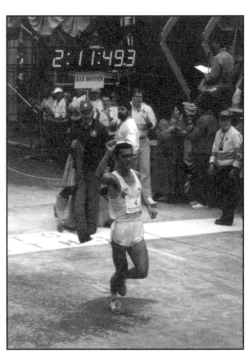

Zanshin… Perfect finish!

Hopefully, this brief digression on various factors that can affect aerobic ability will shake things up a bit, and possibly get the reader thinking in new dimensions about athletic training. Again, everything matters. Everything is interrelated. Life is an interpenetrating and indissoluble unity—so the question of what influences aerobic ability, and how, is never an easy or simple one to answer.

> *The structure of the absolute now is such that the past, present, and future, in an epochal whole… are not arranged in a linear fashion but realized simultaneously in the manner of mutual identity and mutual penetration*
>
> —Dōgen Kigen

Nevertheless, in this country many tend to suppose that athletics is simply what happens in the workouts. There is much to be said for the method of the Australian coach Percy Cerutty, who frequently had athletes reside at Portsea, and also the Japanese coach Kiyoshi Nakamura, who had Toshihiko Seko live with him for a while (Maier, 1981). Why? In order to teach athletes how to live. Most of the things that influence athletes happen in the other 20-plus hours a day spent away from formal training. Everything in life will impact athletic performance, and that certainly includes character development. After attaining victory in a marathon, Seko was taught to erase the ego by meditating in a temple. Too many athletes think the right way to celebrate after a victory is to meditate in a pub and solicit the attention of the opposite sex. Two more contrasting attitudes to the way of athletics cannot be imagined.

Base Period Duration: High School

For young high school athletes (or those whose physical age corresponds to that of a freshman or sophomore), training for the cross-country season should begin with the first day of organized team practice. Make sure that young people enjoy a lengthy period of post-season recovery prior to beginning a new athletic season, since demanding training tends to suppress the natural maturation process, and vice-versa. In the United States, organized cross-country team practice normally begins in mid-August. Young cross-country runners will often desire to peak for their conference and regional championships, during the last two weeks of October. Allowing for an ascent of nine to 10 days and three to four weeks of sharpening work, indicates that the base period should conclude by the end of the third week in September. That normally provides a total of six weeks of base work during the high school cross-country season. During a high school season of 12 weeks, all that a coach can do with young athletes is to bring them into a respectable state of fitness to minimize the risk of injury during competition, and thereby uncover what God has granted in the way of natural talent. It is a much harder job than most imagine.

High school juniors and seniors (or more mature athletes participating in cross-country), would be able to begin the base period in preparation for cross-country around the first of July, and focus on the state cross-country championships generally held in the first week of November. This still permits a month respite after the conclusion of the previous track season. It also provides an additional five to six weeks of preparation prior to the beginning of organized team practice. This effectively doubles the length of the base period for juniors and seniors relative to freshmen and sophomores.

The same prescription holds true for athletes participating in track and field during the spring. Base work for young high school athletes should begin on the first day of organized team practice, which in the United States is generally the first week of March. Most runners will want to deliver optimal performances in the conference and regional championships held during the last two weeks of May. The state championship meets traditionally come in late May or early June. This means that base and hill work must conclude by the end of the third week in April. This allows for roughly seven weeks of base and hill work during a track season lasting approximately 14 weeks. Young high school athletes should take much of the winter season off and engage in some other non-competitive sport or activity. The more mature high school athletes could begin a build-up by the middle of January, which would provide an additional six weeks of preparation for the track and field season. An elite high school athlete participating in the national high school cross-country championships would not finish cross-country until late December, and thus would require a period of post-season recovery extending until the middle of January.

Base Period Duration: Division 1

Collegiate men and women competing in conference track championships in late May should take two to four weeks of post-season recovery, and begin base work for the cross-country season by the first of July. However, athletes competing in the NCAA Track and Field Championships, and the USATF National Championships, might not resume training until the middle of July, after taking two to four weeks of post-season recovery. This presents no problem with regard to their cross-country preparation, since these athletes would focus on the conference championships at the end of October, and in particular, the NCAA Cross-Country Championships in the middle of November. Accordingly, the base and hill periods for collegiate athletes will often extend nearly through the end of September.

Collegiate athletes should take two to four weeks of post-season recovery following the conclusion of the cross-country season. Base and hill work could then begin by the middle of December and continue through the end of January. That would provide three to four weeks of sharpening work prior to taking the nine-to-10-day ascent to a brief plateau of peak performance for the indoor conference track and field championships. Athletes should then return to base and strength work immediately afterwards. To continue with sharpening work and racing would severely compromise competitive results during the outdoor track season. The athletes would then be trying to build on a foundation that was no longer there. However, there is little time to complete regenerative base and hill work. Assuming that the outdoor conference track and field championships come in the third week of May, base and hill work must be completed by the first or second week of April. This only provides time for five or six weeks of base and hill work prior to sharpening for the outdoor conference track and field championships.

Too Many Seasons

Young collegiate athletes commonly ask: is it possible to peak for indoor and outdoor track, and still get optimal results in both? No, it is not possible for a distance runner. Athletes can sharpen up a bit for the indoor season to obtain a respectable result, but if they try to put their eggs in both baskets, they will likely fall between the cracks. The more athletes sharpen for the indoor season, the more they will compromise their performances during the outdoor season. You can only have two optimal competitive seasons during the athletic year at the Division 1 level, that is, cross-country and outdoor track, and even here, one season must have precedence over the other.

Some collegiate athletes do occasionally compete and win multiple titles in cross-country, indoor, or outdoor championships. Realize that they can do this only because they are exceptional—so superior that they do not have to be in their best form to nevertheless dominate the competition. However, the long-term prognosis for these individuals is dim, as most will not be able to survive this treatment for long and enjoy a post-collegiate career. This problem can be aptly described as the "battered athlete syndrome."

Coaches and athletes desiring optimal performances outdoors should then limit the sharpening work for the indoor season to three weeks. Further, the quality of the sharpening work conducted by mature athletes for the indoor season should be reduced on the order of one second/400 meters from the projected goal performance in the main race event for the outdoor season, and nearer two seconds/400 meters for young developing athletes. For example, a mature athlete projecting a 4:00 mile performance outdoors would prepare for 4:04 indoors. An athlete projecting 14:00 for 5,000 meters outdoors would then aim for 14:12 indoors, and so on.

Again, young developing athletes should aim at something closer to outdoor goal pace plus two seconds/400 meters during the indoor season. They should also race infrequently, and if possible, over-distance or under-distance with respect to the main race event. By competing over-distance with respect to the main race event, runners will enhance their endurance and stay relatively close to the base work. This would also enhance their ability to recover from future preliminary rounds, and compete during the outdoor season. Alternately, runners could develop their finishing speed by competing under-distance with respect to the main race event, perhaps in the 400 or 800 meters. If limited, this practice does not sharpen athletes, which is a critical consideration, but rather merely enhances their finishing speed. Coaches and athletes will then be training through the indoor season, while still obtaining respectable results. However, the more frequently athletes race indoors and compete in the main race event, the more they will be sharpened and forfeit optimal performance outdoors. Accordingly, the development of the runners could be compromised, and they might not substantially improve during their collegiate careers.

The hazards presented by the existence of three collegiate competitive athletic seasons leads to an essential point: collegiate distance runners should not compete in three athletic seasons. Once again, it would be best, from the standpoint of both their academic and athletic development, if collegiate distance runners were only granted eligibility to compete in two athletic seasons during the calendar year. Moreover, collegiate distance runners are unable to successfully chase the four rabbits represented by their conference meet, their district qualifying meet, the NCAA Championships, and the USATF National Championships during the outdoor season. The most exciting thing in track and field to happen recently in the United States was the "David versus Goliath" competition of high school athlete Alan Webb against collegiate and world class athletes in the 2001 Prefontaine Classic that resulted in Jim Ryun's high school mile record being broken. Elite collegiate athletes are those who have developed to national class. In truth, the NCAA qualifying marks are nearly the same as those for the USATF National Championships. This redundancy undermines athletic development. The author believes that the quality of the sport would be elevated, and public interest greatly enhanced by combining the NCAA and USATF National Championships.

Base Period Training Prescriptions

The training conducted during the base period should be individualized for athletes having different backgrounds and levels of ability. However, a micro-cycle or weekly training prescription for the base period during the cross-country and track seasons is provided below.

Monday	Passive Recovery
Tuesday	3/4-effort, Anaerobic Threshold Steady-State
Wednesday	Active Recovery
Thursday	1/2-effort, Fartlek + Date Pace
Friday	Active Recovery
Saturday	3/4-effort, Steady-State
Sunday	Easy-effort, Long Run

As discussed in detail in Chapter 1, after two to three weeks of demanding training, athletes need to take a worthwhile break to prevent the onset of residual and chronic fatigue, and also to consolidate the potential created by previous acquisitive work. Further, a controlled time trial at the end of this week will provide a checkpoint with respect to athletic development. The following schedule provides the structure of a micro-cycle corresponding to the worthwhile break.

Monday	Passive Recovery
Tuesday	1/2-effort, Fartlek + Date Pace
Wednesday	Active Recovery
Thursday	Easy Recovery
Friday	Day Before Race Routine
Saturday	Time Trial or Race
Sunday	Easy-effort, Long Run

Obviously, the selection of various days of the week for particular training tasks is somewhat arbitrary. Most important is the pattern and balance of the training being conducted.

Progression of Training Quality

Monday is normally a day of passive recovery with respect to running. It follows the steady-state at 3/4-effort on Saturday, and the long endurance effort on Sunday. The body has a great need to restore muscle glycogen after two days of high caloric expenditure. Sometimes, a complete day off is best, especially in the case of young athletes. Exercise in the form of recreational biking or swimming could also be done. Monday is a preferred day for one of the two or three weight training sessions normally conducted during the week. Any running should have minimal duration and effort, even for mature athletes. After all, Monday is the day of the week that most people are a bit out of whack. Much of this has to do with the weekend's disruption of regular activity cycles, otherwise known as the weekly regime. We owe a certain debt to that regime, as those who have suffered from chronic disruption of daily activity and circadian rhythms can attest. The harmonious movement of biorhythms relates to the question of athletic acquisition, and more generally speaking, to physical and mental health. So, if it can be helped, do not plan demanding running workouts on Monday, especially if you are dealing with a large group of athletes who will necessarily be in different places physically and mentally after the long weekend. Again, both in terms of the quantity and quality undertaken, Monday should be the easiest day of the week. Athletes need one day a week to freshen up in order to better handle the demanding training efforts.

Tuesday is devoted to an anaerobic threshold session conducted at 3/4-effort. The anaerobic threshold session should be reduced about 20% from the duration of the evenly paced steady-state to be conducted on Saturday. If there is a trade off to be made between quantity and quality—for example, either covering six miles at 6:00 minutes/mile pace in the quality workouts and alternately, 10 miles at 7:00 minutes/mile pace during the recovery days, or 10 miles at 6:00 minutes/ mile pace in the steady state and six miles at 7:00 minutes/mile pace on the recovery days—then the latter option is preferable, since more work is being done. On days devoted to high quality training sessions, it is generally best to attempt a longer duration than to break it up into two workouts.

In time, the distance or duration of the Tuesday session will increase, and the athlete will be capable of running the entire workout at a faster pace while maintaining the same level of effort. Perhaps the most important aspect to focus on concerns the duration, frequency, and intensity of the surges within the anaerobic threshold session. In the first week of a two-to-three-week meso-cycle, begin with a relatively high number of shorter segments, then in succeeding weeks gradually increase the distance, while reducing the number and the frequency of the recovery periods. After taking a regenerative worthwhile break at the end of this first meso-cycle, athletes might begin the next meso-cycle by dropping back down to segments nearly as short as those conducted at the beginning of the first cycle, and then proceed with a like progression over a period of weeks.

It is possible to combine short fast segments, and also long slow segments within a given workout, but rather than complicate this presentation, it is presumed that you have already grasped the larger principle. At some point, the length of the surge segments can progress to encompass the duration of a middle distance event. In fact, given a group of middle distance runners, make sure that the anaerobic threshold sessions progress so as to attain and focus on the duration of the middle distance event during the base period, since the athletes will then condition body and mind to later put forth a hard effort over the main race event. In the case of young athletes preparing for 5,000 and 10,000 meters, limit the surges to three to five minutes duration. However, by the end of the base period, elite athletes competing in international cross-country or the marathon may run 3-4 x 5,000 or 2 x 10,000 meters in training to good effect.

Some coaches and athletes also jump all the way up to the distance or duration of the race event and conduct a time trial, then gradually increase the pace over a span of weeks and months (Lydiard, 1970, and Lydiard and Gilmour, 1962). This is fine for mature athletes in a high level of fitness, provided they are running over demanding terrain. However, for a less fit or novice athlete, this might be like trying to carve marble with a large, blunt chisel, when a smaller, sharper instrument could be used to better effect.

Wednesday and *Friday* are both days of active recovery. The anaerobic threshold steady-state, and the evenly paced 3/4-effort steady-state sessions on Tuesday and Saturday are clearly exhausting, and in some sense the hard-day, easy-day rule is being applied. Some athletes tend to muddle up their training and not sufficiently differentiate between high quality training efforts and recovery efforts. Know when to work hard, but also know when to permit your body to recover. Whenever possible on recovery days, mature athletes should undertake a morning run lasting between 10 and 25 minutes. Young high school athletes should waive this requirement, while more mature high school, collegiate, and post-collegiate athletes should cover up to 25 minutes. When athletes undertake two workouts each day during the sharpening and peak periods, it is generally inadvisable to run beyond this duration in the morning, because doing so could trigger an alarm reaction, causing the central nervous system and endocrine system to become over-activated. As a result, the primary workout could suffer due to the athlete's inability to fully recover by the afternoon training session.

To facilitate recovery, the morning training session should include an easy jog with a few easy short accelerations, and also some mild stretching. In lieu of the above, alternate forms of exercise such as biking or swimming are also appropriate. The top priority is to get the metabolism going, since this will provide a faster rate of recovery. Athletes often feel the most sore and sluggish during the morning session since the metabolic by-products of the previous day's high quality effort frequently induce something of a hangover. However, the afternoon training session will be a more pleasant experience as a result.

The afternoon training session on active recovery days should begin with light stretching followed by a good warm-up, then more thorough stretching. In fact, this is a healthy training practice every day. If possible, conduct the warm-up by running barefoot on grass. If a circuit or weight-training session is included, it should then follow directly. Ideally, the active recovery run should be performed over soft rolling terrain, and incorporate some easy short accelerations. A few short hills on a gentle grade can also be included at moderate effort. Barefoot running on grass is desirable during the warm-down, and flexibility exercises should conclude the active recovery workout.

Over time, the duration and pace of the active recovery run will improve, but this is incidental to overall athletic development. The major objective of the Wednesday and Friday active recovery sessions is to help athletes recover in preparation for the high quality training efforts that follow directly—no more, and no less. Make sure that the runners are not attempting too much, too fast—that is, make sure they are recovering! Heart rate monitors can be used to good effect as a governor on quality. Attempt to introduce some variety, and if at all possible, seek out a restorative natural environment.

Thursday's training session of unstructured 1/2-effort fartlek, comes between the 3/4-effort anaerobic threshold steady-state workout on Tuesday, and the 3/4-effort evenly paced steady-state session that follows on Saturday. This schedule provides three to four days for recovery between these two 3/4-effort training sessions. The fartlek workout should be as demanding as possible, but easy as necessary, so as to avoid compromising the quality of either of the two 3/4-effort training sessions. The fartlek format is well suited to serve as a safety valve, since the training structure and effort can be modified according to circumstances at the runner's discretion. The fartlek session should incorporate hilly or otherwise resistant terrain, thus ensure that requisite levels of strength are maintained.

The Thursday training session should also include some date pace work. It is desirable to gradually progress the date pace work to ensure an injury free transition when the sharpening period begins. This will also foster running economy. Athletes specializing in 800 and 1,500 meters are best advised to undertake a brief interval session with reps in the range of 100 to 200 meters, whereas specialists in the 5,000 and 10,000 meters can conduct a brief interval session with reps in the range of 200 to 400 meters. However, at this time, runners should always take ample recovery periods, since the aim of date pace work is not to sharpen for race fitness.

This brings up a question concerning the proper progression of date pace work over the course of an athletic season. The sharpening period will incorporate interval and repetition work at goal pace for the main race event, and will begin approximately five to six weeks prior to the first projected optimal performance during the peak period (Approximately 28 to 33 days of sharpening, plus the nine-to-10-day ascent to the plateau of peak performance = 37 to 43 days). In the meso-cycle immediately preceding the sharpening period, the date pace work should be conducted at goal pace plus one second/400 meters. Likewise, the quality of the date pace work performed in the next preceding meso-cycle should be at goal pace plus two seconds/400 meters, and so on. In short, the date pace work should be increased by one second/400 meters in each consecutive meso-cycle preceding the start of the sharpening period.

In order to attain goal finishing speed during the peak period, a finishing speed progression should be conducted, especially by middle distance runners. The date pace workout formerly conducted on Thursday is then transformed into a finishing speed workout during the sharpening period. Each succeeding week, the number of reps in the range of 100 to 200 meters in the finishing speed progression decreases, but the quality and speed of the reps should increase such that by the end of the progression, three reps between 100 to 200 meters are being run at goal finishing speed. Obviously, long distance runners having a closing speed of 56 seconds over 400 meters do not need a lengthy finishing speed progression. However, athletes competing in the 1,500 meters who need to close in 52 seconds, with the last 200 meters being run under 25 seconds, have a greater need. In this regard, it would not be prudent to progress in only five to six weeks from a goal pace of 59 seconds in the main race event to an exhibited goal finishing speed corresponding to an open 400 meters performance of 49 seconds. Accordingly, individuals competing in the 800 and 1,500 meters should begin their finishing speed progression at the end of the base period. This can take the form of running brief acceleration exercises during the warm-up and warm-down, several times during the week, and some occasional race practice. The essential point is that a foundation of finishing speed work should be provided, or athletes will either not be able to progress to the desired quality, or will get there by assuming too high a risk of injury. Unnecessary risk-taking in a sport with a ten-year developmental period, must be viewed as conducive to a negative outcome. An athlete does not play the odds and win in distance running. It is best to strive towards eliminating any so-called luck or chance from the equation. For detailed date pace and finishing speed progressions see in Chapter 4, Figures 4.2—4.7, and Tables 4.1—4.4, respectively.

Saturday is devoted to conducting an evenly paced 3/4-effort steady-state effort. This will serve to consolidate the potential created by the anaerobic threshold steady-state training session four days previous. At the halfway point of a 3/4-effort workout, an athlete will often have doubt as to the task's completion, but the training session will nevertheless be successfully concluded. It is natural and normal to experience these doubts. Do not attach to them, rather, simply let them pass by in the stream of consciousness.

Some coaches and athletes might seek abstract guidance with respect to predicting the pace at which the steady state effort should be conducted. In this regard, they may wish to study Table 3.2 and Figure 3.3 found in Jack Daniel's fine work entitled *Daniel's Running Formula*, 1998. However, do not become too distracted with trying to determine what abstract level of intensity is correct for you. In truth, there are as many different correct levels of intensity as there are different individuals on a given day. And even the same individual will not be the same from day to day. It is not uncommon for the pace of the steady state run to vary from one week to another by as much as ten or twenty seconds / mile depending upon how an individual feels, and also the environmental conditions. Whether you are a coach or an athlete, the judgments made concerning the distance and pace of the steady state run are not abstract. The training prescription does not suddenly materialize out of the ether. Pay close attention to circumstances. What distance an athlete has covered previously, and at what pace normally provides the most relevant point of reference.

In truth, the correct intensity for the steady-state runs is easy to figure out. You run as hard as you can at a relatively even pace to cover the desired distance-- bearing in mind that you need to be adequately recovered in time for the next 3/4 effort planned three or four days later. If you try for too much your body will let you know. You'll slow down over the second half of the run, or perhaps even have to walk home. "No worries." If that is the biggest mistake you make in Athletics or life, then you're a candidate for sainthood. Do not go out and run at an even pace at some abstractly defined level of intensity on asphalt like a robot. In particular, do not run as if you were an automobile set on cruise control. Whenever possible, run on natural terrain, as this necessarily requires that you maintain a high level of concentration and focus. It will also cultivate subtle variations in your running technique which can significantly enhance your running economy. (See the discussion in Chapter 16).

Moreover, do not underestimate the importance of mental fitness, and conducting race practice even during so-called evenly paced steady state runs. For example, let's say that we have two individuals of equal talent who conduct a steady-state run over a given course and log the same time. One runs at an even pace, and socializes with training partners. The second runs alone, and brings back the second half of the run a bit faster than the fist. And when there is a hill, he picks the pace up. When there is a headwind, he increases his effort. He visualizes competitors on his shoulder. He hears the little voice of temptation say: "Maybe you won't make it... it's OK to slack off a bit" (Elliott, in Meads and Armstrong, 2000). Disgusted at having heard the "little voice," he picks the pace up. With a mile to go he further increases his speed, and with half mile to go—even faster. Then, with four hundred meters to go... he's mentally running the last lap of the biggest race of his life. He finishes past a lamppost as if hitting the tape. Come race day, this second individual will defeat the first by a wide margin.

Over the span of weeks and months, the distance of the steady-state run should be gradually increased. As athletes become more fit, the pace of the training session will also improve when performing at 3/4 effort. In order to monitor progress, it can be helpful to run the steady-state over the same course from time to time, as this will provide a point of reference. The athletes should then merely run at 3/4 effort and note the final result, and guard against turning this progress report into a race. Unless runners are just beginning to train in earnest, they should not expect dramatic improvement from one day to the next, or week-to-week. Improvement is the result of a gradual process that unfolds naturally over months and years. Athletes might have moments of doubt, but they should have faith in themselves and their training, as deeper currents are at work, making steady progress. The direction will be clear when dedicated athletes take a longer look at their training diaries.

Sunday is the longest aerobic training session of the week, and young athletes should always run at a relaxed and easy pace, at less than 1/4-effort. However, mature athletes specializing in the long distance events such as 5,000 and 10,000 meters and the marathon, generally should conduct the Sunday long run at approximately 1/2-effort. This will enhance the ability of the athletes to use fatty acids, as discussed in Chapter 16, devoted to the marathon. The Sunday run also serves as the pathfinder to higher quantity with respect to distances being covered in the individual training sessions during the week. Athletes need to be cautioned to recognize and respect their limitations. In particular, athletes should not go on a binge on Sunday that will knock them flat and compromise the quality of the Tuesday 3/4-effort anaerobic threshold steady-state session. That would not be intelligent or productive. The primary aim is to gradually increase the distance of the long run, but athletes will also find themselves running at a faster pace. The latter should not be striven for, rather, it should just happen.

The requisite level of concentration during more intense training can render athletes semi-oblivious to their surroundings. Athletes should then take care to absorb some of their environment on Sunday, and notice the people and things that normally go by in such a rush. Otherwise, they might look back someday with regret over how much they have missed. Sunday used to be sacred—that is, prior to the invention of football and shopping malls—and it could be that our spiritual needs and limitations were once better observed.

Progression of Training Quantity

It makes little sense to sacrifice quality in favor of quantity. Nevertheless, the tendency is for athletes to play the numbers game with respect to their mileage. Often this is because they do not know what they should be trying to accomplish with respect to quality. And so athletes become obsessed with quantity, as the math is simple and it is something that they do understand. Accordingly, the so-called logic goes, "if so-and-so runs x miles a week, then I must too, and it would no doubt be better to run x + 10 miles a week if I could." If athletes do not know any better, they may sleep well having written "X miles this week" in their training diaries. But it makes no sense to run high mileage just for the sake of doing it, and without an intelligent approach.

Athletes should start with relatively low mileage, and in the first weeks run only to cover the distance, then in following weeks introduce the desired quality. Only when they are running a given level of quantity at the desired quality should

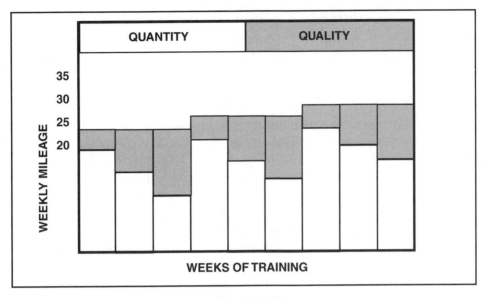

FIGURE 2.12

they again increase their mileage. The athletes should then start all over and merely run to encompass the new level of quantity, then gradually introduce the desired quality until this new level of training is absorbed. If the requisite cycles of acquisition and training periodization are momentarily set aside, the progression of quantity and quality will appear as indicated in Figure 2.12.

Obviously, the more mileage athletes attempt, the longer it will take to assimilate that new level and introduce the desired quality. This is particularly true when athletes are introduced to distance running for the first time. The initial acquisitive effort is always the most costly, both physically and mentally. Again, the ability of the athletes, and their stage of development must always be kept in mind. In order to realize a quantum leap in performance with young athletes, the easiest thing to do is to rapidly increase their mileage. However, long-term development is far more important, so it is best to err with leniency on the side of quality. After a respite from training, mature athletes will be able to reintroduce quantity and quality faster, and with less distress than their younger counterparts. So in some sense it is true: once athletes have done the acquisitive work, they can return to a previously attained level much easier, albeit, it is never truly easy.

It is best to first attempt a given level of weekly mileage in the afternoon training sessions, then gradually introduce easy two-to-four-mile morning runs on the recovery days. In this way, the total mileage can be bumped up to the next level without compromising the desired quality. Now, having attained the desired weekly mileage and quality, via the introduction of morning sessions, athletes are ready for the next level of quantity. For example, if athletes run 35 miles/week in the afternoon workouts and gradually introduce the desired quality, but also five auxiliary morning runs of two miles during the week (35 + (2 x 5) = 45 miles), they would then proceed to the next level of quantity, that is, 45 miles/week, while dropping the auxiliary morning workouts, and then begin the acquisitive cycle all over again. This method provides for gradual transitions of quantity and quality. In keeping with the micro-cycle or weekly training schedule that has been discussed, Table 2.3 provides a progression of quantity over weeks, months, and years of training.

Meso-Cycle Structure of the Base Period

The first training meso-cycle during the base period will be characterized by relatively low intensity and volume. The primary goal is to gradually build up the training volume over a period of several weeks. Reasonably fit young athletes who are not long out of regular training can normally undertake 21 to 28 days of low intensity base work before needing an easy worthwhile break. The second meso-cycle during the base period would then continue to increase in volume, but the focus would then shift towards introducing the desired quality within the base work. This second meso-cycle normally lasts between 14 and 21 days before a worthwhile break is required. Again, as the intensity and effort of the work increases during the course of an athletic season, the length of the training meso-cycles become shorter. A third meso-cycle conducted during the base period would then likely include only 14 days of work followed by a worthwhile break, and this would be the pattern thereafter during the base period.

However, pay close attention to the actual level of effort and response of the individual athlete. If and when the warning signs appear, indicating the need for a worthwhile break, then it should be taken. At the end of each worthwhile break, athletes should conduct a control run or time trial. Sometimes, a road race can be used for this purpose. Table 2.4 indicates the recommended length of the first, second, and possible third control run for athletes competing in various main race events.

Miles per week	25	35	45	55	65	75	85	95	105	115
M	0	2	2	3	4	4	5	6	6	7
T	4	6	7	8	10	12	14	15	16	18
W	3	4	6	7	8	8	9	10	12	13
TH	4	6	7	8	9	10	12	14	16	18
F	3	4	6	7	8	8	9	10	12	13
SA	4	6	8	10	12	14	16	18	20	20
S	6	8	10	12	15	18	20	22	24	26

TABLE 2.3

Main Race Event (Meters)	800	1,500	5,000	10,000
1st	5K	10K	15K	20K
2nd	3K	5K	10K	15K
3rd	1,500	3K	8K	10-12K

TABLE 2.4

Figure 2.13 shows a training progression of quantity and quality for young athletes over two succeeding meso-cycles. Mature athletes normally assume higher training loads, and progress to higher levels of quantity and quality at a faster rate. They also require more numerous and frequent meso-cycles to realize optimal athletic development. Figure 2.14 shows a progression of quantity and quality for mature athletes over three succeeding meso-cycles.

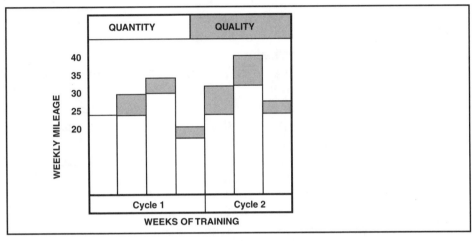

FIGURE 2.13—Young Athletes.

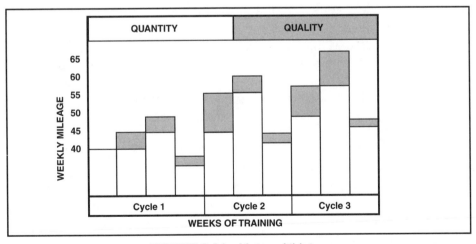

FIGURE 2.14—Mature Athletes.

Heart Rate Response Characteristics

As athletes adapt to training during the course of an athletic season, certain changes in heart rate response will be noted. Let's suppose an athlete started the season with a morning resting pulse of 50 beats per minute (bpm). The morning after a 3/4-effort workout the morning pulse will normally be elevated at least one bpm, more commonly by two, and possibly even three. And so the morning pulse will then likely be 52 bpm. If the morning pulse rises over three bpm, then the athlete may be overtraining. If an athlete's morning pulse remains high on the day of the next planned 3/4-effort workout, reassess the training schedule. The morning following a day of easy active recovery, the athlete's pulse should then recover back to the original baseline of 50 bpm. During the course of any given meso-cycle, the morning pulse will commonly fluctuate between one to three bpm above the original baseline value, and will then return to the baseline value. However, at the end of a worthwhile break, something dramatic normally happens. The morning pulse rate will often drop about two to three bpm, say from 50 bpm to a new level of 47 bpm. That new baseline will then characterize the next meso-cycle, that is, with the morning pulse rising after hard efforts and returning back to normal after recovery days. At the end of that cycle, after taking another worthwhile break, the morning pulse will again drop by about two to three bpm. It is common for an athlete's morning pulse to drop 10 bpm during the course of an athletic season (for example, from 50 to 40 bpm). Obviously, the amount of change will depend on the individual's age, training background, and athletic level.

At the same time, a similar phenomenon occurs at the opposite end of the spectrum with respect to the athlete's heart rate deflection point at the anaerobic threshold, and to a lesser degree, the maximum heart rate. It is not uncommon to see an athlete's deflection point move upwards 3 bpm by the end of the worthwhile break following the first meso-cycle, for example, from 165 to 168 bpm, then from 168 to 171 bpm after the second, then 171 to 174 bpm after the third, and so on. Accordingly, improvement of an athlete's fitness level is normally reflected in the heart rate response characteristics at both ends of the spectrum. Again, the actual heart rate response of different individuals can vary greatly.

Progression of Training Volume by Age, Sex, Athletic Level, and Event

The following abstract training guidelines in no way account for the unique needs and requirements of individual athletes, but rather, indicate the maximum mileage that runners should attempt to undertake. Many individuals may find that they do well with less volume. However, athletes should not be in denial regarding the workloads commonly required to succeed at these levels of athletic competition.

High School Cross-Country

Young female high school athletes competing in cross-country might begin in the low teens, and by the end of their sophomore year be capable of running 30 to 40 miles a week. By their senior year, 40 to 50 miles a week could be possible.

Young male high school athletes might similarly begin in the low 20's, and by the end of their sophomore year be capable of handling 40 to 50 miles a week. By their senior year, 60 to 70 miles a week could be assumed.

High School Track and Field

Mature female high school athletes competing in the 800 meters can normally attempt 30 miles, whereas, those competing in the 1,500 and 3,000 meters can attempt 40 to 50 miles a week by their senior year. Mature male high school athletes competing in the 800 meters can normally attempt 40 to 50 miles, whereas, those competing in the 1,500 and 3,000 meters can attempt 60 to 70 miles a week by their senior year.

Collegiate Women Cross-Country and Track and Field

Collegiate women participating in cross-country could progress from 50 to 90 miles per week over a four-year period. Collegiate women specializing in the 800 meters event might progress from 30 to 70, specialists at 1,500 and 3,000 meters from 40 to 80, and specialists at 5,000 and 10,000 meters from 50 to 90 miles a week over four years.

Collegiate Men Cross-Country and Track and Field

Collegiate men participating in cross-country could progress from 60 to 100 miles per week over four years. Men competing in the 800 meters event might progress from 40 to 80, specialists at 1,500 and 3,000 meters from 60 to 90, and specialists at 5,000 and 10,000 meters from 70 to 100 miles a week over four years.

Elite Women Cross-Country and Track and Field

Elite women competing in international cross-country or the marathon could progress from 90 to 120 miles per week over four years. Women competing in the 800 meters might progress from 70 to 100, specialists at 1,500 and 3,000 meters from 80 to 110, and specialists at 5,000 and 10,000 meters from 90 to 120 miles per week.

Elite Men Cross-Country and Track & Field

Elite men competing in international cross-country or the marathon could progress from 100 to 140 miles per week over four years. Men competing in the 800 meters might progress from 80 to 110, specialists at 1,500 and 3,000 meters from 90 to 120, and specialists at 5,000 and 10,000 meters from 100 to 140 miles per week.

In conclusion, a distance runner must be willing to log thousands of miles and dedicate many years to achieve success at the international level. Accordingly, the pursuit of excellence in distance running is not for the faint of heart or spirit. If you don't experience fear or doubt at some point, then you are not alive.

> *Every morning in Africa a gazelle wakes up. It knows it must outrun the fastest lion or it will be killed. Every morning, in Africa a lion wakes up. It knows it must run faster than the slowest gazelle or it will starve. It doesn't matter whether you're a gazelle or a lion: when the sun comes up, you had better be running.*
>
> —Sheikh Mohammed Bin Rashid Al Maktoum

References

Åstrand, Olaf, and Kaare Rodahl, *Textbook of Work Physiology*, 3rd edition, New York: McGraw-Hill, 1986, pages 458, 652.

Autio, James, *The Digital Mantrap,* eBola Communications, Del Mar, California, 2000.

Becker, Robert, *The Body Electric: Electromagnetism and the Foundation of Life,* New York: William Morrow & Co., 1987.

Bowerman, William J., *Coaching Track & Field,* William H. Freeman, Editor, Boston: Houghton Mifflin Co., 1974.

Cerutty, Percy, *Athletics,* London: The Sportsmans Book Club, 1961.

Cerutty, Percy, *Middle Distance Running*, London: Pelham Books Ltd., 1964.

Cerutty, Percy, *Success: In Sport and Life,* London: Pelham Books Ltd., 1967.

Costill, David L., *Inside Running: Basics of Sports Physiology,* Carmel, Indiana: Cooper Publishing Group, LLP, 1986.

Costill, David L., and Jack Daniels, W. Evans, et. al., "Skeletal Muscle Enzymes and Fiber Composition in Male and Female Track Athletes." *Journal of Applied Physiology*, Volume 40, 1976, pages 149-154.

Coyle, Edward F., "Integration of the Physiological Factors Determining Endurance Performance Ability," *Exercise Sport Science Review*, Volume 23, 1995, pages 25-63.

Daniels, Jack, *Conversation on VO_2 Maximum and Lactate Threshold*, Cortland, New York, 1999.

Daniels, Jack, *Daniels' Running Formula,* Champaign, Illinois: Human Kinetics, 1998.

Dürckheim, Karlfried Graf, *The Call for the Master,* Translated by Vincent Nash, New York: E.P. Dutton, 1989.

Dürckheim, Karlfried Graf, *Hara: The Vital Center of Man,* London: A Mandala Book, 1988.

Fox, Edward, and Donald Mathews, *The Physiological Basis of Physical Education and Athletics,* 3rd Edition, New York: Saunders College Publishing, 1981, page 313.

Goodall, Jane, *Through a Window*, Boston Massachusetts: Houghton Mifflin Company, 1990.

Heads, Ian, and Geoff Armstrong, Editors, *Winning Attitudes*, Introduction by Herb Elliott, Sydney, Australia: Australian Olympic Committee, Mardie Grant Books, 2000.

Janssen, Peter G.J.M., *Training Lactate Pulse-Rate,* 4th Edition. Oulu, Finland: Polar Electro Oy, 1987, pages 16, 23, 25, 28, 58, 61, 82, 89, 91, and 95.

Kim, Hee-Jin. *Dōgen Kigen: Mystical Realist,* Tucson, Arizona: University of Arizona Press, 1987.

Kožík, František, *Zápotek the Marathon Victor*, Prague, Czechoslovakia: Artia, 1954, page 94.

Kraemer, William J., and Steven J. Fleck, "Anaerobic Metabolism and Its Evaluation," *NSCA Journal*, April-May, 1982, page 20.

Lydiard, Arthur, *Arthur Lydiard's Running Training Schedules,* 2nd edition, Los Altos, California: Tafnews Press, 1970.

Lydiard, Arthur, and Garth Gilmour, *Run to the Top,* Auckland, New Zealand: Minerva Ltd., 1962, page 75-77.

Maier, Hanns, "Seko," *Runner's World*, June, 1981.

Maile, Forlence, and Michael Selzer, *The Nuremberg Mind*, Introduction and Rorschach Records by G.M. Gilbert, New York: Quadrangle Books/New York Times Book Company, 1975.

Maktoum, H.H. Sheikh Mohammed Bin Rashid Al, *Quotation from His Webpage*: http://www.sheikhmohammed.co.ae, 2000.

McKenzie, John, "Physical Preparation for Middle Distance and Distance Running," North Texas University, *Unpublished Manuscript*, page 2.

Newsholme, E.A., and A.R. Leech, *Biochemistry for the Medical Sciences,* Chichester, England: John Wiley & Sons, Ltd., 1983.

Newsholme, E.A., and A.R. Leech, Glenda Duester, *Keep On Running,* Chichester, England: John Wiley & Sons, Ltd., 1994.

Noakes, Tim, *Lore of Running,* 3rd Edition, Champaign, Illinois: Human Kinetics, 1991, page 95.

Posterino, G.S., and T.L. Dutka, G.D. Lamb, "L (+)- lactate does not affect twitch and tetanic responses in mechanically skinned mammalian muscle fibers," *Pflugers Archiv: European Journal of Physiology*, Volume 442, Number 2, May, 2001, pages 197-203.

Sparks, Ken, and Garry Bjorklund, *Long Distance Runner's Guide to Training and Racing,* New Jersey: Prentice-Hall, 1984, page 10.

Weissbluth, Marc, *Healthy Sleep Habits, Happy Child,* New York: Fawcett Columbine/Ballantine Books, 1987.

Weissbluth, Marc, "Naps in Children: 6 Months-7 Years," *Sleep*, Volume 18, Number 2, 1995, pages 82-87.

Will-Weber, Mark, Editor, *The Quotable Runner*, Halcottsville, New York: Breakaway Books, 2001.

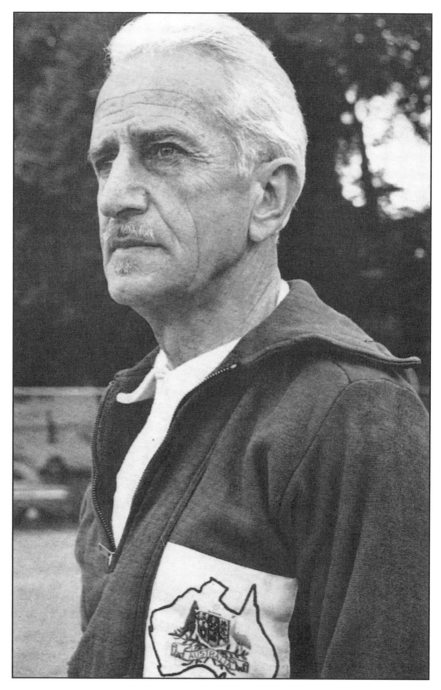

PHOTO 3.1—Percy Cerutty, the controversial and inspiring coach who con-tributed to the golden age of Australian distance running. Photo by M.A. Stratton, from the title page of *Athletics: How To Become a Champion*, London: The Sportsmen's Book Club, 1961, and provided courtesy of Nancy Cerutty.

CHAPTER 3

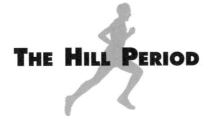

THE HILL PERIOD

The hill period can comprise a distinct training period, but it often takes the form of a training emphasis. This is especially true during the cross-country season, since the nature of the terrain requires considerable specificity of training. When the mileage assumed by the athletes has progressed to a prudent ceiling for the current season, the introduction of hill work can also enhance the quality of their training while simultaneously slowing the pace of the workouts. It can thus prevent the athletes from unwittingly sharpening and accelerating the peaking process. Accordingly, it can be doubly advantageous for elite athletes to train at altitude for at least three weeks at the end of the base and hill periods. The combination of supra-normal training loads provided by the altitude and hill training can elicit substantial improvement in performance potential.

An important aspect of fitness is developed when athletes train near their anaerobic threshold while simultaneously applying muscular strength to overcome the resistance of a supra-normal training load. All other things being equal, athletes who have cultivated greater aerobic ability and strength by incorporating hills or other resistance work in their running program will exhibit less blood lactate accumulation given a sub-maximal work load. Moreover, the athletes will be able to exercise longer while maintaining a higher equilibrium blood lactate level, and their anaerobic threshold will comprise a relatively higher percentage of their maximum oxygen uptake.

Arthur Lydiard advocated up to five weeks of hill training, and noted that within six weeks every Type II fast twitch muscle fiber cell in the body is renewed (Lydiard and Gilmour, 1962, and 1978). During the base period, athletes focus developmental efforts on the aerobic pathway, and predominantly the Type I slow twitch muscle fiber metabolism associated with endurance. Then, during the hill period, the athletes stress the foundation of the anaerobic systems, that is, the Type II fast twitch muscle fiber metabolism associated with speed and strength. The work conducted during the sharpening period then serves to integrate, coordinate, and translate these acquired powers into specific performances during the peak period.

One of the visible physical effects of hill training is a longer and more powerful stride. In particular, the knee-lift, ankle flexion, and hip extension demonstrated by athletes will improve. Speed flows from strength, and one of the aims of the hill period is to enhance muscular strength in preparation for the subsequent sharpening work. Athletes will also obtain the durability required to avoid injury.

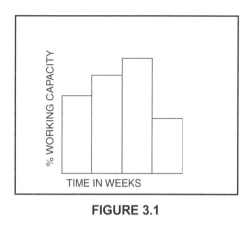

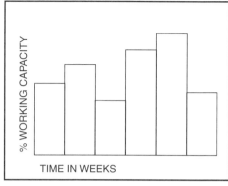

FIGURE 3.1   FIGURE 3.2

Meso-Cycle Structure of the Hill Period

The following discussion will address the meso-cycle structure of the hill period. When Arthur Lydiard suggested five weeks of hill work, people generally inferred that this should be conducted in a continuous five-week training block. However, this would generally constitute a training overload. It is not advisable to conduct more than three consecutive weeks (21 days) of hill work without taking an easy week or worthwhile break. Obviously, meso-cycles lasting less than three weeks can be conducted without hazard, given the adoption of sound training practices. For example, it is possible to conduct seven, 10, or 14 days of hill work prior to taking an easy week. Again, the worthwhile break normally concludes with a control run, time trial, or athletic competition that stabilizes and consolidates the runner's athletic level. The meso-cycle indicated in Figure 3.1 can be described as a hill period lasting for a total duration of four weeks, including three progressive workweeks of hill training followed by an easy week or worthwhile break.

To avoid confusion when discussing the various hill training scenarios, this text will always refer to the total number of workweeks. The possible desire to conduct more than one time trial, control run, or athletic competition over the duration of a month generally leads to the construction of a hill period comprising two consecutive meso-cycles. At an absolute maximum, the total duration of the hill period, including these two meso-cycles, should not exceed six weeks. For example, two weeks of hill work might be followed by a worthwhile break, and conclude in an athletic competition. Then, two additional weeks of hill work would follow, and a second easy week or worthwhile break would conclude in a second athletic competition, as shown in Figure 3.2.

Figure 3.2 illustrates a hill period having a total duration of six weeks, including four weeks of hill work and two worthwhile breaks. It is not advisable to conduct more than six weeks of focused hill training, and generally, four weeks will provide optimal results for high school and collegiate athletes. In the United States, novice high school athletes (or those whose physical age corresponds to that of a freshman or sophomore) would not likely begin base work until the first day of organized cross-country team practice in mid-August. These athletes would then not begin base work for the spring track and field season until the start of organized team practice in the first week of March. Generally, they would enjoy a relatively short athletic season, as few will normally be competing after their conference championships. Since they have an abbreviated season and no pre-season training, novice athletes can make best use of the available time by conducting base work. They should generally avoid demanding hill training sessions for which their relatively immature bodies are ill prepared. With reference to the cross-country and track and field seasons, they are generally best advised to proceed with easy base work for the better part of the athletic season, and should then conduct only three weeks of sharpening work prior to the beginning of the peak period.

In the United States, the more mature high school athletes (those whose physical age corresponds with the average junior and senior) can be expected to begin a pre-season training program of base work for the cross-country season in the first week of July. This provides for a month of post-season recovery after the conclusion of the outdoor state track and field championships, normally held in late May or the first week of June. Following the state cross-country championships, normally held in the first week of November, another extended period of post-season recovery should be taken. However, if high school athletes also qualify and compete in the national cross-country championships, then their athletic season could be extended until December. In any case, at least a month of post-season recovery should be taken between the cross-country and track seasons. The more mature high school athletes would then commence pre-season training for the track season by mid-January. Given their more extensive preparation, they will normally be able to conduct three to four workweeks of hill training during the cross-country and track and field seasons. For example, three workweeks could be followed by a worthwhile break, or four workweeks could be broken up into two meso-cycles which end in worthwhile breaks, but all within a hill period lasting a total of four to six weeks.

Collegiate athletes in the United States face a challenge when participating in three competitive athletic seasons. The summer provides the only time for extensive base work for athletes who are expected to compete well during the cross-country, indoor, and outdoor track seasons. Given the proximity of the indoor and outdoor track seasons, it would only be possible to undertake a hill training period during the fall cross-country season. Nevertheless, a hill training emphasis could be included within the base period during the build-up for the track and field seasons. Again, an athletic year consisting of two athletic seasons is far better for athletic development than one including three athletic seasons. Because of this, coaches and athletes are generally best advised to de-emphasize or train through the indoor season to realize optimal performances during the outdoor track and field season. In this case, it would be possible to undertake distinct hill periods in preparation for both the cross-country and outdoor track and field seasons.

Depending on their body type and relative strengths, individual athletes can benefit by placing greater or lesser emphasis upon hill training. Physically weaker athletes generally benefit from a longer hill period. For this reason, collegiate women should normally assume three to four workweeks of hill training, and if need be, at the expense of a week of sharpening work. Accordingly, mature high school boys and collegiate men normally undertake three workweeks of hill training and four workweeks of sharpening, whereas women often assume four workweeks of hill training and only three workweeks of sharpening during an athletic season.

With particular reference to the cross-country season, three to four workweeks of hill training and only three workweeks of sharpening is advised for both genders, since the terrain and expected weather conditions will test their strength. This prescription can also apply to long distance runners who conduct relatively high quality base and hill work. However, with respect to middle distance athletes, competitive requirements normally dictate more extensive hill training and sharpening work. Accordingly, mature specialists at 800 and 1,500 meters can often, to good effect, assume a hill period lasting a total of six weeks, comprising four workweeks and two worthwhile breaks. However, to go beyond this duration could result in diminished returns, because other aspects of fitness would then be sacrificed.

Transitions and the Hill Period

A number of common questions arise concerning the transition from the base period to the hill period. For example, how much should an athlete's training-volume or mileage decrease? Due to the more exhaustive nature of the hill work, the training volume should normally decrease in mileage relative to that attained during the previous base period. Just how much of a reduction depends on a number of things, including the athlete's event, age, sex, and athletic level. The following guidelines may help:

The specialist at 10,000 meters should reduce volume by 10 to 15%. Thus, if the athlete had attained 100 miles per week in the workweeks during the base period, the athlete would drop down to about 85 to 90 miles per week during the workweeks in the hill period.

The specialist at 5,000 meters should reduce volume by 10 to 15%. Thus, if the athlete had attained 85 to 90 miles per week in the workweeks during the base period, the athlete would drop down to about 75 to 80 miles per week.

The specialist at 1,500 meters should reduce volume by 15 to 20%. Thus, if the athlete had attained 75 to 85 miles per week in the workweeks during the base period, the athlete would drop down to about 65 to 75 miles per week.

The 1,500-meter sided 800-meter specialist should reduce volume by 20 to 25%. Thus, if the athlete had attained 65 to 75 miles in the workweeks during the base period, the athlete would drop down to about 55 to 60 miles per week.

The 400-meter sided 800-meter specialist should reduce volume by 25 to 30%. Thus, if the athlete had attained 50 to 60 miles in the workweeks during the base period, the athlete would drop down to about 40 to 45 miles per week.

Another question concerns just which training elements are retained, and which are dropped during the hill period? Essentially, in the present training prescription, the Sunday long run (LR), the Monday passive recovery day (PR), and the active recovery days (AR), placed after the 3/4 and 1/2-effort workouts, remain unchanged.

A 3/4-effort hill circuit then replaces the 3/4-effort Anaerobic Threshold Steady State (ATSS) on Tuesday. This actually represents a subtle change, as the ATSS can also be conducted during the base period on a loop containing a series of hills. However, if more than three workweeks of hill training are to be undertaken, or if the total duration of the hill period (including worthwhile breaks) extend beyond four weeks, it is best to alternate running the ATSS over a hilly route with an evenly paced Steady State (SS) in the Tuesday training session on succeeding weeks. This ensures that an athlete's aerobic ability will be maintained at a high level prior to commencing the sharpening period.

The fartlek workout conducted on Thursday during the base period would then be retained during the hill period, and continue to include date pace work that would progress in quantity and quality. Some finishing speed work could also be introduced on this day, depending upon the athlete's main race event and any special needs and requirements (See Chapter 1 and Chapter 4). A more significant change made during the transition between the base and hill periods, is that a structured hill workout will replace the Steady State (SS) on Saturday.

The changes made in the content of the high quality training sessions during the transition from the hill period to the sharpening period are more dramatic. Once again, little if anything changes with respect to the Long Run (LR), the day of Passive Recovery (PR) or days of Active Recovery (AR). To help maintain aerobic fitness, the athlete should maintain the same volume of training on these days as during the hill period. Nevertheless, the overall net effect will often slightly decrease the athlete's training volume during the sharpening period relative to the preceding hill period. However, during the sharpening period, the 3/4-effort hill workouts on Tuesday and Saturday will be replaced by high quality sharpening workouts. In this prescription, the 1/2-effort fartlek workout on Thursday is retained in order to help maintain the athlete's aerobic ability and muscular strength. The portion of the fartlek workout formerly devoted to Date Pace (DP) work is dropped, since the athlete has progressed to Goal Pace (GP) work during the sharpening period. Instead, after a warm-up and stretching, the athlete will conduct Finishing Speed (FS) work and then conclude the Thursday session with a 1/2-effort fartlek session. Coincidentally, this will help the athlete recover from the preceding finishing speed work.

Cross-Country: Weekly Structure of the Hill Period

The competitive distances in cross-country (3,000 to 5,000 meters for high school girls, 5,000 meters for high school boys and collegiate women, 8,000-10,000 meters for collegiate men, and 12,000 meters for men competing at the international level) place similar demands on athletes who are nevertheless at different levels of development. Table 3.1 provides a typical micro-cycle or weekly schedule for the hill period in which the Tuesday and Saturday sessions can be interchanged.

Again, in order to freshen up and avoid chronic fatigue, after anywhere between two to three weeks of progressive hill training, athletes will require an easy week. At the end of this worthwhile break, a check should be made on the fitness of the athletes by conducting a 3/4-effort control run, time trial, or an actual competition. This also serves to consolidate their new performance potential. Table 3.2 provides a typical schedule for a worthwhile break to set up athletes for a time trial on Saturday.

The coach and athlete should both appreciate how much race performance will be suppressed during the hill period. Peter Snell, a former world record holder at 800 and 1,500 meters, could only run 800 meters in 2:02 during his hill training. However, Lydiard's hill training program was more intensive than anything advocated here. Nevertheless, it can be destructive to an athlete's confidence to compete in the main race event, or for an athlete to expect a level of performance that cannot be delivered at this time. As a rule of thumb, expect performances to be suppressed on the order of at least two seconds/400 meters (thus, four seconds in the 800 meters, eight seconds in the 1,500 meters and 16 seconds in the 3,000 meters).

Track and Field: Weekly Structure of the Hill Period

The hill period for specialists at 5,000 and 10,000 meters during the track and field season is nearly identical to that undertaken during the cross-country season. However, during the track and field season, middle distance runners will focus upon events between 800 to 3,000 meters. Athletes competing in the 800 and 1,500 meters must place greater emphasis on strength development and hill training. The more a given race event requires strength, power, and explosive speed, or the greater the deficiency of athletes in this regard, the greater should be the hill training emphasis. Keep in mind the particular needs of individual athletes and the specific training required for their race events when planning the hill training sessions.

Table 3.3 provides a typical micro-cycle or weekly training schedule for workweeks within the hill period during the track and field season.

Table 3.4 provides a typical micro-cycle or weekly training schedule for worthwhile breaks during the hill period to set up athletes for a Saturday competition. For a detailed discussion regarding the use of time trials to set up athletes for optimal performance in a given race event, see Chapters 4 and 5.

Hill Running Technique

Athletes should perform most of the hill work using their normal running technique, but some variety is good from time to time. For example, the Lydiard style of hill bounding and also skip bounding can sometimes be introduced. However, these forms of bounding are too stressful for novice athletes to safely assume. Even mature men and women can be exposed to a high risk of injury

Monday	Passive Recovery
Tuesday	3/4 Effort, Hill Circuit
Wednesday	Active Recovery
Thursday	1/2 Effort, Fartlek + Date Pace
Friday	Active Recovery
Saturday	3/4 Effort, Hill Workout
Sunday	Easy Effort, Long Run

Table 3.1

Monday	Passive Recovery
Tuesday	1/2 Effort, Fartlek + Date Pace
Wednesday	Active Recovery
Thursday	Easy Recovery
Friday	Day Before Race Routine
Saturday	3/4 Effort, Time Trial
Sunday	Easy Effort, Long Run

Table 3.2

Monday	Passive Recovery
Tuesday	3/4 Effort, Hill Workout
Wednesday	Active Recovery
Thursday	1/2 Effort, Fartlek + Date Pace
Friday	Active Recovery
Saturday	3/4 Effort, Hill Workout
Sunday	Easy Effort, Long Run

Table 3.3

Monday	Passive Recovery
Tuesday	1/2 Effort, Fartlek + Date Pace, or 3/4 Effort, Time Trial in an Under-Distance Event
Wednesday	Active Recovery
Thursday	Easy Recovery
Friday	Day Before Race Routine
Saturday	Race
Sunday	Easy Effort, Long Run

Table 3.4

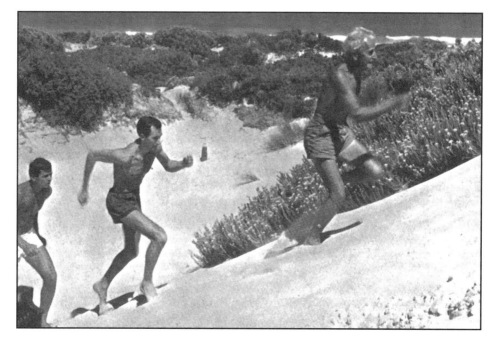

PHOTO 3.2—Percy Cerutty and Herb Elliott running in the sand dunes at Portsea, Australia. Photo from *Middle Distance Running*, Great Britain: Pelham Books, Ltd., 1964, and provided courtesy of Nancy Cerutty.

with hill bounding. It can be beneficial, but not in the doses originally prescribed by Lydiard. One of his strongest pupils, Peter Snell, apparently came to the same conclusion, as recorded in his athletic memoirs (Snell, 1965).

Hill bounding must be performed on a natural grass or earthen surface, as asphalt surfaces impart high shock loads, and can greatly increase the risk of injury. However, beware of wet or slippery conditions—including loose bark dust, mud, or snow, because these can cause a short, sudden, and apparently minor slip during toe off. This can result in an injury, particularly to the area of the hip joint. The precise location can often be found at approximately the 10 o'clock position when the afflicted athlete stands sideways facing the viewer's right. Perhaps the ideal physical environment for conducting hill training is on sand dunes, as was the practice of the Australian coach Percy Cerutty.

> *If you die, I will bury you in the sandhills with all the other runners.*
>
> —Percy Cerutty, greeting a visitor to Portsea

If coaches or athletes desire to include another form of bounding in the hill training program, then skip bounding can also be incorporated. Skip bounding is perhaps more rhythmic than other bounding styles, and rhythmic movement should be cultivated, especially by the sprinter. However, coaches should first attempt skip bounding, because they need to appreciate how exhausting it is before prescribing it to athletes. Skip bounding should be done for height as opposed to distance, thus to cover just 60 meters would completely exhaust the ATP-PC energy system. The skip bounding training session is then best suited to sprinters and middle distance runners, as opposed to long distance runners. An effective way to train the ATP-PC and ATP-Lactic Acid systems on a short hill is to skip bound 60 meters, then sprint the last 40 meters. Athletes will then be too exhausted to sprint at anything faster than 3/4-speed, and so they will not be sharpening. Physiologically, and certainly by way of subjective feeling, the sprint segment run on the ATP-Lactic Acid system is probably the closest thing to simulating the last 100 meters of the 400 meters event. The advantages are that this does not require a long hill, and the relatively slow speeds fully stress the anaerobic systems without substantially sharpening the athletes. Nevertheless, bear in mind the effect of this anaerobic work upon the balance of the training being conducted during the athletic season.

Sprint coaches sometimes advocate downhill running. The primary aim being to enhance speed. This activity is then most often performed during the sprinter's sharpening and peak periods. However, if downhill running is planned for the sharpening period, then some downhill running should also be done at controlled speeds during the hill period, because the potential for injury at a later date would otherwise be exceptionally high. In any case, the quantity of downhill sprint training should be low and the grade of the hill slight—less than three percent. Otherwise, the risk of injury to an athlete's lower back and hamstrings would be great.

The Long Sprint Events

Quantity will tend to compromise and suppress quality, and the converse is also true. The shorter the duration of the main race event (or the greater the athlete's deficiency of requisite strength), the more should hill training incorporate quality at the expense of quantity. Although training for the 400 meters is not the focus of this text, it will be briefly discussed vis-á-vis middle distance running, since 400 meters constitutes the under-distance event relative to the 800 meters.

The hill training progression for specialists at 400 meters should include a maximum of six to eight structured hill training sessions conducted during three to four workweeks within a hill period lasting between four to six weeks. In contrast with middle distance and distance runners, specialists at 400 meters will not normally include a hill circuit in their training program. Table 3.5 provides a hill training progression for athletes preparing for 400 meters. They should begin with more numerous short reps, and then progress to fewer reps and greater distances.

The grade of the hill and length of the recovery periods also affect the quality of the hill training, as do the technique and running speed of the athletes. Obviously, the shorter the main race event, the more explosive the hill repetitions should be. For athletes training for 400 meters, the recovery period can be a full downhill walk or jog and need not be otherwise controlled, so long as their resting

Distance (meters)	Number
100	10
150	8
200	6
300	5
400	4
500	3
600	2

TABLE 3.5

pulse does not fall below 120 bpm between repetitions (which could indicate a loss of sufficient warm-up). Pay close attention to the duration of the hill repetitions since the distance covered can be a deficient measure of the work actually being done.

Middle Distance Events

This discussion will focus on preparing athletes for 800 and 1,500 meters. Again, a maximum of four workweeks and two regenerative weeks can be assumed by mature athletes within a hill period of four to six weeks. Given that only two 3/4-effort training sessions are possible over a seven day period, a maximum of six to eight 3/4-effort training sessions are possible during the hill period. Obviously, any competitions or time trials undertaken must be counted against this total.

Middle distance runners could perform a 3/4-effort hill circuit on Tuesday, four days previous to a more highly structured 3/4-effort hill repetition workout on Saturday, or vice-versa. Accordingly, during a typical workweek, a training session including continuous running on a hill circuit alternates with another including shorter and faster hill repetitions. The hill circuit can be one continuous loop or can comprise a smaller closed loop. For example, a 3,000 meters loop could be run two to four times with five minutes of easy running recovery between each hill circuit. The objective would be to run all of the circuits in approximately the same time during any given 3/4-effort training session. In succeeding weeks, athletes will naturally post faster times over the hill circuit.

In the more structured hill workout, normally conducted on Saturday, the duration or distance of the hill repetitions would be gradually progressed. Table 3.6 provides a hill training progression suitable for mature specialists at 800 and 1,500 meters.

The specialist at 800 meters will normally assume fewer hill repetitions, but will conduct them at greater speed than the specialist at 1,500 meters. The same is true of the specialist at 1,500 versus 3,000 meters. When conducting the longer hill repetitions, a segment of controlled downhill running can be incorporated to enhance the quality of the recovery period. To better facilitate recovery, athletes can also run two easy accelerations between 100 and 200 meters in length at the top and bottom of the hill.

Distance (meters)	Number
100	20
200	16
300	12
400	10
600	8
800	6
1,200	4

TABLE 3.6

Generally, novice runners are not physically or mentally capable of handling a high quality recovery period. Most are not yet mature enough to endure high intensity levels, nor should they be expected to. If and when athletes are ready to make a 3/4-effort in training—well, then they are ready. Most people are never ready. This is not to say they should be. It simply is the natural order of things. Normally, the number of hill repetitions and the training volume for young athletes should be reduced by at least 25%. Novice high school athletes will be doing all they can, both physically and mentally, to simply run to the top of the hills. The next step in improving quality would be for them to run through the top of the hills and then at least 20 to 30 meters beyond. This causes a cardiovascular and respiratory adjustment that affects the heart, diaphragm, and breathing pattern in a way that is often experienced as distressful. Athletes should not clench their teeth and resist the pain, rather embrace it and instead maintain their concentration.

Long Distance Events

When preparing for long distance events, athletes are not so concerned with training the anaerobic energy systems and muscle fiber types for explosive power. Instead, the objective is to further enhance their aerobic ability with the use of supra-normal training loads, but without inducing a substantial sharpening effect. Again, an important aspect of fitness is developed when athletes train near their anaerobic threshold while simultaneously applying muscular strength to overcome the resistance of a supra-normal training load. All other things being equal, athletes who have cultivated greater strength and aerobic ability by incorporating hills or other resistance work in their running program will exhibit less blood lactate accumulation while performing a given sub-maximal work load. Moreover, the athletes will be able to exercise longer, while maintaining a higher equilibrium blood lactate level, and their anaerobic threshold will then comprise a higher percentage of their maximum oxygen uptake.

Running in the mountains at altitude provides at least two different stimuli for imposing supra-normal training loads. Further, the following athletes performed fartlek training while running fully clothed in ankle deep snow: Gunder Haegg, the former World Record holder in the mile, Emil Zatopek, the 1952 Olympic Champion at 5,000 meters, 10,000 meters and the marathon, and Lasse Viren, the 1972 and 1976 Olympic Champion at both 5,000 and 10,000 meters. Running barefoot in sand dunes also imposes a similar supra-normal training load. The Australian coach Percy Cerutty, and Herb Elliott (the 1960 Olympic Champion at 1,500 meters) often trained barefoot in the sand dunes surrounding Portsea, Australia. Here in the United States, Bill Dellinger, Bronze Medallist in the 5,000 meters at the 1964 Olympic Games, once measured the distance of intervals by counting strides on his fingers as he ran barefoot along the beach. Pat Porter, the United States National Cross-Country Champion for nearly a decade, utilized both altitude and sand dunes when training in Alamosa, Colorado. Joan Benoit Samuelson, the 1984 Olympic Champion in the marathon, once lived in Florence, Oregon and sometimes trained in the Oregon Dunes National Recreation Area. When injured, she was capable of riding an exercise bicycle for over an hour with the resistance put at the highest setting (Sevene, 1985). In brief, athletes who desire to achieve supra-normal levels of athletic performance are well advised to assume supra-normal training loads. Accordingly, aspiring national or international class athletes should seek out and incorporate challenging physical environments into their training programs.

Given the weekly training schedule provided herein, long distance runners competing in events ranging from 3,000 meters to the marathon are advised to conduct a 3/4-effort hill circuit, or a continuous run over demanding terrain on Tuesday, four days prior to a more highly structured 3/4-effort hill repetition workout on Saturday, or vice-versa. Given the relatively flat terrain of the Midwest region of the United States, a hill circuit on a demanding short course can provide a second best solution in lieu of a continuous run over equally challenging terrain on a long course. The Kenyan's have a demanding 21-kilometer route that climbs from approximately 5,000 to 8,500 feet of elevation, and similar courses exist in Boulder, Colorado.

Once again, the 3/4-effort workout, including a hill circuit or continuous run over demanding terrain, can be alternated with a more highly structured 3/4-effort hill repetition workout within a typical workweek during the hill period. The distance of the hill repetitions should gradually increase over succeeding weeks. With middle distance runners, it is sometimes possible to progress the distance or duration of the repetitions to equal the main race event. Of course, not many long distance runners will have a five to 10 kilometer hill in their backyard. The caveat being that if athletes are training at altitude, then they may indeed have a five to 10 kilometer hill in their backyard, and could then perform both the hill circuit and repetitions workouts over suitable long courses.

However, when conducting long repetitions, there is clearly a point of diminishing returns. After all, what goes up must come down. Unless an athlete has some means of quickly getting back to the bottom of a hill, thus permitting a recovery period of reasonable duration, the goal of the training session can be compromised. Introducing a segment of gentle downhill running can strengthen the abdominals and can also serve as a partial solution to the problem of exorbitant recovery. However, while downhill running does condition the abdominals and diaphragm, the shock associated with this activity can be injurious to the legs and lower back. Regardless of the efficiency of an athlete's downhill running technique, it is prudent to guard the quantity and quality being assumed.

One-half to three quarters of a mile normally represents the practical limit with respect to the hill repetitions conducted by long distance runners, but consider the following true story: On Highway 96 near the St. Croix river just outside of Stillwater, Minnesota, there is a demanding hill 1,200 meters long that levels off slightly over an additional 400 meters. To run a full uphill mile and then all the way back down five times would be ten miles. And who needs all that recovery? The coach (or chauffeur) on the scene piled a number of athletes into the back of a subcompact car and dropped them off at the bottom of the hill. The coach then drove to the top of the hill where he would wait for the athletes with a stopwatch. Of course, the athletes would then crawl into the back seat once again to be whisked off to the base of the hill in something less than a three-minute recovery period before the next repetition. Some might question the prudence of this practice, but most of the Midwest region in the United States is notoriously flat. And in the winter months, when road conditions in Minnesota prohibit quality hill work, dedicated athletes can sometimes still be found running up various parking ramps, or dashing up the stair wells of tall buildings, only to take the elevator back down to start the next repetition. Table 3.7 provides a progression of hill repetitions suitable for use by mature athletes.

Athletes can acquire some important physical and mental skills by running hill repetitions approximately a mile long. These skills relate to the manner in which they impart muscular force, and endure physical and mental fatigue. Running long hill repetitions provides a mental exercise in concentration. Athletes must focus on breathing and bodily relaxation while simultaneously delivering near-maximal effort. On hills shorter than a half mile in length, it is still possible for athletes to will themselves with their egos and force their way up with relatively inefficient running technique and energy expenditure. Athletes can then still mentally attach to the effort and pain, but overcome it by an act of will. However, superior performances are not attained by the ego and will. They are achieved by surrendering the ego, and concentrating on the moment. Running on long hills provides such a lesson in non-attachment. If athletes apply the same willful technique to running long hill repetitions, they will not be able to complete them well. When half way up the hill, athletes must learn to not attach to the pain they have experienced, rather they must let it go. In addition, they must learn to not attach to the pain waiting for them further up the hill, rather they must concentrate on their breathing and the immediate biofeedback of the moment. Athletes must be able to relax and minimize muscle tension while simultaneously putting forth a near maximal running effort, as this will permit them to best employ their aerobic ability. Many individuals have unconsciously learned to resist pain or fatigue by increasing muscular tension. With respect to distance running, this is dysfunctional. Tension induced by fear and a lack of focus results in the degradation of a runner's aerobic ability.

Distance (meters)	Number
200	16
300	12
400	10
600	8
800	6
1,200	5
1,600	4

TABLE 3.7

Structure and Athletic Maturity

Novice athletes lack the knowledge and experience required to successfully perform athletic training in a completely unstructured environment. In the absence of guidance, they will train unintelligently, and so injure or exhaust themselves. Because of this, young athletes initially require education, and need a teacher or coach. In fact, they will often demand structure to clarify the training task: What hill? How many times? How Fast? In time, as the athletes gain understanding and experience, and acquire a better feel for their abilities, they will eventually desire and should be granted relative freedom.

> *Overtraining is the biggest problem incurred by runners who lack the experience or discipline to cope with their own enthusiasm.*
>
> —Marty Liquori

Ultimately, the aim of the coach should be to liberate young athletes from the structure that was once provided out of necessity. In fact, during the first few days of practice at the beginning of a season, it is appropriate for a coach to conduct several one-hour classes on the subject of athletic training. At the end of this exercise, each athlete should leave the classroom with a calendar including a schedule for the entire season written in their own hand. As the season progresses, the coach can then work with each athlete individually, and communicate at a mature level. The results will reflect it.

When a coach plays a dominating or controlling role, and athletes simply glance at the workout schedule each day, something is fundamentally wrong. That kind of coach/athlete relationship does not truly involve education, nor does it yield the best results. Unfortunately, it is common to see mutual dependency needs played out between athletes and their coaches. The athletes want their coaches to play the role of their father or the Almighty, and the coaches want the athletes to make them feel like it. This situation is not healthy for either party.

Accordingly, the training of mature athletes should not be regimented. Rather, the coach (who at this point has become something of an advisor) guides the athletes towards the training task. Relative freedom is granted with the certain knowledge that the quality of the training will be enhanced over and above the more highly structured methods that may have been necessary in their youth. The mature athlete will then plan a progression of workouts, some highly structured, and some not, adapting them to circumstances. In no event will the schedule serve as more than a guide. When in doubt, listen to your body and the whisper of intuition.

The gift of enlightenment is a partial product of cultivating wholeness. This entails being receptive to alternative ways of knowing, and striking a balance between head and heart—thinking and feeling, judging and perceiving, feeling and intuition. The knowledge gained thereby can contribute to the ability to make accurate plans and predictions. However, life is characterized by change, spontaneity, and uncertainty. Even with the best-laid plans, it is necessary for athletes to correctly interpret their status at any point in time, and prudently modify their training program.

> *A constant vigilance and attention to the train of things as they successively emerge, and to act on what they direct, are the only sure courses... Circumstances give to each act its distinguishing color and discriminating effect.*
>
> —Edmund Burke

References

Burke, Edmund, *Reflections on the Revolutions in France, III,* 1790.

Cerutty, Percy, *Athletics,* London: The Sportsman's Book Club, 1961.

Cerutty, Percy, *Audio Tape Recording,* 1970's.

Cerutty, Percy, *Middle Distance Running,* Great Britain: Pelham Books, Ltd., 1964.

Cerutty, Percy, *Success: In Sport and Life,* London: Pelham Books, Ltd., 1967.

Lydiard, Arthur, and Garth Gilmour, *Running the Lydiard Way,* Mountain View, California: World Publications, Inc., 1978, pages 37-41.

Lydiard, Arthur, and Garth Gilmour, *Run to the Top,* Auckland, New Zealand: Minerva Ltd., 1962, pages 52-54.

Sevene, Bob, Conversation on Distance Running, Eugene, Oregon, 1985.

Snell, Peter, and Garth Gilmour, *No Bugles, No Drums,* Auckland, New Zealand: Minerva, 1965.

Will-Weber, Mark, Editor, *The Quotable Runner*, Halcottsville, New York: Breakaway Books, 2001.

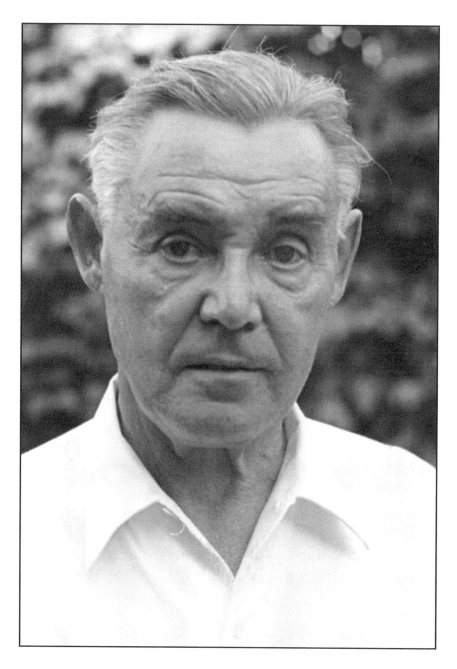

PHOTO 4.1—Woldemar Gerschler, who with the assistance of exercise physiologist Dr. Herbert Reindell, was the pioneer of modern interval training. Gerschler was an educator at the University of Freiburg, and influenced former 800 meters World Record holders Rudolf Harbig, and also Roger Moens. Photo courtesy of Dr. Klaus-Jürgen Müller, University of Freiburg, Germany.

CHAPTER 4

THE SHARPENING PERIOD

The sharpening period is a time of specific conditioning for athletic performance in the selected main race event. The preceding base and hill periods are devoted to general conditioning, which primarily enhance an athlete's aerobic ability and muscular strength. However, it is during the sharpening period that the athlete's acquired powers are truly integrated and translated into the ability to sustain a desired goal pace over the duration of the main race event.

Duration of the Sharpening Period

Arthur Lydiard of New Zealand is credited with identifying the various athletic training periods and addressing many of their governing principles. Extensive physiological studies have confirmed what Lydiard learned through experimentation: The human body requires no more than approximately four weeks of sharpening work (Lydiard and Gilmour, 1962, and 1978). Nevertheless, many variables must be considered when planning the actual duration of the sharpening period for an individual athlete. As can be expected, the mature athlete who enjoys a higher aerobic ability, and more extensive training background will require and be able to sustain a longer sharpening period. Female athletes normally require about 30% less sharpening work than men. This reflects the difference in their relative aerobic ability. On the other hand, female athletes often benefit from roughly 30% more strength training and hill work than men, due to the relative difference in their natural endowment (Åstrand, 1986). That is why women should generally assume four workweeks of hill training and only three weeks of sharpening work, whereas the normal prescription for men is just the opposite.

The nature of the competitive season and racing distance being assumed must also be considered. As a rule, athletes do not need to sharpen as much for cross-country as they do for the track and field season, nor do they have to sharpen as much for the 10,000 meters as for the 800 or 1,500 meters. And the more muscular type who drives into the running surface often requires a bit more sharpening work than the lighter type whose technique seems to carry them over the ground. Again, consider the athlete's age and level of development, because young athletes will not require or be able to sustain as much sharpening work. For example, a high school athlete attempting to run five minutes for the mile does not require the same amount of sharpening as an athlete attempting to run a sub-four-minute mile. High school boys with a physical age corresponding to the freshman and sophomore years should not attempt more than three weeks of sharpening work. The same holds true for all high school girls, with the exception

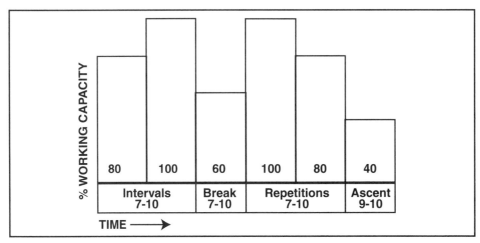

FIGURE 4.1—Mesocycle structure of the sharpening period

of mature juniors and seniors competing at 400 meters, 800 meters, or 800-meter sided competitors at 1,500 meters. Mature high school boys normally benefit from four weeks of sharpening work.

The prescription for collegiate men and women is essentially the same, but with the addition of approximately five days—that is, the possible addition of one or two sharpening efforts. Normally, a total of five quality sharpening sessions at 3/4-effort, and two competitions over a four to five week period is sufficient for athletes to attain peak competitive fitness. Even world-class athletes must be careful when attempting to go beyond four weeks (28 days) of sharpening work, because 33 to 35 days probably represents an absolute maximum before such work proves counterproductive.

The Sharpening Period Meso-Cycles

This is a brief review of the discussion found in Chapter 1. It would be unwise to attempt three to four weeks of the most demanding work of the athletic season without taking a worthwhile break. The sharpening period therefore includes a worthwhile break of seven to 10 days, which divides it into two meso-cycles.

As previously noted, it is advantageous to increase the training loads (as in the Matveyew model), during the first seven-to-10-day sharpening meso-cycle, when interval work predominates. Then follows an easy week or worthwhile break, conducted at no more than 60% of working capacity. This break normally includes an under-distance time trial or competition three to five days prior to performance in the main race event, and serves to consolidate the athlete's fitness. The second seven-to-10-day sharpening meso-cycle is then character-ized by decreasing training loads (as in the Vorobyew model). Accordingly, the overall training load begins at 100% of working capacity, but then decreases to 80%, and finally, to less than 60% during the second worthwhile break. This second break may last between seven to 14 days, and normally, nine to 10 days is optimal for high school and collegiate athletes. This worthwhile break corresponds to the so-called taper or ascent to the plateau of peak performance that follows directly.

The reduced effort of the training loads undertaken near the end of the second sharpening meso-cycle can facilitate respectable, even if not optimal competitive performances within the nine-to-10-day ascent to peak performance. During the worthwhile break and ascent, the residual fatigue induced by previous hard training will clear, and the athlete's energy will rebound.

Again, counting back approximately nine to 10 days from the first desired performance on the plateau of peak performance marks the beginning of the ascent. Then count back three to four weeks to establish the beginning of the sharpening period.

Micro-Cycle or Weekly Structure of the Sharpening Period

The basic micro-cycle structure of the sharpening period is consistent with that outlined in Chapter 1. Given the complexity of the sharpening period, numerous training schedule examples for cross-country and track and field have been provided later in this chapter, and in Appendix I. An abstract model and schedule suited for middle distance events during the sharpening period is provided below. However, the proximity of the 3/4-effort workout in the second meso-cycle, only three days after a competition in the main race event, renders this schedule unsuitable for athletes in the long distance events. Obviously, substantial variation can exist between different individuals and competitive schedules. Nevertheless, carefully study the training schedules provided. In particular, notice the pattern and alternation of sharpening work for the main race event, over-distance, under-distance, the wide separation of sharpening efforts, and the placement of the major competitions.

End of the Hill Period / Start of the Sharpening Period
First Meso-Cycle

Monday	Passive Recovery
Tuesday	3/4-Effort, Intervals for the Main Race Event
Wednesday	Active Recovery
Thursday	1/2-Effort, Fartlek + Finishing Speed
Friday	Active Recovery
Saturday	3/4-Effort, Intervals for the Over-Distance Event
Sunday	Easy Effort, Long Run

Worthwhile Break

Monday	Passive Recovery
Tuesday	3/4-Effort, Time Trial in the Under-Distance Event
Wednesday	Active Recovery + Finishing Speed
Thursday	Easy Recovery
Friday	Day Before Race Routine
Saturday	Race the Main Race Event
Sunday	Easy Effort, Long Run

Second Meso-Cycle

Monday	Passive Recovery
Tuesday	3/4-Effort, Repetitions for the Main Race Event
Wednesday	Active Recovery
Thursday	1/2-Effort, Fartlek + Finishing Speed
Friday	Active Recovery
Saturday	3/4-Effort, Repetitions for the Main Race Event
Sunday	Easy Effort, Long Run
Monday	Passive Recovery
Tuesday	1/2-Effort, Fartlek + Finishing Speed
Wednesday	Active Recovery
Thursday	3/4-Effort, Repetitions for the Over-Distance Event

End of the Sharpening Period / Beginning of the Ascent

The first time trial or competition, within the nine-to-10-day ascent to the plateau, would not be conducted sooner than four to five days after the last quality 3/4-effort repetition session shown above. This time trial or competition is then used to set up athletes for their first true peak performance in the main race event some three to five days later. Accordingly, with high school and collegiate athletes, the last high quality training effort of the sharpening period will normally fall nine to 10 days prior to the first peak performance. Elite athletes who regularly undertake 100+ miles per week, enjoy a greater load and recovery capability, and therefore, can sometimes assume a worthwhile break lasting only seven days.

The Main Race Event and Goal Performance

By the end of the base and hill periods, athletes must make a final decision and select the athlete's main race event. Ideally, this decision will be made prior to the athletic season. In addition, a realistic goal for optimal performance in the main race event should be set. If athletes try for too little, they will miss out on what they might have accomplished. On the other hand, if runners overestimate their ability and try for too much, they will get into trouble when attempting the quantity and quality called for in the sharpening workouts, and over-train.

Athletes should avoid unnecessarily testing themselves in the course of training: that reflects a lack of confidence, and ultimately compromises training, thus proves counterproductive. Athletes who unduly test themselves could reach a less than optimal so-called peak relatively early in the season, or suffer chronic fatigue and succumb to the so-called "burnt out" syndrome. Testing can also lead to mental gratification and satisfaction due to workout results—instead of race results. From the standpoint of mental preparation, athletes might then find themselves with insufficient emotional gumption to achieve peak performance when it counts.

The primary factor limiting how much quantity and quality can be assumed during the sharpening period is the aerobic ability and strength of the individual. If an athlete enters the sharpening period with the aerobic ability to run a 4:10 mile (as predicted by a clinical test of their VO_2 maximum, anaerobic threshold, and running economy), then sharpening work can be conducted to realize that potential performance. However, no amount of sharpening work will enable that athlete to raise his aerobic ability sufficiently to run a 4:00 minute mile. No amount of wishful thinking will alter this fact of life. Many are misled by the fact that when athletes begin to conduct sharpening workouts, their performances begin to improve dramatically. Coaches and athletes might then assume that sharpening is the "right thing," and should be done all the time—the more the better. This is a grave error—a mistake that destroys more young athletes than any other. Sharpening an athlete for optimal performance can be like putting a point on a pencil. No amount of sharpening will transform a 2B lead, suitable for taking exams, into a 4B lead used in drawing. You can sharpen the pencil, but you cannot change the material of which the pencil is made, and would only consume it by making the attempt. When prescribing sharpening work to young athletes, always err on the side of leniency.

Once you have established a realistic goal performance in the main race event, you can determine the pace at which sharpening work should be conducted. It is simply done: The projected goal performance in the main race event determines the goal pace, and also substantially defines the training progression undertaken during the sharpening period. This agrees with the specificity of training principle, but physiologically speaking, why is this so?

Again, muscle fiber type has for many years been differentiated into fast-twitch Type II fibers (associated with explosive power) and slow-twitch Type I fibers (associated with endurance). More recently, so-called swing fibers have been recognized (that is, fast-twitch Type IIc fibers that can take on qualities of the slow-twitch). In truth, muscle fiber types are largely determined by their metabolic characteristics and enzyme profiles. Although the ratio of fast to slow twitch fibers appears to be genetically determined, the enzyme profiles among fast twitch Types II a/b/c fibers will adapt specifically in response to the nature of the training load (Åstrand, 1986). Muscle glycogen is also stored and summoned specifically by the local energy demands of previous exhaustive efforts. Neuro-muscular learning, coordination, and running economy also improve with specific training. For any given individual, an ideal mix of physiological attributes exists that is most conducive to optimal performance over a specific racing distance. In the words of the Australian coach Percy Cerutty: "Muscles are educated by movement" (Cerutty, 1967).

Date Pace and Finishing Speed Progressions

During the preceding base and hill periods, athletes will normally conduct date-pace work once a week in conjunction with a fartlek session. In the course of this work, athletes will have also instilled a dominant sense of pace, that is, a mental clock, or habit associated with a neuromuscular stereotype.

In the course of an athletic competition, conscious control gives way to an instinctive, intuitive and unconsciously conscious mode of functioning that might be described as a special form of automatism. In fact, if a letting-go of the attachments of the ego during the competition does not occur, a superior performance will not be delivered!

So, sound training habits are extremely important. We are all familiar with the athlete who eases up in the last five to 10 meters of a race and is defeated because that same easing of effort has occurred many times in the training. It has become the dominant habit, and closely resembles a conditioned response. Pace sense is a similar phenomenon. If athletes do not have that internal clock, then they will waver in competition as though lost, unless another competitor assumes the lead and does all the work—thus they are incapable of delivering a superior performance alone, or from the lead. Therefore, athletes need to enter the sharpening period having already conducted the date pace work required to facilitate sharpening work and performance at goal pace in the main race event, because the requisite physical and mental adaptations normally take approximately three months to instill.

Bill Bowerman's training prescription for date pace work represented a progression in quality of one second / 400 meters during the course of each succeeding monthly training cycle. Thus, in the four weeks preceding the sharpening period, date pace work would be conducted at projected goal pace for the main race event plus one second / 400 meters. In the month previous to that, the work would be done at goal pace plus two seconds / 400 meters, and so on. By the time athletes begin the sharpening period, they would then be sufficiently conditioned to goal pace so as to begin the sharpening work with minimal risk of injury (Bowerman, 1974).

This is a prudent training practice. However, in the context of this presentation, it would be more precise to say that the date pace work is reduced in quality by one second / 400 meters from goal pace during the first meso-cycle preceding the start of the sharpening period. The quality of date pace work then further reduces by an additional one second / 400 meters in each preceding meso-cycle. Again, during the course of an athletic season, the succeeding meso-cycles will decrease in length—from approximately 28 to 21 days, then to 14 days, and finally to between seven to 10 days—as the quality and intensity of the training increases.

The training schedule for an athletic season should indicate the progression of the athlete's fitness level in the goal main race event. The coach and athlete would also benefit from having an indication of the athlete's equivalent level of performance with respect to over-distance and under-distance events at any point in time. In addition, the date pace progression for the athlete's main race event should also be provided. The quality of the time trials or races conducted at the end of each meso-cycle will then directly correspond to the quality of the date pace work conducted during that meso-cycle. In addition, a sound progression of finishing speed work is required during the athletic season, and in particular, for those competing in the middle distance events. It is advisable to gradually progress the quality of finishing speed work by meso-cycle, but beginning with the worthwhile break that comprises the nine to 10 day ascent to the plateau.

Figures 1.27, 1.28, 1.29, and Tables 1.2 and 1.3 from Chapter 1 have been reproduced here for the sake of convenience, and now appear as Figures 4.2, 4.4, 4.5, and Tables 4.1 and 4.3, respectively. Figures 4.6 and 4.7 and Tables 4.2 and 4.4 also provide additional training schedules corresponding to the performance level of talented high school boys and girls. In addition, for possible use as worksheets, Figure 4.3, and Table 4.5 provide blank versions of the date pace and finishing speed progressions.

Abstract Sharpening Work Progression

If the coach and athlete have projected a realistic goal performance in the main race event and have properly conducted date pace work during the base and hill periods, then the next issue is how to best progress the sharpening work over the limited three to four week duration of the sharpening period. Previous discussion of training load tolerances suggested a maximum of two quality sessions at 3/4-effort, and one quality session at 1/2-effort in the course of any given week. That simple observation would establish an absolute limit of eight 3/4-effort training sessions over a four-week sharpening period, and any time trials or competitions must be further subtracted from this total.

In the training schedule examples provided later in this chapter, the actual number of possible 3/4-effort training sessions often total seven. Conducting a time trial and a competition during the worthwhile break taken between the two sharpening meso-cycles, thus reduces to five the number of 3/4-effort training sessions for the sharpening period. This will normally suffice to accomplish all the sharpening work required.

The fact that approximately five 3/4-effort training sessions constitute the primary training progression within the sharpening period should provide a sobering realization: make every training session count, and conduct the training progression so as to permit the athletes to assume optimal levels of quantity and quality. In practice, this suggests that they begin their sharpening work with interval training:

- Interval training workouts generally include a relatively large number of selected distances run in a series at equal to, or slower than goal pace in the main race event. These workouts also utilize a continuous jog or running recovery period of less than 2:30 duration, which substantially retains the venous preload on the heart and workload on the diaphragm.

- Repetition workouts generally include two or more selected distances, run at equal to, or faster than goal pace in the main race event. These workouts include a continuous jog or running recovery period equal to or greater than 2:30 duration. Repetition workouts normally come late in the sharpening period. In this treatment, the progression of sharpening work makes the point of transition between the conduct of intervals and repetitions difficult to discern.

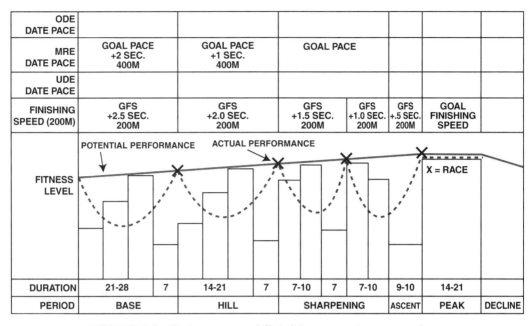

ODE DATE PACE									
MRE DATE PACE	GOAL PACE +2 SEC. 400M		GOAL PACE +1 SEC. 400M		GOAL PACE				
UDE DATE PACE									
FINISHING SPEED (200M)	GFS +2.5 SEC. 200M		GFS +2.0 SEC. 200M		GFS +1.5 SEC. 200M	GFS +1.0 SEC. 200M	GFS +.5 SEC. 200M	GOAL FINISHING SPEED	

POTENTIAL PERFORMANCE   ACTUAL PERFORMANCE

FITNESS LEVEL

X = RACE

| DURATION | 21-28 | 7 | 14-21 | 7 | 7-10 | 7 | 7-10 | 9-10 | 14-21 | |
| PERIOD | BASE | | HILL | | SHARPENING | | | ASCENT | PEAK | DECLINE |

FIGURE 4.2—Date pace and finishing speed progressions

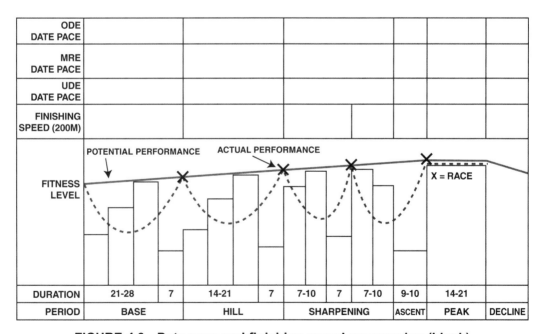

ODE DATE PACE									
MRE DATE PACE									
UDE DATE PACE									
FINISHING SPEED (200M)									

POTENTIAL PERFORMANCE   ACTUAL PERFORMANCE

FITNESS LEVEL

X = RACE

| DURATION | 21-28 | 7 | 14-21 | 7 | 7-10 | 7 | 7-10 | 9-10 | 14-21 | |
| PERIOD | BASE | | HILL | | SHARPENING | | | ASCENT | PEAK | DECLINE |

FIGURE 4.3—Date pace and finishing speed progression (blank)

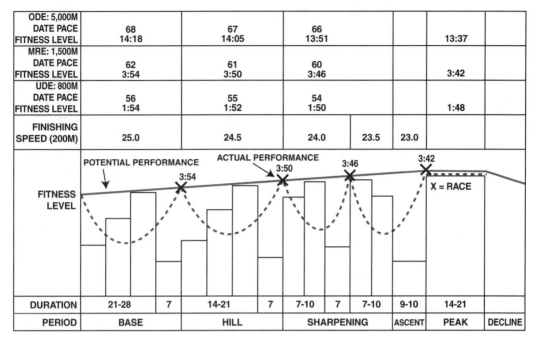

FIGURE 4.4—Schedule for a 1,500 meters performance of 3:42

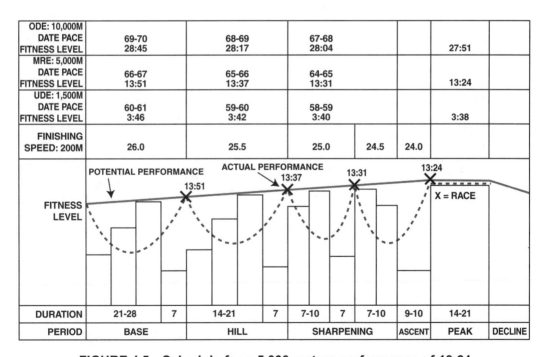

FIGURE 4.5—Schedule for a 5,000 meters performance of 13:24

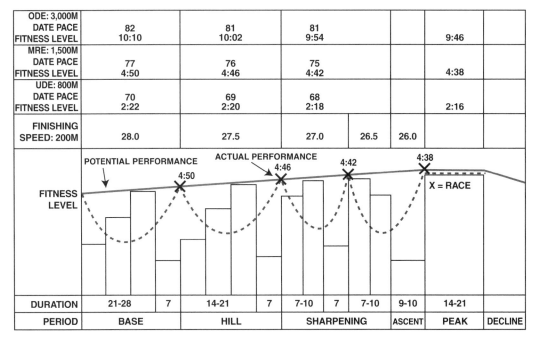

FIGURE 4.6—Schedule for a 1,500 meters performance of 4:38

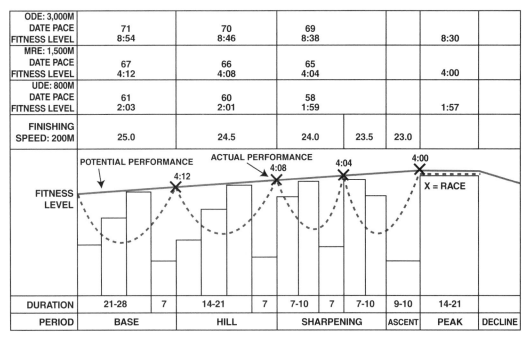

FIGURE 4.7—Schedule for a 1,500 meters performance of 4:00

TRAINING PERIOD	800 METERS	1,500 METERS	3,000 METERS	5,000 METERS	10,000 METERS
BASE	26.0 5x150	27.0 5x200	28.0 5x200	29.0 5x200	30.0 5x200
HILL	25.5 5x100	26.5 5x150	27.5 5x200	28.5 5x200	29.5 5x200
SHARPENING PART 1	25.0 4x100	26.0 4x150	27.0 4x200	28.0 4x200	29.0 4x200
SHARPENING PART 2	24.5 4x60	25.5 4x100	26.5 4x150	27.5 4x200	28.5 4x200
ASCENT	24.0 3x60	25.0 3x100	26.0 3x150	27.0 3x200	28.0 3x200

TABLE 4.1—Finishing speed progression for world class women by event

TRAINING PERIOD	800 METERS	1,500 METERS	3,000 METERS	5,000 METERS
BASE	27.0 5x150	28.0 5x200	29.0 5x200	30.0 5x200
HILL	26.5 5x100	27.5 5x150	28.5 5x200	29.5 5x200
SHARPENING PART 1	26.0 4x100	27.0 4x150	28.0 4x200	29.0 4x200
SHARPENING PART 2	25.5 4x60	26.5 4x100	27.5 4x150	28.5 4x200
ASCENT	25.0 3x60	26.0 3x100	27.0 3x150	28.0 3x200

TABLE 4.2—Finishing speed progression for national class high school girls

TRAINING PERIOD	800 METERS	1,500 METERS	3,000 METERS	5,000 METERS	10,000 METERS
BASE	23.0 5x150	24.0 5x200	25.0 5x200	26.0 5x200	27.0 5x200
HILL	22.5 5x100	23.5 5x150	24.5 5x200	25.5 5x200	26.5 5x200
SHARPENING PART 1	22.0 4x100	23.0 4x150	24.0 4x200	25.0 4x200	26.0 4x200
SHARPENING PART 2	21.5 4x60	22.5 4x100	23.5 4x150	24.5 4x200	25.5 4x200
ASCENT	21.0 3x60	22.0 3x100	23.0 3x150	24.0 3x200	25.0 3x200

TABLE 4.3—Finishing speed progression for world class men by event

TRAINING PERIOD	800 METERS	1,500 METERS	3,000 METERS	5,000 METERS
BASE	24.0 5x150	25.0 5x200	26.0 5x200	27.0 5x200
HILL	23.5 5x100	24.5 5x150	25.5 5x200	26.5 5x200
SHARPENING PART 1	23.0 4x100	24.0 4x150	25.0 4x200	26.0 4x200
SHARPENING PART 2	22.5 4x60	23.5 4x100	24.5 4x150	25.5 4x200
ASCENT	22.0 3x60	23.0 3x100	24.0 3x150	25.0 3x200

TABLE 4.4—Finishing speed progression for national class high school boys

TRAINING PERIOD	800 METERS	1,500 METERS	3,000 METERS	5,000 METERS	10,000 METERS
BASE					
HILL					
SHARPENING PART 1					
SHARPENING PART 2					
ASCENT					

TABLE 4.5—Finishing speed progression (blank)

As can be gleaned from these figures and tables, the aim of the training progression undertaken during the sharpening period should be to provide just that—a true progression and continuity—so that athletes are, in the words of Lydiard, "training and not straining" their way to higher levels of fitness.

There are a number of reasons for beginning the sharpening period with interval training. It will be difficult enough for middle distance and distance runners to undertake intervals between 100 to 400 meters in the first session, since they are not yet fully accustomed to the quality associated with goal pace. Physiologically, interval training brings the heart and diaphragm to a higher level of fitness, thus enhancing the quality of the repetition training later on. In contrast with repetition training, which is more highly anaerobic, properly conducted interval training will normally not so greatly stress an athlete's metabolism.

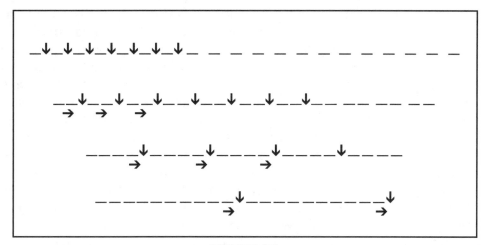

FIGURE 4.8

When performing interval training, athletes should run the desired pace—no faster or slower—and take up any slack in the effort of the workout by pushing or squeezing the recovery periods. Avoid unevenness in the pacing of the interval training, since one of its purposes is to instill a mental clock, or pace sense, needed for later repetition training and competition. Nevertheless, the exclusive conduct of interval training during the sharpening period would bring undesirable consequences.

Both Arthur Lydiard and Percy Cerutty criticized the intensive interval methods prevalent in their day by observing that the body and mind become conditioned to expecting an interval recovery that never comes in the race (See Lydiard, 1962, and Cerutty, 1961). Keep in mind this simple fact: the ultimate goal of the training progression is to physically and mentally condition the athletes to later execute a single repetition at projected goal pace in the main race event. This means that recovery periods must be either progressively absorbed by increased physical and mental conditioning, or likewise, deferred until after the training or racing effort.

For example, the training progression during the sharpening period could begin with an interval session with distances between 100 to 400 meters. An athlete would then be capable of handling a greater number of quality intervals at 800 meters sometime later. Then, after conducting the session at 800 meters, the athlete could better handle quality one-mile repetitions at a later date, as opposed to trying these repetitions immediately. Thus, a true progression permits the assumption of optimal levels of quantity and quality.

Therefore, in the training progression of the sharpening period, the distances being run tend to become fewer and longer, and incorporate like recovery periods. This sometimes makes it difficult to determine where the gradual transformation from interval to repetition training format actually takes place. The sharpening period training progression is constructed to condition the body and mind to make fewer and more maximal efforts, as the recovery periods are progressively absorbed by improved physical and mental conditioning, or deferred until after the training and racing effort. This principle is illustrated in Figure 4.8.

Again, in the early stages of the training progression athletes need to push or squeeze the recovery periods, since the ultimate aim is to eliminate them, that is, absorb and defer them until after the single repetition that constitutes the main race event. The quality of the recovery period is the most critical part of the interval sessions. However, as the sharpening period progresses, the recovery period becomes less and less important, and rather, the quality of the repetitions become the preeminent concern. To insure the desired quality of the repetitions, the recovery periods should then be extended as necessary. So, whereas an athlete might risk the quality of the series being run for the recovery period when doing intervals—just the opposite is true when conducting repetitions. Ultimately, when an athlete later runs a single repetition in the form of the main race event the recovery period is irrelevant. It does not matter whether the athlete lies spread-eagle on the grass afterwards. Of course, the caveat being that it *does* matter if the athlete needs to weather multiple qualifying heats. Accordingly, a runner needs to be specifically conditioned to meet the competitive demands.

The Need for Variation

The above discussion addresses an important characteristic, but threatens to oversimplify the training progression undertaken during the sharpening period. In the sharpening period, the meso-cycle structure defines the pattern of training loads and worthwhile breaks. This larger framework defines the number, placement, and characteristics of the quality training workouts. However, conducting sharpening work is not the only task to be accomplished at this time. To deliver optimal performances, it will be necessary to devote some time to maintaining previously acquired powers. The aerobic ability developed during the base period must be maintained by at least one long training run, conducted at less than 1/4-effort, over any given seven-to-10-day period. To facilitate recovery from sharpening·work and maintain acquired strength, an athlete should occasionally conduct a 1/2-effort fartlek workout on hills, and also run over rolling terrain on the recovery days. The fitness of the heart and diaphragm can be maintained by running a series of 100-meter cross-field accelerations, incorporating a brief 50-meter jog-recovery during the warm-up and warm-down.

The key point: Do not let the structural emphasis of the training lead you to believe that various components of fitness, once acquired, are forever locked away for safekeeping. In this regard, without the conduct of suitable maintenance work, an athlete would begin to lose substantial aerobic ability after three weeks. The loss of significant levels of acquired strength would only take two weeks. And the loss of substantial fitness acquired via sharpening work would only take a week. This is relatively how fast an athlete would lose these components of fitness. However, considerably less time and energy is needed to maintain any given component of athletic fitness. But without maintenance work, the accumulated powers drain away, and subsequent training will then be building on quicksand.

Further, the sharpening work will not normally progress as indicated in Table 4.10, that is, with all of the quality sharpening workouts being run at goal pace for the main race event. Athletes preparing for the 800 meters can often conduct their sharpening work this way, but it does not provide for optimal results in the long distance events. This degree of specificity is generally counterproductive for three reasons:

- Athletes must be capable of executing surges, a breakaway, and a finishing kick if they expect to compete at the highest level. This makes some under-distance and finishing speed work necessary.

- Runners must also maintain their stamina and endurance to handle preliminary qualifying rounds in championship competitions. And that would suggest conducting some anaerobic threshold and over-distance work, even during the sharpening period.

- Undertaking a gauntlet of sharpening work at goal pace for the main race event can produce adverse side-effects in the form of habituation, stagnation, and delayed recovery from exercise.

In addition, a fundamental training principle here defined as the principle of equilibrium needs to be examined.

The Principle of Equilibrium

The word equilibrium is used to describe the harmony amongst various components of fitness required for optimal performance. Disequilibrium then refers to administering these various components in a manner that is disproportionate or possibly even destructive to an athlete's requirements for optimal performance in a specific competitive event (See the discussion in Chapter 8 on strength training). The primary components of equilibrium are commonly assumed under the somewhat generic labels:

- Endurance
- Strength
- Speed

The most important thing to realize: the better one can read the needs and requirements governing the maintenance of equilibrium, the higher the quantity and quality an athlete can productively assume in training. When the training induces a state of disequilibrium, an athlete will experience higher levels of physical and mental fatigue. Remarkably, we could take the same athlete and with a properly composed training prescription, perhaps considerably increase the overall training load, yet find the individual both physically and mentally fit. The various physical and mental stimuli (and would-be stressors) tend to cancel out one another when equilibrium is maintained. Successful mature athletes develop a sixth sense in this regard, which is partly why they can sustain such heavy training loads. It is difficult to describe to one who has not had the experience.

In order to attain optimal competitive results, the coach and athlete must develop an intuitive sense for the athlete's needs when implementing the training program. Moreover, maintaining equilibrium is critical when attempting to extend

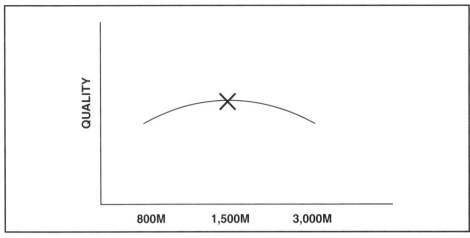

FIGURE 4.9

the plateau of peak performance by undertaking an extended or multiple-peak period. This is not to advocate the principle of equilibrium with the simple premise that more work is better. Given common practice of the day, often less work is in order. The essential point being: "Work does things, but intelligent work does things better" (Cerutty, 1961).

Equilibrium and the Concept of Balance

Whereas the word equilibrium describes the harmony between sometimes opposing aspects of fitness that contribute to optimal performance in the main race event, balance refers more specifically to an athlete's over-distance versus under-distance ability. Equilibrium must be maintained, thus enabling a proper balance to be achieved. Clearly, the athlete should be balanced with respect to the main event. Inferior speed in the under-distance event ultimately acts as a governor on performance in the main race event. Inferior over-distance ability would suggest insufficient stamina to weather preliminary rounds of competition. The word balance has been employed, because if one were to graph the relative quality of an athlete's performances at various distances, it would resemble a balance, with the main race event placed at the fulcrum as shown in Figure 4.9.

Event	Under	Main Event	Over
400	40%	30%	30%
800	50%	40%	10%
1,500	30%	40%	30%
5,000	40%	30%	20%
10,000	60%	30%	10%

TABLE 4.6

Balancing the Training Prescription

The question of equilibrium and balance presents itself throughout the athletic season, but it becomes particularly important during the sharpening and peak periods. Table 4.6 shows an abstract prescription regarding the balance of over-distance and under-distance work conducted during the sharpening and peak periods for various race events.

Take these estimations with a large grain of salt, since the actual training prescription for individual athletes will vary considerably. Nevertheless, this table provides abstract percentages relating to the sharpening work and racing conducted in various events. Young athletes, or those in early development, should fully develop their speed ability, thus assume more under-distance work when preparing for any given main race event. They should not rapidly move up to the 5,000 and 10,000 meters, as the rate of this transition could determine the ultimate length of their athletic careers. Also, the prescription for female athletes should be shifted slightly towards over-distance work because of the longer relative duration associated with competition in any given race event. However, the relative strengths and weaknesses of each individual athlete provide the main criteria for determining questions of equilibrium and balance. As shown in Table 4.7, it is possible to plan the balance of training during the sharpening and peak periods by recording the sessions under the following descriptive categories:

- Under-Distance Event (UDE)
- Over-Distance Event (ODE)
- Main Race Event (MRE)

Moreover, when making a plan or assessment, it is also possible to weigh the effort of the training sessions. The final percentages provided in Table 4.7 represent an abstract training prescription for a 400-meter sided competitor at 800 meters. However, apply only the training principles and general methodology, rather than use any example as an ideal prescription. As illustrated in the sharpening period model provided earlier, the preferred method for conducting sharpening work is to alternate between sessions that are directed under-distance, over-distance, and towards the main race event. *The decision analysis governing the composition of the training sessions and the athletic competitions should aim to maintain equilibrium and achieve optimal balance with respect to the main race event.* If an athlete is weaker on the speed (or under-distance) side of the main race event, they should conduct a larger proportion of under-distance work. If an athlete is weaker on the stamina (or over-distance) side, they should conduct a greater proportion of over-distance work to bring this aspect of fitness up to par, thus enhance later performance in the main race event. The coach and athlete then select how much under or over, and the specifics with regard to quantity (volume, duration) and quality (intensity, density and frequency), depending on the magnitude of the deficiency. For example, Table 4.7 shows calculations and ratios with respect to the various types of high-quality training sessions and competitions that could be assumed by an 800 meters specialist during the sharpening and peak periods.

800 Meters			
Sharpening Period Training	**UDE**	**MRE**	**ODE**
3(4 x 300) meters	0	1	0
2(4 x 400) meters	0	0	1
4 x 400 meters	0	1	0
2 x 600 meters	0	1	0
2 x 1,000 meters	0	0	1
4 x Finishing Speed	4	0	0
Sharpening Period Time Trials or Racing			
	2	1	0
Peak Period Training			
2 x Finishing Speed	2	0	0
Peak Period Time Trials or Racing			
	2	4	0
Totals	**10**	**8**	**2**
Percent	**50 %**	**40 %**	**10 %**

TABLE 4.7

Balance and Equivalent Performances

If an athlete will normally alternate between sessions geared for the over-distance, under-distance, and main race events, what is the appropriate quality of the over-distance and under-distance work? This question introduces the concept of equivalent performance(s) in the over-distance and under-distance events: It is best to direct over and under-distance work at the corresponding performance levels indicated by the projected goal performance in the main race event.

Table 4.8 provides formulas for calculating equivalent performances that can be easily memorized. They will enable a coach or athlete to quickly convert a given competitive result or performance prediction into its corresponding over-distance and under-distance equivalent (Fišer, 1965, Noakes,* 1991). These formulas presuppose comparable quality of preparation for the events, and are directed towards mature athletes. In most cases, the under-distance performance is a reliable indicator of performance in the immediate over-distance event. Obviously, the further away you project from a given performance, the less reliable the estimate can be. Nevertheless, the remarkable accuracy of these formulas to predict equivalent performances can be tested against the present world records, and an athlete's personal best performances (For prediction of athletic performance based on maximum oxygen uptake, see Daniels and Gilbert, 1979, and Daniels, 1998). Table 4.9 indicates equivalent athletic performances in the 800-10,000-meter events predicted from the formulas provided in Table 4.8 (Fišer, 1965).

Calculating Equivalent Performances 800 Meters - Marathon	
Event(s)	**Formula(s)**
800 to 1,500m	2 (800m P.R.) + 6-8 seconds
1,500 to 3,000m	2 (1,500m P.R.) + 28 seconds
1,500 to 5,000m	5 (1,000m split from the 1,500m P.R.) +15-16 seconds
3,000 to 5,000m	5 (1,000m split from the 3,000m P.R.) + 3 seconds
5,000 to 10,000m	2 (5,000m P.R.) + 63-68 seconds
10,000 to 20,000m	2 (10,000m P.R.) + 2 minutes
10,000 to Marathon	5.48 (10,000m P.R.) ⪅ 28 minutes*

TABLE 4.8

Given a demonstrated performance, a coach or athlete can use the information provided in Tables 4.8 and 4.9 in order to determine the equivalent level of performance to attempt when competing in other events. This information is also needed to determine the appropriate level of quality to assume within the over-distance and under-distance training sessions relative to the goal performance in the main race event. In this regard, the predicted over-distance and under-distance performance establishes the pace (quality) at which the corresponding sharpening work should be conducted.

The Sharpening Work: Quantity

The preceding discussion has addressed the question of quality. It is now possible to consider appropriate levels of quantity that might be assumed during the sharpening period. Table 4.10 provides a progression of training sessions for various main race events, and also the equivalent progression of over-distance and under-distance training sessions. The indicated number of reps would be suitable for mature athletes. Generally, the training prescription for female or young athletes should be reduced by 30% across the board. Note that the main race event and the respective over-distance and under-distance sessions constitute equivalent training efforts at any given point in time within the progression. These can then be interchanged, depending on the individual athlete's requirements for maintaining equilibrium and proper balance. If an athlete appears to need more under-distance work at some point during the sharpening period, that would suggest the conduct of the equivalent under-distance workout corresponding to the training session indicated for the main race event, at that point in the training progression. The same kind of determination would also be made at any point if the question concerned the proper selection of an over-distance versus under-distance competition. Thus, one should follow the area of relative weakness and assume training or racing efforts that will best serve to maintain equilibrium and optimal balance.

The relative quantity athletes can assume in the equivalent under-distance training session is normally greater than their load tolerance in the over-distance sessions. For example, the specialist at 1,500 meters will normally be able to

Table Of Equivalent Performances

800m	1,500m	1,600m	3,000m	3,200m	5,000m	10,000m
1:40	3:26	3:44	7:22	7:55	12:45	26:33
1:41	3:28	3:46	7:26	7:59	12:52	26:46
1:42	3:30	3:48	7:30	8:03	12:58	26:59
1:43	3:32	3:50	7:34	8:07	13:07	27:12
1:44	3:34	3:52	7:38	8:11	13:11	27:25
1:45	3:36	3:54	7:42	8:15	13:18	27:38
1:46	3:38	3:56	7:46	8:19	13:24	27:51
1:47	3:40	3:58	7:50	8:23	13:31	28:04
1:48	3:42	4:00	7:54	8:27	13:37	28:17
1:49	3:44	4:02	7:58	8:32	13:44	28:31
1:50	3:46	4:04	8:02	8:36	13:51	28:45
1:51	3:48	4:06	8:06	8:40	13:57	28:59
1:52	3:50	4:08	8:10	8:44	14:05	29:13
1:53	3:52	4:10	8:14	8:44	14:12	29:26
1:54	3:54	4:12	8:18	8:52	14:18	29:39
1:55	3:56	4:14	8:22	8:56	14:25	29:52
1:56	3:58	4:16	8:26	9:00	14:31	30:05
1:57	4:00	4:18	8:30	9:04	14:38	30:19
1:58	4:02	4:20	8:34	9:08	14:45	30:33
1:59	4:04	4:22	8:38	9:13	14:52	30:49
2:00	4:06	4:24	8:42	9:17	14:58	30:59
2:01	4:08	4:26	8:46	9:21	15:05	31:12
2:02	4:10	4:28	8:50	9:25	15:11	31:25
2:03	4:12	4:30	8:54	9:29	15:17	31:38
2:04	4:14	4:32	8:58	9:33	15:24	31:51
2:05	4:16	4:34	9:02	9:37	15:30	32:04
2:06	4:18	4:36	9:06	9:41	15:37	32:17
2:07	4:20	4:38	9:10	9:44	15:45	32:32
2:08	4:22	4:40	9:14	9:49	15:52	32:47
2:09	4:24	4:43	9:18	9:54	15:59	33:00
2:10	4:26	4:45	9:22	9:59	16:05	33:13
2:12	4:30	4:49	9:30	10:07	16:18	33:39
2:14	4:34	4:53	9:38	10:15	16:31	34:05
2:16	4:38	4:57	9:46	10:23	16:45	34:33
2:18	4:42	5:01	9:54	10:31	16:58	34:59
2:20	4:46	5:06	10:02	10:40	17:11	35:25
2:22	4:50	5:10	10:10	10:48	17:24	35:51
2:24	4:54	5:12	10:18	10:56	17:38	36:19
2:26	4:58	5:16	10:26	11:04	17:51	36:45
2:28	5:02	5:20	10:34	11:12	18:05	37:13
2:30	5:06	5:26	10:42	11:20	18:18	37:39

TABLE 4.9

Equivalent Sharpening Training Progressions

200 Meters **Under-Distance**	**400 Meters** **Main Race Event**	**800 Meters** **Over-Distance**
Starts x 10	8-10 x 100m	3-4 (4 x 200m)
8-10 x 60m	6-8 x 150m	2-3 (4 x 300m)
4-6 x 100m	4-6 x 200m	4-5 x 400m
3 x 150m	3 x 300m	3 x 500m
2 x 300m ODE	2 x 500m ODE	2 x 600m

400 Meters **Under-Distance**	**800 Meters** **Main Race Event**	**1,500 Meters** **Over-Distance**
8-10 x 100m	3-4 (4 x 200m)	3-5 (4 x 200m)
6-8 x 150m	2-3 (4 x 300m)	2-3 (5 x 300m)
4-6 x 200m	4-5 x 400m	8-10 x 400m
3 x 300m	3 x 500m	4-6 x 600m
2 x 500m ODE	2 x 600m	2 x 800m

800 Meters **Under-Distance**	**1,500 Meters** **Main Race Event**	**5,000 Meters** **Over-Distance**
3-4 (4 x 200m)	3-5 (4 x 200m)	4 (5 x 200m)
2-3 (4 x 300m)	2-3 (5 x 300m)	3-4 (5 x 400m)
4-5 x 400m	8-10 x 400m	6-8 x 800m
3 x 500m	4-6 x 600m	5-6 x 1,000m
2 x 600m	2 x 800m	3-4 x 1,600m

1,500 Meters **Under-Distance**	**5,000 Meters** **Main Race Event**	**10,000 Meters** **Over-Distance**
3-5 (4 x 200m)	4 (5 x 200m)	4 (5 x 400m)
2-3 (5 x 300m)	3-4 (5 x 400m)	8-10 x 800m
8-10 x 400m	6-8 x 800m	6-8 x 1,000m/CR
4-6 x 600m	5-6 x 1,000m	5-6 x 1,600m/CR
2-3 x 800m	3-4 x 1,600m	2-3 x 3000m

TABLE 4.10

Typical Duration of Recovery Periods

200 Meters	Recovery Period
Starts x 10	walk full recovery
8-10 x 60m	walk full recovery
4-6 x 100m	walk/jog full recovery
3 x 150m	walk/jog full recovery
ODE 2 x 300m	walk/jog full recovery

400 Meters	Recovery Period
8-10 x 100m	1-3 minutes walk/jog recovery
6-8 x 150m	3-5 minutes walk/jog recovery
4-6 x 200m	5-7 minutes walk/jog recovery
3 x 300m	7-10 minutes walk/jog recovery
ODE 2 x 500m	10-15 minutes walk/jog recovery

800 Meters	Recovery Period
3-4(4 x 200m)	100m jog recovery; 400m jog recovery at series break
2-3(4 x 300m)	100m jog recovery; 400m jog recovery at series break
4-5 x 400m	400-800m jog recovery (5-7 minutes)
3 x 500m	600-800m jog recovery (7-10 minutes)
2 x 600m	800-1200m jog recovery (10-15 minutes)

1,500 Meters	Recovery Period
3-5(4 x 200m)	100m jog recovery; 400m jog recovery at series break
2-3(5 x 300m)	150m jog recovery; 400m jog recovery at series break
2(4-5 x 400m)	200m jog recovery; 400m jog recovery at series break
4-6 x 600m	300-400m jog recovery (3-5 minutes)
2 x 800m	800-1200m jog recovery (10-15 minutes)

5,000 Meters	Recovery Period
4(5 x 200m)	100m jog recovery; 200m jog recovery at series break
3-4(5 x 400m)	100m jog recovery; 400m jog recovery at series break
6-8 x 800m	200m jog recovery; 400m jog recovery at series break
5-6 x 1,000m	200-400m jog recovery (2-5 minutes)
3-4 x 1,600m	400-800m jog recovery (5-10 minutes)

10,000 Meters	Recovery Period
4(5 x 400m)	100m jog recovery; 200m jog recovery at series break
8-10 x 800m	200m jog recovery; 400m jog recovery at series break
6-8 x 1,000m	200-400m jog recovery (2-5 minutes)
5-6 x 1,600m	400m jog recovery (3-5 minutes Controlled Recovery)
2-3 x 3000m	800m jog recovery (5-10 minutes Controlled Recovery)

TABLE 4.11

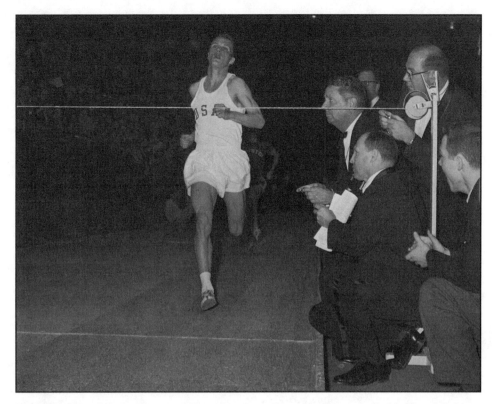

PHOTO 4.2—Bill Dellinger setting the American 3-mile record, Madison Square Garden, 1959. Copyright Otto Bettmann/CORBIS. Reprinted with permission.

assume the maximum quantity indicated in the equivalent 800 meters training progression, but will likely only be able to undertake the minimum quantity indicated in the equivalent 5,000 meters progression. ODE stands for Over-Distance Event, and here indicates the quality at which the particular training session is conducted. The designation CR refers to Controlled Recovery, that is, an optional high quality running recovery period. This can be advantageous when athletes are training for 5,000 and 10,000 meters, since it extends the quality of the training effort over a longer duration. The CR does this by maintaining a high internal load during the would-be recovery period. This is necessary because, it is not possible to cover much quantity at quality in the long distance events, whereas this is clearly possible in the middle distance events. In contrast, the athlete competing at 10,000 meters cannot prudently attempt much more quantity in the training sessions at goal pace than the racing distance (See Dellinger and Beres, 1978). Table 4.11 indicates the recovery period typically associated with various training sessions.

TRAINING SCHEDULES BY EVENT

The following training schedules for events between 400 and 10,000 meters are provided for the sharpening period.

Beginning of the Sharpening Period

First Meso-Cycle
Monday	Passive Recovery
Tuesday	3/4-Effort, 4-5 x 200m at 400m Goal Pace
Wednesday	Active Recovery
Thursday	1/2-Effort, 4 x 60m Starts
Friday	Active Recovery
Saturday	3/4-Effort, 3 (3 x 300m) at 800m Goal Pace
Sunday	Easy Effort, Long Run, 30-40 minutes

Worthwhile Break
Monday	Passive Recovery
Tuesday	Race 100m and 200m
Wednesday	Active Recovery
Thursday	Easy Recovery + 3 x 60m Starts
Friday	Day Before Race Routine
Saturday	Race 400m, 200m
Sunday	Easy Effort, Long Run, 30-40 minutes

Second Meso-Cycle
Monday	Passive Recovery
Tuesday	3/4-Effort, 3 x 500m at 800m Goal Pace
Wednesday	Active Recovery
Thursday	1/2-Effort, 3 x 60m Starts
Friday	Active Recovery
Saturday	3/4-Effort, 3 x 300m at 400m Goal Pace
Sunday	Easy Effort, Long Run, 30-40 minutes
Monday	Passive Recovery
Tuesday	1/2-Effort, 3 x 60m Starts
Wednesday	Active Recovery
Thursday	3/4-Effort, 2 x 600m at 800m Goal Pace

End of the Sharpening Period / Beginning of the Ascent

Beginning of the Sharpening Period

First Meso-Cycle

Monday	Passive Recovery
Tuesday	3/4-Effort, 3(4 x 300m) at 800m Goal Pace
Wednesday	Active Recovery
Thursday	1/2-Effort, Fartlek + 4 x 100m at Finishing Speed
Friday	Active Recovery
Saturday	3/4-Effort, 2(4 x 400m) at 1,500m Goal Pace
Sunday	Easy Effort, Long Run, 40-60 minutes

Worthwhile Break

Monday	Passive Recovery
Tuesday	Race 400m and 200m
Wednesday	Active Recovery + 4 x 100m at Finishing Speed
Thursday	Easy Recovery
Friday	Day Before Race Routine
Saturday	Race 800m, 400m
Sunday	Easy Effort, Long Run, 40-60 minutes

Second Meso-Cycle

Monday	Passive Recovery
Tuesday	3/4-Effort, 4 x 400m at 800m Goal Pace
Wednesday	Active Recovery
Thursday	1/2-Effort, Fartlek + 4 x 100m at Finishing Speed
Friday	Active Recovery
Saturday	3/4-Effort, 3 x 500m at 800m Goal Pace, or Race 2 x 400m
Sunday	Easy Effort, Long Run, 40-60 minutes
Monday	Passive Recovery
Tuesday	1/2-Effort, Fartlek + 4 x 60m Starts
Wednesday	Active Recovery
Thursday	Time Trial(s) 600m, full recovery, then 300m

End of the Sharpening Period / Beginning of the Ascent

Beginning of the Sharpening Period

First Meso-Cycle

Monday	Passive Recovery
Tuesday	3/4-Effort, 3(4 x 300m) at 1,500m Goal Pace
Wednesday	Active Recovery
Thursday	1/2-Effort, Fartlek + 4 x 150m at Finishing Speed
Friday	Active Recovery
Saturday	3/4-Effort, 6 x 800m at 3,000m Goal Pace
Sunday	Easy Effort, Long Run, 60-80 minutes

Worthwhile Break

Monday	Passive Recovery
Tuesday	Race 800m and 400m
	or Time Trial 1,000m, full recovery, then 300m
Wednesday	Active Recovery + 4 x 150m at Finishing Speed
Thursday	Easy Recovery
Friday	Day Before Race Routine
Saturday	Race 1,500m
Sunday	Easy Effort, Long Run, 60-80 minutes

Second Meso-Cycle

Monday	Passive Recovery
Tuesday	3/4-Effort, 2(4 x 400m) at 1,500m Goal Pace
Wednesday	Active Recovery
Thursday	1/2-Effort, Fartlek + 4 x 100m at Finishing Speed
Friday	Active Recovery
Saturday	Time Trial or Race 2 x 800m, or 800m and 400m
Sunday	Easy Effort, Long Run, 60-80 minutes
Monday	Passive Recovery
Tuesday	1/2-Effort, Fartlek + 4 x 100m at Finishing Speed
Wednesday	Active Recovery
Thursday	3/4-Effort, 4 x 1,000m at 3,000m Goal Pace

End of the Sharpening Period / Beginning of the Ascent

Beginning of the Sharpening Period

First Meso-Cycle
Monday	Passive Recovery
Tuesday	3/4-Effort, 3(4 x 300m) at 1,500m Goal Pace
Wednesday	Time Trial or Active Recovery
Thursday	1/2-Effort, Fartlek + 4 x 200m at Finishing Speed
Friday	Active Recovery
Saturday	3/4-Effort, 6 x 800m at 3,000m Goal Pace
Sunday	Easy Effort, Long Run, 60-80 minutes

Worthwhile Break
Monday	Passive Recovery
Tuesday	Time Trial or Race 800m, 400m
Wednesday	Active Recovery + 4 x 150m at Finishing Speed
Thursday	Easy Recovery
Friday	Day Before Race Routine
Saturday	Race 3,000m
Sunday	Easy Effort, Long Run, 60-80 minutes

Second Meso-Cycle
Monday	Passive Recovery
Tuesday	3/4-Effort, 2(4 x 400m) at 1,500m Goal Pace
Wednesday	Active Recovery
Thursday	1/2-Effort, Fartlek + 4 x 150m at Finishing Speed
Friday	Active Recovery
Saturday	Time Trial or Race 2 x 800m
Sunday	Easy Effort, Long Run, 60-80 minutes
Monday	Passive Recovery
Tuesday	1/2-Effort, Fartlek + 4 x 150m at Finishing Speed
Wednesday	Active Recovery
Thursday	3/4-Effort, 4 x 1,000 at 3,000m Goal Pace

End of the Sharpening Period / Beginning of the Ascent

In this 3,000 meters schedule, the 2(4 x 400m) and 3 x 1,600m workouts in the second meso-cycle may have to be moved and delayed a day depending upon the recovery status of the athlete from the 3,000m race in the preceding week.

Beginning of the Sharpening Period

First Meso-Cycle

Monday	Passive Recovery
Tuesday	3/4-Effort, 3(4 x 300m) at 1,500m Goal Pace
Wednesday	Active Recovery
Thursday	1/2-Effort, Fartlek + 4 x 200m at Finishing Speed
Friday	Active Recovery
Saturday	3/4-Effort, 6 x 800m at 3,000m Goal Pace
Sunday	Easy Effort, Long Run, 60-90 minutes

Worthwhile Break

Monday	Passive Recovery
Tuesday	Time Trial 1,200m, full recovery, then 300m
Wednesday	Active Recovery + 4 x 200m at Finishing Speed
Thursday	Easy Recovery
Friday	Day Before Race Routine
Saturday	Race 5,000 meters
Sunday	Easy Effort, Long Run, 60-90 minutes

Second Meso-Cycle

Monday	Passive Recovery
Tuesday	1/2-Effort, Fartlek + 4 x 200m at Finishing Speed
Wednesday	Active Recovery
Thursday	3/4-Effort, 2(4 x 400m) at 1,500m Goal Pace
Friday	Active Recovery
Saturday	1/2-Effort, Fartlek + 4 x 200m at Finishing Speed
Sunday	Easy Effort, Long Run, 60-90 minutes
Monday	Passive Recovery
Tuesday	3/4-Effort, 4 x 1,200m at 5,000m Goal Pace

End of the Sharpening Period / Beginning of the Ascent

This 5,000 meters schedule provides 5 days between the 5,000m competition and the following 2(4 x 400m) sharpening workout to permit adequate recovery.

Beginning of the Sharpening Period

First Meso-Cycle
Monday	Passive Recovery
Tuesday	3/4-Effort, 2-3 (5 x 300m) at 1,500m Goal Pace
Wednesday	Active Recovery
Thursday	1/2-Effort, Fartlek + 4 x 200m Finishing Speed
Friday	Active Recovery
Saturday	3/4-Effort, 6-8 x 800m at 5,000m Goal Pace
Sunday	Easy Effort, Long Run, 80-100 minutes

Worthwhile Break
Monday	Passive Recovery
Tuesday	Time Trial 1,200m, full recovery, then 300m
Wednesday	Active Recovery + 4 x 200m Finishing Speed
Thursday	Easy Recovery
Friday	Day Before Race Routine
Saturday	Race–men 8,000m, women 5,000m
Sunday	Active Recovery + 6-8 x 200m at 1,500m Goal Pace

Second Meso-Cycle
Monday	Easy Effort, Long Run, 80-100 minutes
Tuesday	Passive Recovery
Wednesday	3/4-Effort, 2(4 x 400m) at 1,500m Goal Pace
Thursday	Active Recovery
Friday	1/2-Effort, Fartlek + 4 x 200m at Finishing Speed
Saturday	Active Recovery
Sunday	3/4-Effort, 4-5 x 1,600m at 10,000m Goal Pace
Monday	Active Recovery
Tuesday	Easy Effort, Long Run, 70-90 minutes
Wednesday	Passive Recovery
Thursday	3/4-Effort, 4-5 x 1,000m at 5,000m Goal Pace

End of the Sharpening Period / Beginning of the Ascent

Comparison of Sharpening Work
Track & Field Events 400-10,000 Meters

KEY TO ABBREVIATIONS

AR	Active Recovery	**MRE**	Main Race Event
ER	Easy Recovery	**ODE**	Over-Distance Event
PR	Passive Recovery	**UDE**	Under-Distance Event
LR	Long Run	**XUDE**	X Under-Distance Event
TT	Time Trial	**@ 1/4**	1/4 Effort
F	Fartlek	**@ 1/2**	1/2 Effort
FS	Finishing Speed	**@ 3/4**	3/4 Effort
DBR	Day Before Race Session		

400m	800m	1,500m	5,000m
PR	PR	PR	PR
MRE 4-5 x 200m	MRE 3(4 x 300m)	MRE 3(4 x 300m)	UDE 3(4 x 300m)
AR	AR	AR	AR
4 x 60m Starts	F + FS 4 x 100m	F + FS 4 x 150m	F + FS 4 x 200m
AR	AR	AR	AR
ODE 3(3 x 300m)	ODE 2(4 x 400m)	ODE 6 x 800m	MRE 6-8 x 800m
LR	LR	LR	LR
PR	PR	PR	PR
Race 100m / 200m	Race 400m / 200m	Race 800m / 400m	TT 1,200m / 300m
AR	AR & FS 4 x 100m	AR & FS 4 x 150m	AR & FS 4 x 200m
ER & Starts	ER	ER	ER
DBR	DBR	DBR	DBR
Race 400m / 200m	Race 800m / 400m	Race 1,500m	Race 5,000m
LR	LR	LR	LR
PR	PR	PR	PR
ODE 3 x 500m	MRE 4 x 400m	MRE 2(4 x 400m)	F + FS 4 x 200m
AR	AR	AR	AR
3 x 60m Starts	F + FS 4 x 100m	F + FS 4 x 100m	UDE 2(4 x 400m)
AR	AR	AR	AR
MRE 3 x 300m	MRE 3 x 500m	TT 2 x 800m	F + FS 4 x 200m
LR	LR	LR	LR
PR	PR	PR	PR
3 x 60m Starts	F + 4 x 60 Starts	F + FS 4 x 100m	MRE 4 x 1,200m
AR	AR	AR	
ODE 2 x 600m	TT 600m / 300m	ODE 4 x 1,000m	

TABLE 4.12

100m	200m	300m	400m	500m	600m	800m	1,000m
10.5	21.0	31.5	42				
10.75	21.5	32.25	43				
11.0	22.0	33.0	44	54.0			
11.25	22.5	33.75	45	56.25			
11.5	23.0	34.5	46	57.5	69.5		
11.75	23.5	35.25	47	58.75	1:10.5		
12.0	24.0	36.0	48	60.0	1:12.0		
12.25	24.5	36.75	49	61.25	1:13.5	1:38	
12.5	25.0	37.5	50	62.5	1:15.0	1:40	
12.75	25.5	38.25	51	63.75	1:16.5	1:42	2:07.5
13.0	26.0	39.0	52	65.0	1:18.0	1:44	2:10.0
13.25	26.5	39.75	53	66.25	1:19.5	1:46	2:12.5
13.5	27.0	40.5	54	67.5	1:21.0	1:48	2:15.0
13.75	27.5	41.25	55	68.75	1:22.5	1:50	2:17.5
14.0	28.0	42.0	56	70.0	1:24.0	1:52	2:20.0
14.25	28.5	42.75	57	71.25	1:25.5	1:54	2:22.5
14.5	29.0	43.5	58	72.5	1:27.0	1:56	2:25.0
14.75	29.5	44.25	59	73.75	1:28.5	1:58	2:27.0
15.0	30.0	45.0	60	75.0	1:30.0	2:00	2:30.0
15.25	30.5	45.75	61	76.25	1:31.5	2:02	2:32.5
15.5	31.0	46.5	62	77.5	1:33.0	2:04	2:35.0
15.75	31.5	47.25	63	78.75	1:34.5	2:06	2:37.5
16.0	32.0	48.0	64	1:20.0	1:36.0	2:08	2:40.0
16.25	32.5	48.75	65	1:21.25	1:37.5	2:10	2:42.5
16.5	33.0	49.5	66	1:22.5	1:39.0	2:12	2:45.0
16.75	33.5	50.25	67	1:23.75	1:40.5	2:14	2:47.5
17.0	34.0	51.0	68	1:25.0	1:42.0	2:16	2:50.0
17.25	34.5	51.75	69	1:26.25	1:43.5	2:18	2:52.5
17.5	35.0	52.5	70	1:27.5	1:45.0	2:20	2:55.0
17.75	35.5	53.25	71	1:28.75	1:46.5	2:22	2:57.5
18.0	36.0	54.0	72	1:30.0	1:48.0	2:24	3:00.0
18.25	36.5	54.75	73	1:31.25	1:49.5	2:26	3:02.5
18.5	37.0	55.5	74	1:32.5	1:51.0	2:28	3:05.0
18.75	37.5	56.25	75	1:33.75	1:52.5	2:30	3:07.5
19.0	38.0	57.0	76	1:35.0	1:54.0	2:32	3:10.0
19.25	38.5	57.75	77	1:36.25	1:55.5	2:34	3:12.5
19.5	39.0	58.5	78	1:37.5	1:57.0	2:36	3:15.0
19.75	39.5	59.25	79	1:38.75	1:58.5	2:38	3:17.5
20.0	40.0	60.0	80	1:40.0	2:00.0	2:40	3:20.0
20.5	41.0	61.5	82	1:42.5	2:03.0	2:44	3:25.0
21.0	42.0	63.0	84	1:45.0	2:06.0	2:48	3:30.0
21.5	43.0	64.5	86	1:47.5	2:09.0	2:52	3:35.0
22.0	44.0	66.0	88	1:50.0	2:12.0	2:56	3:40.0
22.5	45.0	67.5	90	1:52.5	2:15.0	3:00	3:45.0
23.0	46.0	69.0	92	1:55.0	2:18.0	3:04	3:50.0
23.5	47.0	70.5	94	1:57.5	2:21.0	3:08	3:55.0

TABLE 4.13—Pace Schedules, 100-1,000 meters

100m	200m	300m	400m	500m	600m	800m	1,000m	1,500m	1,600m	3,000m	3,200m	5,000m	10,000m
10.5	21.0	31.5	42										
10.75	21.5	32.25	43										
11.0	22.0	33.0	44	54.0									
11.25	22.5	33.75	45	56.25									
11.5	23.0	34.5	46	57.5	69.5								
11.75	23.5	35.25	47	58.75	1:10.5								
12.0	24.0	36.0	48	60.0	1:12.0								
12.25	24.5	36.75	49	61.25	1:13.5	1:38							
12.5	25.0	37.5	50	62.5	1:15.0	1:40							
12.75	25.5	38.25	51	63.75	1:16.5	1:42	2:07.5						
13.0	26.0	39.0	52	65.0	1:18.0	1:44	2:10.0						
13.25	26.5	39.75	53	66.25	1:19.5	1:46	2:12.5						
13.5	27.0	40.5	54	67.5	1:21.0	1:48	2:15.0	3:22.5	3:36				
13.75	27.5	41.25	55	68.75	1:22.5	1:50	2:17.5	3:26.2	3:40				
14.0	28.0	42.0	56	70.0	1:24.0	1:52	2:20.0	3:30.0	3:44				
14.25	28.5	42.75	57	71.25	1:25.5	1:54	2:22.5	3:33.7	3:48				
14.5	29.0	43.5	58	72.5	1:27.0	1:56	2:25.0	3:37.5	3:52	7:15.0	7:44		
14.75	29.5	44.25	59	73.75	1:28.5	1:58	2:27.5	3:41.2	3:56	7:22.5	7:52		
15.0	30.0	45.0	60	75.0	1:30.0	2:00	2:30.0	3:45.0	4:00	7:30.0	8:00	12:30.0	
15.25	30.5	45.75	61	76.25	1:31.5	2:02	2:32.5	3:48.7	4:04	7:37.5	8:08	12:42.5	
15.5	31.0	46.5	62	77.5	1:33.0	2:04	2:35.0	3:52.5	4:08	7:45.0	8:16	12:55.0	25:50
15.75	31.5	47.25	63	78.75	1:34.5	2:06	2:37.5	3:56.2	4:12	7:52.5	8:24	13:07.5	26:15
16.0	32.0	48.0	64	1:20.0	1:36.0	2:08	2:40.0	4:00.0	4:16	8:00.0	8:32	13:20.0	26:40
16.25	32.5	48.75	65	1:21.25	1:37.5	2:10	2:42.5	4:03.7	4:20	8:07.5	8:40	13:32.5	27:05
16.5	33.0	49.5	66	1:22.5	1:39.0	2:12	2:45.0	4:07.5	4:24	8:15.0	8:48	13:45.0	27:30
16.75	33.5	50.25	67	1:23.75	1:40.5	2:14	2:47.5	4:11.2	4:28	8:22.5	8:56	13:57.5	27:55
17.0	34.0	51.0	68	1:25.0	1:42.0	2:16	2:50.0	4:15.0	4:32	8:30.0	9:04	14:10.0	28:20
17.25	34.5	51.75	69	1:26.25	1:43.5	2:18	2:52.5	4:18.7	4:36	8:37.5	9:12	14:22.5	28:45
17.5	35.0	52.5	70	1:27.5	1:45.0	2:20	2:55.0	4:22.5	4:40	8:45.0	9:20	14:35.0	29:10
17.75	35.5	53.25	71	1:28.75	1:46.5	2:22	2:57.5	4:26.2	4:44	8:52.5	9:28	14:47.5	29:35
18.0	36.0	54.0	72	1:30.0	1:48.0	2:24	3:00.0	4:30.0	4:48	9:00.0	9:36	15:00.0	30:00
18.25	36.5	54.75	73	1:31.25	1:49.5	2:26	3:02.5	4:33.7	4:52	9:07.5	9:44	15:12.5	30:25
18.5	37.0	55.5	74	1:32.5	1:51.0	2:28	3:05.0	4:37.5	4:56	9:15.0	9:52	15:25.0	30:50
18.75	37.5	56.25	75	1:33.75	1:52.5	2:30	3:07.5	4:41.2	5:00	9:22.5	10:00	15:37.5	31:15
19.0	38.0	57.0	76	1:35.0	1:54.0	2:32	3:10.0	4:45.0	5:04	9:30.0	10:08	15:50.0	31:40
19.25	38.5	57.75	77	1:36.25	1:55.5	2:34	3:12.5	4:48.7	5:08	9:37.5	10:16	16:01.5	32:05

TABLE 4.14—Pace Schedules, 100-10,000 meters

800m	1,600m	3,000m	5,000m	10,000m
1:50	4:04	8:02	13:51	28:45
1:48	4:00	7:54	13:37	28:17
1:46	3:56	7:46	13:24	27:51
1:44	3:52	7:38	13:11	27:25
1:42	3:48	7:30	12:58	26:59
1:40	3:44	7:22	12:46	26:34

TABLE 4.15

Career Progression of Quantity and Quality

Up to this point, relatively little has been said about the progression of sharpening work over years of training and development. A young athlete initially exhibits relatively rapid improvements in performance, and the quality of the sharpening work should be modified accordingly. However, an improvement in pace of approximately one second / 400 meters is normally all a mature distance runner can hope to safely assume within a calendar year. This sounds precious little, but given the passage of time, the practical result is dramatic. Remember, a ten-year developmental period is normally required for elite performance in the distance events. Table 4.15 illustrates the annual progression of performance associated with an improvement in pace of approximately one second / 400 meters in the 800-to-10,000-meter events.

The length of the recovery periods taken by different athletes in any given sharpening workout will vary considerably, depending upon their age and level of development, but the need to provide a recovery period that permits the pulse rate to return to 120 bpm remains nearly constant. The exceptions would be those workouts intended to develop the anaerobic ATP-lactic acid system (often used in training athletes for 800 meters), and the controlled recovery (CR) sessions (often used in training athletes for 5,000 and 10,000 meters). Otherwise, any reduction in the duration of the recovery periods should for the most part just happen with an athlete's improved aerobic ability and anaerobic power over time—it should not be aggressively pursued. Training frequency will also increase, because mature athletes will often undertake two-a-day workouts, and sometimes conduct quality training and racing efforts in closer proximity. This reflects their superior load and recovery capacity. The quantity assumed in the sharpening period will also progress over time:

- The volume assumed in the individual workouts will increase.

- The balance of the training for any given event often shifts towards the over-distance side, since higher levels of competition are associated with more numerous preliminary heats, which place greater demands on an athlete's stamina.

- Having fully developed their potential at the shorter race events, athletes will move up to the next over-distance event.

However, from the standpoint of optimal development, it is a mistake for athletes to rapidly advance to the longer distances without fully developing their potential in the middle distance events. This practice would shorten the length of their competitive careers and limit their ultimate level of performance.

Race Practice and Callusing

The race will be what the training has been. In practice, this means that the physical and mental conditioning being instilled by the training loads must be addressed from three perspectives.

The first is called the micro-view: regard each rep as a compressed form of the main race event. Earlier, reference was made to the example of an athlete with the habit of slowing down during the last five to 10 meters of a race. This weakness was acquired by the repetition of a thousand such lapses during the course of previous training. From the micro-view perspective, it is easy to see how such habits can be instilled—both good and bad. Therefore, athletes are well advised to make a habit of running the second half of their workouts faster than the first. Moreover, they should always finish off the individual reps within an interval or repetition workout forcefully and completely.

The second perspective is called the exploded view: Regard the entire training session, including the reps and recoveries, as an exploded view of the main race event. By stressing various parts of the larger workout, it is possible to acquire competitive abilities, and eliminate areas of weakness. When the micro and exploded views are combined, the physical and mental conditioning can be shaped dramatically.

The third perspective is called the macro-view: It refers to the dynamic movement of the larger training progression.

All three perspectives can be used to effect substantial physical and mental conditioning. Sometimes an athlete exhibits an area of weakness in the main race event that needs to be addressed. On the other hand, sometimes certain competitive strengths need to be cultivated. The portrait of the main race event revealed by taking splits then needs to be put to good use. By applying the insights provided by the micro, exploded, and macro-views, the individual sessions and larger training progression can be designed to eliminate evident weaknesses and instill formidable competitive abilities. For example, let's suppose an athlete has recently exhibited weakness in the fifth and sixth laps of the 3,000 meters event, and the next workout in the training progression is 5 x 1,000 meters at 3,000-meter goal pace with a 400 meters jog recovery. How could this training session be redesigned to remedy the athlete's area of weakness?

First, conceive of each 1,000 meters repetition as a condensed version of the main race event (micro-view). In this case, stress the third quarter of each 1,000 meters repetition to bring the athlete up to par both physically and mentally. But also view the entire 5 x 1,000 meters workout as an exploded view of the main race event. Therefore, you should also stress the third quarter of the training session when taken as a whole. Thus, in some sense, you can work at the problem from two angles.

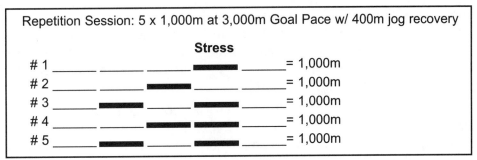

FIGURE 4.10

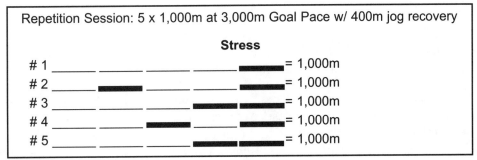

FIGURE 4.11

Figure 4.10 indicates 200-meter segments within the individual repetitions of the larger 5 x 1,000 meters training session. Darker lines represent heavily stressed segments where the athlete would run faster than goal pace. Obviously, the faster the stressed segments are run, the more difficult it will be to maintain goal pace over the entire workout. Ideally, it would be desirable to have the total time of the unevenly paced 1,000 meters repetitions come out at goal pace, but since this represents a significant improvement in the quality of the training, only mature athletes should make the attempt. If an athlete exhibited weakness in the last 800 meters of the 3,000 meters event, it would be prudent to conduct stressed segments in the manner shown in Figure 4.11.

Many individuals hold the misconception that weakness exhibited in the final stages of a competition means that a runner's finishing speed is inadequate. If this truly is the case, the problem can be easily diagnosed by timing the athlete over a few reps at 100 to 200 meters distance. However, more often the runner lacks sufficient stamina and over-distance ability. When this is the problem, conducting under-distance work is just the opposite of what the athlete needs. But what if, by all indications, the individual's stamina and raw speed are adequate for the task? In this case, the athlete is insufficiently conditioned or callused to finish well (For a discussion of the callusing effect see Dellinger and Beres, 1978). Accordingly, attempting to improve an athlete's kick by sprinting 100 to 200 meters is not going to solve the problem either—that is, unless those sprints are placed at the end of longer repetitions, thereby simulating race conditions.

These conditioning methods can be used to prepare athletes for particular courses, or other environmental factors which are anticipated in championship competitions. For example, a common practice would be to condition athletes for especially demanding hills and terrain on a given cross-country course. Again, athletes will race as they have trained.

As previously discussed, athletes must be conditioned by pace work to develop a dominant neuromuscular stereotype, or mental clock, that will sustain them through the later stages of a competition. However, unless an individual is superior enough to sustain an even pace that none can follow, some other competitive abilities are required. To enjoy success athletes must acquire the ability to:

- Surge
- Make the breakaway
- Execute an effective finishing kick

All of these abilities are developed by race-practice, and in fact, this is the only kind of practice that athletes should ever conduct! Figure 4.12 shows another single training session structured to induce determinate physical and mental effects. By employing the macro perspective, you can similarly structure the entire training progression for the athletic season. In the course of the date pace work or the early interval sessions, it is undesirable to do anything counterproductive to the task of instilling a dominant pace sense. Further, intervals often have too short a duration to lend themselves to the segmentation that is possible with the later repetition workouts. So, with the early interval training, it is most effective to stress the recovery periods and stack the density of the workout in the desired areas, rather than to disturb the even pacing of the series. For example, Figure 4.12 illustrates the possible modification of an interval workout for a mature athlete who exhibits weakness in the third quarter of the 5,000 meters (Note: the presence of a circle indicates shortening of the associated recovery period).

Accordingly, you can structure the entire training progression to instill various competitive abilities, or eliminate evident areas of weakness. In all race practice, the relative effort and mode of conditioning is of primary importance. In this respect, the times posted are secondary to the manner in which the training sessions are conducted. However, mature athletes can eventually progress to conduct the training sessions in a manner that will not compromise either aspect. It can be advantageous for middle distance runners to compete in the main race event during the worthwhile break that is placed in the middle of the sharpening period. This can provide an indication with respect to any areas needing special attention prior to the repetition workouts, which are especially suitable for the task of callusing. Figure 4.13 provides an example of a training progression for an athlete whose athletic level corresponds to 13:20 for 5,000 meters.

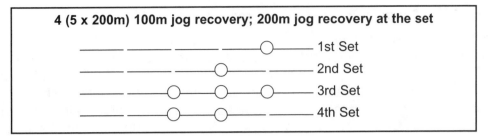

4 (5 x 200m) 100m jog recovery; 200m jog recovery at the set

—————— —————— —————— ——————○—————— 1st Set
—————— —————— ——————○———— —————— 2nd Set
—————— ——————○——————○——————○—————— 3rd Set
—————— ——————○——————○———— —————— 4th Set

FIGURE 4.12

Session 1: 4 (5 x 400m), 100m jog recovery; 400m jog recovery at series break

1st Set	66	64	66	64	66
2nd Set	64	66	64	66	64
3rd Set	66	63	66	63	66
4th Set	66	64	66	63	60

Session 2: 2(4 x 800m), 200m jog recovery; 400m jog recovery at series break

1st	2:10	65	65
2nd	2:08	33/31	33/31
3rd	2:10	65	65
4th	2:08	33/31	31/33
5th	2:08	33/31	33/31
6th	2:08	33/31	31/33
7th	2:08	31/33	31/33
8th	2:02	31/31	30/30

Session 3: 5 x 1,200m, 400m Controlled Recovery in 90-120 Seconds

1st	63	65	65	3:13
2nd	65	31/33	31/33	3:13
3rd	65	62	65	3:12
4th	65	30/33	30/33	3:10
5th	65	64	31/29	3:09

Session 4: 4 x 1,600m, 400m jog recovery

1st	66	66	66	64	4:22
2nd	65	31/33	31/33	63	4:18
3rd	65	65	61	65	4:16
4th	65	65	64	60	4:14

FIGURE 4.13

Mega-Cycle Progression and Race Practice

Certain measures relating to achieving peak performance in the last year of a multiple year developmental cycle have been addressed in Chapter 1. Obviously, the initial requirement with respect to sharpening work is to assume the necessary quantity in the training sessions. Accordingly, the workouts should first be conducted at goal pace in an evenly paced manner before attempting any callusing work. Race practice and callusing work should then be emphasized in the latter portion of a multiple year developmental and peaking scenario, such as the junior and senior year of a high school or collegiate career. Athletes desiring to peak in the fourth year of a developmental cycle for the Olympic Games should introduce the required callusing work in the third year, and then polish their skills during the Olympic year.

In closing this treatment of the sharpening period and race practice, athletes would do well to consider the advice of an individual who placed fifth in the modern Pentathlon at the 1912 Olympic Games—who fell unconscious at the finish of the cross-country event.

> *Do not regard what you do as only preparation for doing the same thing more fully or better at some later time. Nothing is ever done twice. There is but one time to do a thing that is the first and last... there is no next time... Everything is a final heat. There are no practices...*
>
> —George S. Patton

References

Åstrand, Per Olaf, and Kaare Rodahl, *Textbook of Work Physiology, 3rd Edition,* New York: McGraw-Hill, 1986, pages 33-39, 332 and 345.

Bowerman, William J., *Coaching Track & Field,* William H. Freeman, Editor, Boston, Massachusetts: Houghton Mifflin Company, 1974.

Cerutty, Percy, *Athletics,* London: The Sportsmen's Book Club, 1961, pages 23 and 86.

Cerutty, Percy, *Success: In Sport and Life,* London: Pelham Books Ltd., 1967, page 126.

Daniels, Jack, *Daniels' Running Formula,* Champaign, Illinois: Human Kinetics, 1998.

Daniels, Jack, and Jimmy Gilbert, *Oxygen Power,* Tempe, Arizona: Published Privately, 1979.

Dellinger, Bill, and George Beres, *Winning Running,* Chicago, Illinois: Contemporary Books, Inc., 1978, pages 7-10, and 128-130.

Fišer, Ladislav, *Mílaři a Vytrvalchi,* Prague: Sportovní a Truistické Nakladatelství, 1965, pages 41-44.

Kim, Hee-Jin, *Dogen Kigen: Mystical Realist,* Tuscon, Arizona: University of Arizona Press, 1987, page 156.

Lydiard, Arthur, and Garth Gilmour, *Running the Lydiard Way,* Mountain View, California: World Publications, Inc., 1978.

Lydiard, Arthur, and Garth Gilmour, *Run to the Top,* Auckland, New Zealand: Minerva, Ltd., 1962, page 105.

Noakes, Tim, *Lore of Running*, 3rd Edition, Champaign, Illinois: Human Kinetics, 1991, page 52.

Patton, George S., *The Patton Papers,* Martin Blumenson, Editor, 2 Volumes, Boston, Massachusetts: Houghton Mifflin Company, 1972, pages 167 and 170.

Pedemonte, Jimmy, "Updated Acquisitions About Training Periodization," *NSCA Journal*, October-November, 1982.

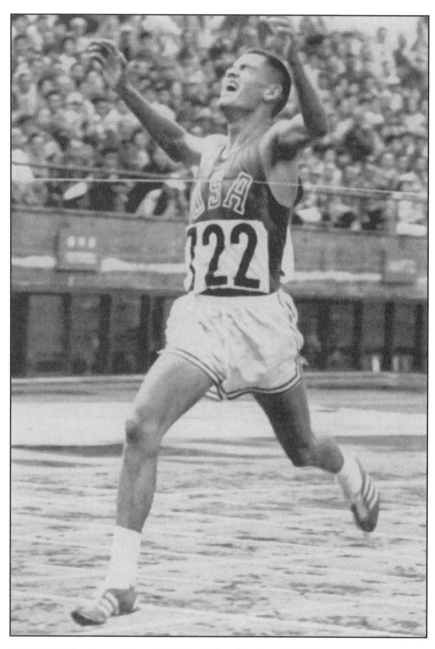

PHOTO 5.1—An exhilarated Billy Mills wins the 10,000 meters at the 1964 Olympic Games. The Marine Lieutenant of Native American ancestry had a vision. Considered far out of his class in this event, he upset the favorites while achieving the exact time he had foreseen and posted above his bed nearly a year before. Photo from AP/ Wide World Photos.

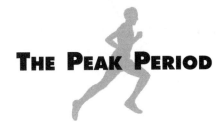

CHAPTER 5

THE PEAK PERIOD

Athletes will be able to compete and perform at the highest level during the peak period. Since the truly hard work is all but done, it can also be the most enjoyable time of the athletic season. If the training has been faithfully executed, athletes will gather themselves with confidence for the approaching contests. But beware: Nemesis punishes man by fulfilling his dreams, hopes, and desires too completely. Success can magnify character flaws. It can lead athletes on like an intoxicant into an abyss. Training is building. Each workout is a brick in the wall, a gathering of physical and mental powers. Racing takes away. The moment of achievement has the two faces of Janus: It places a capstone upon an edifice that has been months or years in the making, but at the same time shatters the edifice.

> *In the moment of victory I did not realize that the inner force, which had been driving me to my ultimate goal, died when I became the world's fastest miler.*
>
> —Derek Ibbotson

The Short Peak Period

There are essentially three types of peak periods: the short peak period, the extended peak period, and the multiple peak period. These three variations differ greatly in length and complexity. The short peak period consists of three distinct phases that differ in duration depending on the athlete's physical age, training age, sex, aerobic ability, and the nature of the preceding training program.

- **The Ascent**
- **The Plateau of Peak Performance**
- **The Descent**

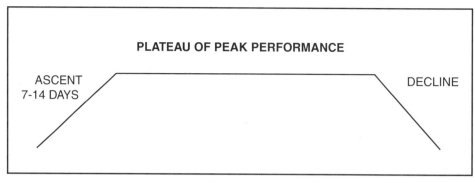

Figure 5.1

The Ascent to the Plateau of Peak Performance

The peak period begins immediately after the last 3/4-effort sharpening workout. It starts with an ascent, or so-called taper, that corresponds to a worthwhile break lasting seven to 14 days. During this time, athletes train at less than 60% of their maximal working capacity. The ascent leads to a relatively brief plateau of peak performance, and competition in the main race event for the seasonal goal performance. The duration of the ascent largely depends on the ability of the athletes to recover from the demanding sharpening work which has preceded. Normally, high school and collegiate athletes will require an ascent, or worthwhile break, lasting nine to 10 days. However, elite athletes who train upwards of 100 miles a week sometimes only require seven days, due to their superior load and recovery capabilities. Obviously, the training activity conducted during the ascent can significantly determine the quality of the performances delivered on the plateau.

Once athletes begin the ascent and enter the peak period, absolutely no exhaustive work should be done. This cannot be overemphasized. Athletes should not perform demanding interval or repetition training as during the sharpening period, or the anaerobic threshold, steady state, or hill training sessions as during the base and hill periods. Further, athletes will normally not engage in over-distance time trials at this time, unless their buildup to the peak period was, for some reason, compromised by lost training time due to illness or injury. In general, demanding efforts including substantial quantity (volume and duration), will suppress quality (performance). Such efforts could knock athletes flat and incapable of performing at a high level. In this case, some part of the nine-to-10-day ascent would have to be repeated all over again, and generally not without some loss of performance potential. In sum, by the time athletes enter the peak period, "the hay should be in the barn." If the hay is not in the barn, then nothing can be done about it. Any work attempted at this time (insofar as it is work) will only serve to suppress performance.

The Plateau of Peak Performance

The duration of the plateau depends upon a number of factors, including an athlete's physical age, training age, sex, aerobic ability, the nature and content of the training program, and the momentum gathered during the preceding athletic season. The plateau enjoyed by female athletes is generally 20 to 30% shorter than that of males at a comparable level of development. This reflects the differences in their relative aerobic ability and strength. Mature athletes who possess a higher aerobic ability and also a more extensive training background will enjoy a longer plateau of peak performance.

The quantity, volume, or mileage undertaken in training has a direct impact on the length of the plateau. All things being equal, athletes who have introduced higher levels of quantity in training (without compromising quality) will recover faster from training and racing efforts. These athletes will be able to compete and deliver superior performances in closer proximity, and potentially enjoy a longer period of peak performance. Obviously, those athletes who need to undertake numerous preliminary trials will require superior powers of recovery, and must prepare themselves accordingly. The following provides some guidelines with respect to the duration of the peak period.

- Mature high school boys can hold the peak for a full 14 days, whereas girls must subtract three to four days (20-30%), and thus have approximately 10 days.

- Mature collegiate men and women can be considered elite national and international class athletes (See below).

- Elite men can maintain peak performance for about three weeks, whereas the duration for women is unlikely to exceed two weeks.

The duration of the short peak period consists of a seven-to-14-day ascent to a plateau of peak performance lasting approximately two to three weeks. Keep in mind that respectable performances are possible during the ascent to the plateau. However, competition during the descent associated with declining powers should be avoided. Accordingly, the total duration of the short peak period is approximately four weeks for high school athletes, and closer to six weeks for mature collegiate athletes and elite post-collegiate athletes.

The Descent from the Plateau of Peak Performance

A descent characterized by a decline in fitness follows the plateau of peak performance. The duration of the descent approximately corresponds to that of the ascent. However, much depends on the quality of decision-making with respect to maintaining equilibrium and balance during the peak period. The physical decline will be characterized by a gradual dwindling, as opposed to being a dramatic event. It results from the inevitable loss of the fitness attained through previous training, since athletes cannot maintain accumulated physical powers for an indefinite period of time. The cessation of hard work was necessary to enable optimal performance, but in time, the momentum gathered will run its course, and the fitness of the athletes will begin to decline. The risk of injury, both physical and mental, would be greatly increased by engaging in competition during the descent. If athletes have peaked properly, the decline of physical powers is never

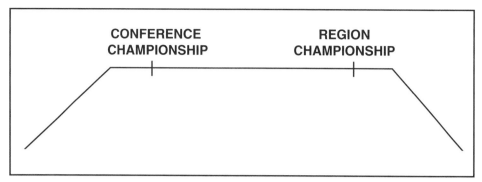

FIGURE 5.2—Plateau for young high school athletes

seen. It should not be. Rather, the athletes should fulfill their goals and expectations for the competitive season within the plateau of peak performance when it counts! This being the case, it would be physically and mentally difficult to proceed further. Frankly, it should not be attempted, lest the athletes suffer needless frustration. It is better to finish with exhilaration, and the feeling that greater things are still possible. There is a physical peak and an emotional peak, and both must happen at the right time and place. It is important to know when to persevere, but also when to quit.

Considerations For Young Versus Mature Athletes

High school athletes normally attempt a short peak period, consisting of a single ascent and plateau of peak performance, and then focus on one or two relatively closely spaced competitions. Remember, as a general rule, high school athletes can only maintain the plateau for approximately two weeks. Young athletes should normally focus on the conference championship and region championship (sometimes the latter is also called the district, or sectional championship). They should then properly position these competitions on the plateau so they can qualify for the state championship (as shown in Figure 5.2).

More mature athletes should position the region and state championships on the plateau, and then compete in the conference championships on the fifth to seventh day of the ascent—that is, when not at their full performance potential. During the conference championships in track and field, mature athletes generally should compete in either their over-distance or under-distance event, since they will face numerous contests in the main race event during the upcoming region and state championships. Figure 5.3 shows the general structure of the peak period for these athletes.

The same kind of accommodation must be made with respect to collegiate athletes. In collegiate cross-country, young athletes will focus on the conference and region championships. Because these events normally fall two weeks apart, they can bridge the gap and place both competitions on the plateau of peak performance (as shown in Figure 5.4).

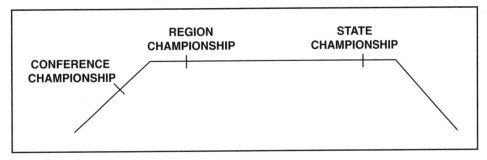

FIGURE 5.3—Plateau for mature high school athletes

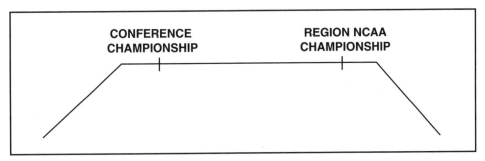

FIGURE 5.4—Collegiate Cross-Country: Young Athletes

The Extended Peak Period

High school athletes participating in cross-country or track and field sometimes use an extended peak period when they compete in conference, region, and state championships, which are separated by three or more weeks. Collegiate athletes in cross-country or track and field also use it when they must compete in relatively widely separated conference, region, or national championships. Elite athletes preparing for a national championship meet in which team selection for the World Championships or Olympic Games is on the line, also sometimes use an extended peak period. This can provide them with a preliminary indication of their fitness and enable fine-tuning before the qualifying competition.

When conducting an extended peak period, athletes normally begin with a short peak period scenario—an ascent consisting of a worthwhile break lasting seven to 14 days that includes an under-distance time trial placed three to four days prior to the first competition on the plateau. During the cross-country season, it may not be possible for athletes to vary the distance of their races. However, during the track and field season, athletes would be able to compete over-distance or under-distance relative to the main race event in this first competition on the plateau of peak performance. For example, specialists at 10,000 meters could race 3,000 or 5,000 meters, two or three weeks prior to a major 10,000 meters competition. Specialists at 5,000 meters could similarly race 1,500 or 3,000 meters, and specialists at 1,500 meters could compete at 800 meters. Thereafter, the athletes could recover four to five days, and then conduct one or more stabilizing training sessions during a seven-to-14-day micro-cycle. In any case, the last 3/4-effort training session should be performed at least seven to 10 days before the goal main race event. An under-distance time trial should then be conducted three to five days prior to the competition to set the athletes up for optimal performance.

The extended peak period conducted by collegiate cross-country athletes merits further discussion. In the United States, the various collegiate conference cross-country championships are normally held two weeks prior to the regional championships, and the national championship is normally contested nine days later. Given sound preparation, mature male collegiate athletes will not have a problem bridging this three-to-four-week gap. However, sometimes it is prudent to compete in the conference championships while still within the nine-to-10-day ascent to ensure that the athletes will be able to maintain their momentum all the way through to the national championship. If young collegiate athletes are being relied upon in order to advance a team from the regional to the national championship, then certain adjustments should be made. In this regard, young male athletes, mature male 1,500-meter sided athletes, and female competitors should be held out of either the conference or regional championships, and instead, other athletes should be rotated into the lineup. If this is not possible, they should compete in the conference championship while still within the nine-to-10-day ascent to the plateau of peak performance. Figure 5.5 shows this particular example of an extended peak period.

In collegiate track and field, only mature athletes will be capable of qualifying for the national championship on the basis of their individual performances. Young athletes should then focus exclusively on the conference championship, and can use either the short or the extended peak period models, as desired. Mature male athletes can normally hold peak fitness for three weeks. If their conference championship is scheduled less than two weeks prior to the regional qualifier, and the NCAA championships less than two weeks later, they will be able to bridge the gap, provided that they are well prepared and do not over-race. However, they are best advised to compete in the conference championship during the ascent to the plateau in order to ensure optimal performance at the NCAA championships, as shown in Figure 5.6. Mature collegiate women should adopt the model shown in Figure 5.6, or alternatively, that shown in Figure 5.7.

The Multiple Peak Period

The necessity of achieving optimal results during several widely separated peak periods within a single athletic season poses a difficult challenge. In the United States, high school athletes face this situation when, after their state cross-country championships, they attempt to qualify for the national championship in San Diego, California. This could require athletes to maintain peak fitness over a span of nearly two months. A multiple peak period is also required by elite athletes who qualify in mid-June or July at their national track and field championship for competition in the World Championships or Olympic Games in August or September.

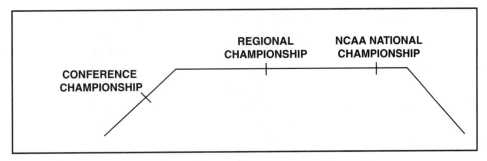

FIGURE 5.5—Collegiate cross-country

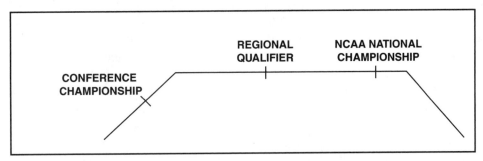

FIGURE 5.6—Collegiate track and field: mature male athletes

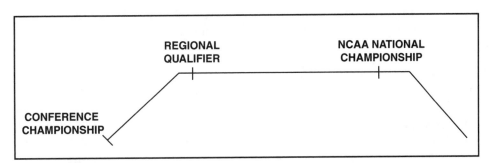

FIGURE 5.7—Collegiate track and field: mature female athletes

The multiple peak period is an infrequent case, but certainly the most complex. When conducting a simple peak period, the athletes ascend to the plateau of peak performance and race off of the momentum gathered during the preceding athletic season. During this time, they enjoy a respite from acquisitive work. But when trying to bridge a wide gap between major competitions, athletes will need to withdraw from the plateau in order to recharge and prepare themselves for further competition.

The multiple peak period begins with a short peak period, or alternatively, an extended peak period, as described above. However, the athletes must withdraw from the first plateau of peak performance, and then engage in acquisitive, regenerative, or stabilizing work. It is relatively uncommon to conduct acquisitive work in the midst of a multiple peak period, since truly hard work tends to suppress performance. Acquisitive work should only be done if the two succeeding peak periods are widely separated, or if an athlete suffers inadequate preparation and fitness due to a preceding illness or injury. Normally, athletes undertake one or more meso-cycles of regenerative work. The aim of a regenerative meso-cycle is to rebuild and restore certain aspects of fitness. Accordingly, the training loads undertaken during a regenerative meso-cycle do not attempt to break any new ground. Within a multiple peak period, the training conducted in the course of one or more regenerative meso-cycles will often briefly recapitulate the work performed during the base, hill, and sharpening periods, and in like sequence. The multiple peak period therefore resembles a miniature athletic season. For example, during a regenerative meso-cycle following the first plateau, several weeks of base and hill work could be performed. The athletes could then sharpen over the next seven to 14 days, and then assume a seven-to-10-day worthwhile break and thereby ascend to the second plateau of peak performance. This second plateau could comprise another short or extended peak period. Obviously, the longer athletes try to extend themselves, the higher the risk of injury and loss of peak fitness.

Young high school competitors trying to bridge the gap between their state meet and the national championship in cross-country should conduct regenerative and stabilizing work. Figure 5.8 shows a multiple peak period model for high school athletes who need to maintain a high fitness level for their state, regional, and national cross-country championships.

In a regenerative meso-cycle, athletes could repeat select training sessions previously conducted during the buildup to the first plateau of peak performance. In fact, when performing regenerative or stabilizing work, it is generally best to reduce the effort of the workouts relative to the original acquisitive training sessions. The emphasis is on maintaining and refining previously acquired powers. Repeating previous workouts that are slightly reduced in both quantity and quality will be less stressful, both physically and mentally, than the original acquisitive effort. This training practice can cause stagnation of athletic performance, but that is entirely consistent with the goal of maintaining peak fitness.

The challenge faced by elite athletes who need to qualify at their national track and field championships for an international competition such as the World Championships or Olympic Games will now be addressed. For example, at least six weeks generally separate the USATF National Track and Field Championship from the World Championships or Olympic Games. Six weeks is too long for athletes to maintain their peak fitness by merely continuing to race and recover. If they continue to race in the weeks following their national championship (and perhaps travel extensively in order to do so), they could lose their peak form and be heading downhill before the World Championships or Olympic Games.

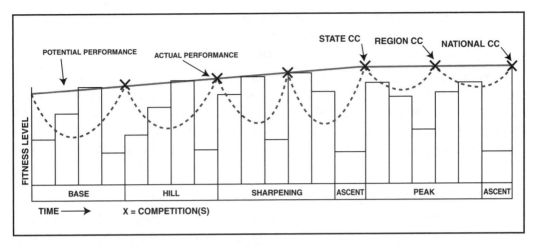

FIGURE 5.8—Multiple peak period for cross-country

It would better for athletes to conduct at least two weeks of base and strength work after their national track and field championships. Thereafter, they would need at least two or three sharpening workouts to regain peak fitness. However, the training sessions should then constitute regenerative or stabilizing efforts. Specifically, the training sessions would essentially repeat select workouts conducted previously, but with some reduction in effort. Again, athletes should not attempt dramatic aquisative efforts at this time. For example, athletes should not attempt to attain a new and improved working capacity by any of the following: increase their weekly mileage; extend the distance of their long run; conduct a particular workout at a faster pace; or undertake a new type or style of workout, possibly including more reps or shorter recovery periods. All of these variables are commonly used to raise an athlete's working capacity and performance potential. Acquisitive training efforts often have the short-term effect of suppressing athletic performance, and this would be clearly undesirable heading into the World Championships or Olympic Games.

After conducting one or more regenerative meso-cycles, a seven-to-10-day ascent would be undertaken prior to the second plateau of peak performance for the World Championships or Olympic Games. Table 5.2 provides examples of training schedules for possible use between the respective dates of the USATF Championships and the World Championships. Obviously, these schedules are only meant to illustrate key training principles, since the particular information in a given model year is unique. A number of assumptions have been made in drafting these particular schedules. The model year 1995 was used to derive the actual date of the events, and the men's track and field competition schedules were used. The schedules also assume that elite athletes would compete at the Bislett Games in Oslo, Norway, which fell approximately three weeks prior to the 1995 World Championships in Gothenburg, Sweden. In order to achieve optimal results, some athletes should avoid competition in such high level events prior to a World Championships or Olympic Games. Nevertheless, the schedules were written to accommodate both the Bislett Games and the World Championships. This introduces greater complexity and risk, but may serve to impart a better understanding of certain training principles.

The multiple peak period scenario is not easy to accomplish without making a fundamental mistake. Obviously, many other solutions are possible, but for every viable solution, there are a dozen alternatives that simply do not add up. When drafting a multiple peak period schedule, coaches and athletes should carefully count backwards and forwards from each date of competition, and study every interrelationship.

The Control and Refinement of Peak Fitness

The specific conditioning required to bring an athlete to a high level of fitness for competition in the main race event is largely conducted during the sharpening period. At that time, decisions concerning the quantity and quality of the work aim at maintaining equilibrium and balance relative to the desired goal performance in the main race event. Again, once within the peak period, no exhaustive training sessions of any kind should be undertaken. During the peak period, athletes essentially compete on the momentum created during the course of the athletic season. But that momentum can either be preserved or dissipated by the quality of decisions made regarding the composition of the training and racing program during the peak period. The fitness level of the athletes can be greatly influenced by both the selection of the time trials and races, and also the manner in which they are conducted. In this regard, the time trials and competitions should be carefully composed and placed so as to enable athletes to always be on the crest of the supercompensation from the preceding effort when the next is being assumed. To do this, the load and recovery capacity of each individual athlete needs to be appreciated, and then a series of training or racing efforts must be conducted in a way to permit the supercompensation effects to build upon one another without a miss. This can be accomplished by prudently modulating quantity (volume, duration) and quality (frequency, density, and intensity). More-over, a series of succeeding time trials and competitions should be conducted that will best serve to maintain optimal balance with respect to the main race event. At this time, the competitions and time trials are almost the only high quality efforts that can induce significant changes in the fitness of the athletes. Essentially, they will be racing and recovering during the peak period. However, the length of the peak period can be extended by regenerative or stabilizing work aimed at maintaining endurance, strength, and speed.

The coach and individual athlete should develop a select training schedule for the peak period that can be used and refined over succeeding seasons. This provides a basis for comparison, analysis and interpretation that would otherwise not be possible. In this case, the coach and athlete not only have a way of knowing the athlete's response at any given time, but of viewing present circumstances in light of experience. They will then be able to read the athlete's status at any point in time with greater clarity, and thus better address outstanding needs and requirements. This will enhance their ability to control the acquisition of peak fitness, and permit greater fine-tuning of performance. Athletes have a tremendous edge when they approach the starting line with the confidence of knowing that they are ready to deliver their best personal performance at that time and place.

The practical effects of various time trials and races depend upon their quantity (volume, duration) and quality (frequency, density and intensity). Peak fitness can be more rapidly attained and ultimately exhausted by increasing the quality of the training sessions, time trials, and races. In the course of a given athletic season, the fastest way to sharpen is to frequently engage in competition. However, the inherent physical and mental liabilities associated with this practice normally induce a peak relatively early in the athletic season, and at less than optimal performance levels. Likewise, the fastest way to consume and exhaust fitness during the peak period is to engage in frequent competition. Quantity tends to suppress quality, and vice-versa. The lesser the quantity and higher the quality, the greater the sharpening and peak accelerating effect. Conversely, the greater the quantity and lesser the quality, the lesser the sharpening and peak accelerating effect. For example, a long easy run can boost the length of the peak period, whereas a day off can freshen up an athlete and permit the benefits of preceding quality efforts to arrive. Running 3,000 meters at 3/4-effort does not sharpen or peak an athlete as rapidly as performing 2 x 1,500 meters at the same effort. Running 1,500 meters at 3/4-effort does not sharpen an athlete as quickly as 2 x 800 meters at the same effort. Clearly, various combinations of quantity and quality can be used to induce similar sharpening effects.

Within the peak period, there is less disparity in training between athletes of various levels than at any other time in the season. For this reason, the most productive way to address questions concerning athletic development and the means of controlling the peaking process is to discuss the individual training sessions during the peak period.

The "Day Off" is a form of passive recovery, and serves to slow the rate at which athletes reach peak form. A day off allows the preceding quality work to take effect and the athletes to freshen up. For this reason, many misinterpret the practical effect of a day off as accelerating the rate of reaching peak fitness. A day off is most appropriate in the days following an intense competition that may have resulted in a severe depletion, such as after competition in 5,000 or 10,000 meters; numerous prelims in middle distance events; and, always after contests held in conditions of extreme temperature and humidity. A day off also permits the restoration of energy stores, and can serve as the stitch in time that saves athletes from a dangerous level of residual fatigue.

During the peak period, young athletes would do well to take a day off occasionally. They enjoy a shorter plateau of peak performance, and a day off helps to extend their range, thus preventing a decline as the championship meet approaches. Psychologically, the same holds true, because physical and mental states are interdependent. Mature athletes, as a result of superior physical and mental conditioning, tend to better weather the stress associated with championship competitions. Nevertheless, a day off between succeeding championship competitions would be highly desirable even for mature athletes. Despite their feelings of elation following a successful outcome, they have faced a long and hard season. This drains them emotionally. Athletes should beware if they often find themselves thinking: "I'll be glad when it is over." A day off can go far to restore the athletes' perspective—and potential for optimal performances. They will then clearly see how much they desire to excel in the coming contest.

The "Passive Recovery" options in the training schedules can be taken as a complete day off from all athletic activity. However, when athletes can benefit from speeding up their metabolism and recovery rate, a morning run or swim can be conducted. Running or swimming at this time should always be at an easy effort and limited to 10 to 25 minutes. If athletes need a mental break from training, the passive recovery day can provide an opportunity for a non-exhaustive form of recreation.

The "Easy Recovery" option includes 20 to 40 minutes of easy running during a single training session. Since an easy recovery day will often fall two days prior to a time trial or competition, athletes should then stretch thoroughly, because extensive stretching should not be done the day before a major competition. If a morning running session has been the habit, it would be dropped on this day.

The "Active Recovery" session normally follows a demanding training or racing effort. When the athletes' level of development permits, that is, by the time they qualify as mature high school athletes, an easy morning run should be added on days of active recovery. During the morning run, the athletes only need to elevate their metabolism by conducting an easy 10-to-25-minute warm-up. By speeding up their metabolisms in the morning, the athletes will accelerate their rate of recovery, and the practical effect will be as if they had an additional half-day of recovery. Morning runs are also the most constructive and painless way to control any undesired weight gain, since the metabolism will be increased by 10 to 15%, and more calories will be burned in the course of a day. As an alternative, an easy swim can sometimes be more beneficial than a morning run. The afternoon training session on days of active recovery could last from 20 to 70 minutes, depending on the athletes' level of development. During the peak period, this session should not generally exceed 40 to 50 minutes, because energy stores could otherwise become too depleted. Athletes should conduct a pre warm-up, light stretching and flexibility work, then a full warm-up and a running session over gentle rolling terrain. In the course of the run, athletes should perform about a dozen 50-to-100-meter accelerations at speeds approaching that of the training effort conducted on the preceding day. Otherwise, their recovery rate will be slowed due to the lack of specific use of affected muscle groups, and their metabolism will remain relatively dormant. Sometimes it helps to run the accelerations up and down a gentle incline, since this tends to ensure successful completion of the task. The active recovery session concludes with light stretching and flexibility work, and whenever possible, some easy barefoot jogging on grass.

The "Long Easy Run" is done to maintain equilibrium and balance with respect to the endurance required for the main race event. For this reason, it is good to maintain an aerobic session once a week throughout the peak period. Depending on the ability of the athletes and their particular main race event, the long easy run will normally last 30 to 90 minutes during the ascent to the plateau of peak performance. Nevertheless, once upon the plateau, even mature specialists at 10,000 meters should reduce the long run to 80 minutes maximum. Otherwise, their energy reserves can become too depleted. However, a longer run can sometimes be performed during a regenerative or stabilizing meso-cycle within an extended or multiple peak period. Provided the athletes are not hung over from a demanding race or suffering extremely low energy reserves, a long easy run can allow athletes to recharge and refit themselves for competition—but only if it is not *too* long, and is actually easy. In many instances, a long easy run can better recharge athletes than taking a day off, but sometimes they need to get away from training altogether. In any case, a restorative environment is extremely important at this time. If possible, go to a natural environment alone or with select company.

The "Finishing Speed" sessions put the final edge on the capability of the athletes to perform their finishing kick. At this time, the aim is purely to enhance their speed and efficiency. In no way should the athletes become fatigued by doing hard work. The finishing speed sessions normally include relatively few repetitions between 50 and 300 meters in distance, and should be conducted at 3/4 to 7/8ths of an individual athlete's maximum speed, but without any indication of pressing. The athlete's speed should flow and be controlled, as opposed to being forced. Given the speeds assumed, athletes would not do well to extend the distance beyond 300 meters, since they would then move away from primary use of the ATP-PC energy system, and instead tap into the ATP-Lactic Acid system, which could introduce residual fatigue. The recovery periods provided within the session must also be complete. The athletes can take walking recoveries as long as they do not lose sufficient warm-up, thus perhaps begin to cool off and tighten-up. It is unwise to place a finishing speed workout less than three days prior to a competition, because any possible stiffness and soreness would be most apparent on the second day following the session (Liquori with Parker, 1980).

The "Time Trials" are normally conducted three to five days before a major competition, and permit athletes to arrive on the day of the contest while on the resulting crest of supercompensation. If athletes do not undertake such an effort after enjoying a relatively long recovery from a preceding competition, then they will become flat and lose peak fitness. The placement of the time trial depends largely on the individual's athletic level, and any special needs that arise in the light of circumstances. Trade-offs are then made between the quantity and quality most suitable for a given athlete and competitive event.

Mature athletes normally require a time trial at 3/4-effort approximately three to four days prior to a major competition. Alternately, they can sometimes time trial or race approximately 1/3rd the distance of the main race event at full effort four to five days prior to competition.

- Mature athletes normally require a volume of 2,000-3,000 meters at 3/4-effort 3-4 days prior to a 10,000 meters competition, but could run a 3,000-meter race approximately 4-5 days prior to the competition to achieve the same result.

- Mature athletes normally require a volume of 1,000-2,000 meters at 3/4-effort 3-4 days prior to a 5,000-meter competition, but could run a 1,500-meter race approximately 4-5 days prior to the competition to achieve the same result.

- Mature athletes normally require a volume of 600-1,000 meters at 3/4 to full-effort 3-4 days prior to a 1,500-meter competition, but could run a 1,000-to-2,000-meter race 4-5 days prior to the competition to achieve the same result.

- Mature athletes normally require a volume of 300-500m 3 days prior to an 800 meters competition, but could run a 400m race to achieve the same result.

The time trials can be used to maintain equilibrium and optimal balance. For example, if a specialist at 1,500 meters is weaker on the over-distance side, a 2,000-meter race could be run four to five days prior to the competition to better balance the athlete. Alternately, if a specialist at 1,500 meters athlete was weaker on the under-distance side, then something between 600 to 1,000 meters could be run three to five days prior to the competition. Given like circumstances, the same principle would apply to athletes competing in other events. An athlete's schedule can then be planned in advance to coordinate a string of competitive opportunities to be used for the purposes just described.

If desired, the time trials can alternately take the form of the 50-60 drill or 30-40 drill to accelerate the athletes' rate of peaking. In particular, middle distance athletes can use the 50-60 drill (alternating 50 meters sprint with 60 meters float, for two to three laps), and long distance athletes can use the 30-40 drill (alternating 200 meters in 30 seconds with 200 meters in 40 seconds in a continuous manner for less than 3,200 meters).

Young athletes must err on the side of leniency regarding the quantity, quality and proximity of the time trials so they can deliver superior performances in the main race event. To permit an adequate recovery and rebound of performance, these athletes can move the time trial back a day relative to mature athletes, and also conduct an easier time trial. Most importantly, young athletes should guard against racing in practice when running the time trials. It is fine for athletes to run a personal best in a time trial, so long as it is incidental. Athletes should not emotionally spend themselves by getting "psyched" for training sessions and then deliver their best performance in practice. It is best for athletes to save themselves and build up internal pressure of a constructive kind that will enable then to prove all things at the right time and place.

> *I think there's a great temptation for an athlete to test himself. It's a weakness in every one of us. We like to know if everyday we're improving. That's part of human nature. If a guy decides to go on a crash diet, he doesn't want to see that scale a couple pounds lighter in three week's time. He's got to be bloody lighter by tomorrow or to hell with it.*
>
> *The athlete has the same sort of tendency when he's training. There is a terrific temptation to test yourself and to measure your improvement and I believe that's a weakness. I think that you have to resist that temptation and have confidence in yourself and the toughness of your training and know within yourself that is going to produce results...*
>
> *This is why Lasse Viren seems to save himself up for a specific event... When he actually gets into the event that he's saved himself for, maybe for three years, there's a tremendous internal pressure. He hasn't proved himself to himself or the world by continually doing fast times. . .the pressure that has built up inside him is enormous. If he has the ability to transfer that pressure into performance, then he's going to have a great performance...*
>
> *So I'm a great believer in resisting the temptation to keep proving yourself to yourself.*
>
> —Herb Elliott

The "Day Before Race" (DBR) training session is required when no preliminary rounds are run prior to a final. Without undertaking a stimulating cardiovascular activity within 48 hours of a major competition, optimal performance will not be possible. Something must then be done to elevate the readiness of cardiovascular system. Obviously, the day before a major competition it is desirable to jolt the cardiovascular system into a high state of readiness with the least expenditure of energy, and also while incurring the least possible fatigue. An advisable method would be to conduct the following session:

- A full warm-up followed by light stretching
- 4-6 x 100 meters stride-outs
- A hollow 400 meters with the first 100 meters consisting of a gradual acceleration to 75% of full speed for 400 meters, then float 200 meters, and finish the last 100 meters at 75% of full speed, but without any evidence of pressing or engaging the kick reserved for competition

When dealing with relatively young and fit athletes, within 10 seconds, their 10-second pulse reading after completing the hollow 400 meters should be at least 160+ bpm, thus indicating that their pulse was actually near 180 bpm during the exercise, as desired. If not, after a full recovery, 300 meters should then be run in the same manner. Mature high school boys will normally run the hollow 400 meters at least in the low 60's, and girls in the high 60's to low 70's, depending on

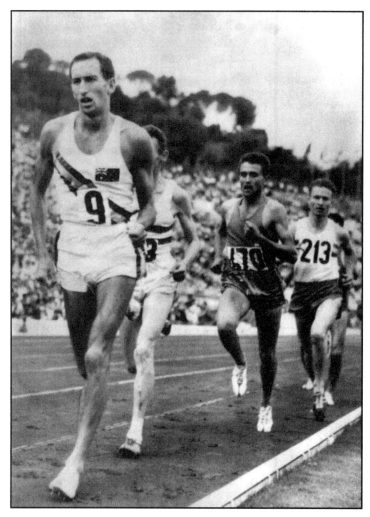

PHOTO 5.2—Herb Elliott breaks away from the field en route to a World Record in the 1,500 meters at the Olympic Games, 1960. Photo from Keystone Germany.

their level of ability. Again, four to six gradual 100 meters stride-out, some light stretching and flexibility work, and a good warm-down conclude the DBR session. Elite athletes who have recently traveled might wish to run a few reps at goal pace between 100 to 400 meters in distance (depending on their competitive event), but with full recovery periods.

The "Race Day" routine should be planned far in advance of a major competition. In order to be prepared for optimal performance, athletes should awaken at least four hours prior to a morning competition. Further, athletes should awaken at that time at least one day before the race, and train at the appointed hour of the race to set their circadian rhythm. However, if significant travel across time zones will take place, then at least seven to 10 days are required for adaptation.

When a preliminary round is conducted prior to a final, it is extremely important that athletes assume easy training sessions twice a day to speed recovery. The most desirable activity for the evening or morning after a preliminary round is 20 to 30 minutes of easy swimming. Packing the athletes' quads, hamstrings, and calves with ice for 20 minutes in the evening following a preliminary round will also facilitate recovery. Ingesting at least a liter of fluid such as a citrus juice (which serves as natural buffer), or a commercially available electrolyte replacement drink, will also enhance recovery. Fluid replacements should be ingested within 20 minutes of the exhausting effort, thus before the body registers the full extent of the athletes' fatigue, and possible symptoms of shock appear. To enhance recovery, athletes should consume a simple form of sugar, but also some protein shortly after a preliminary round.

Whenever possible, athletes should run for 10 to 20 minutes in solitude the morning before a major race. During the easy morning run the athletes should center themselves, and visualize the coming day of competition. Afterwards, a light meal should be taken, and the remainder of the day spent in a positive environment. Some athletes need to be around the hype attending competitions to reach an optimal performance state, but most need to be kept away from it. Recognize the particular needs of individual athletes so that they will be able to compete to the best of their ability.

Athletes must prepare for weather conditions. For example, they should:

- In hot weather—take a cool shower, have ice water with them at all times, and stay out of the sun and heat
- In frigid weather—dress appropriately prior to competition, allow for a preliminary warm-up indoors, then a longer warm-up outdoors

Expect the unexpected in the way of mix-ups. Do not become frazzled by the difficulties that always attend major competitions. Be polite with officials, but otherwise give nothing away. Athletes should keep to themselves and not permit coaches, athletes, or members of the media to distract them by making conversation, or any form of physical contact. Athletes are best advised to avoid these situations whenever possible. Otherwise, their physical and mental powers could be greatly compromised.

Peak Period Training Schedules

Training schedules for various events during the peak period are provided below for young and mature high school, collegiate, and elite distance runners, in events from 400 to 10,000 meters.

High School Track and Field / Cross-Country

The first Thursday in the provided schedules indicates the last 3/4-effort sharpening workout and the end of the sharpening period. Using this day as a starting point (or day zero), and then counting forwards, athletes will assume a worthwhile break and normally complete their ascent to the plateau of peak performance by the ninth to 10th day. The finals in the state meet can also serve as an origin (day zero), when counting backwards. These two counting methods can produce an overlap, as shown in the schedule. Whether planning the training schedule forwards or backwards, everything must add up and make sense in both directions. This method encourages coaches and athletes to think critically about the workouts, the number and distance of the races, and the impact that all of these will have on the primary competition and ultimate outcome of the athletic season.

Clearly, high school athletes should not race the same main race event over three succeeding weeks in the conference, regional and state championships during the track and field season. For optimal performance in the state championships, moderation must be exercised regarding the number of events contested during the earlier conference and region championships. Some high school coaches might be tempted to "sacrifice," or overuse a talented athlete to elevate the team point total in the conference championship. They might imagine that the individual will still be able to shine in the regional and state championships. This is a big mistake. *When coaches find themselves asking whether or not to risk overextending an athlete, whether in training or competition: the mere posing of the question provides the answer. And the answer is no, do not do it.*

The awful truth in distance running is—greed is not good. A decision to overextend an athlete for a team point total is fundamentally different from a decision based upon prudence, such as, recognizing that an athlete is only capable advancing to the conference meet, and then training the athlete to peak at that time. It is not possible to compromise without losing something—the athlete's development, and possibly the outcome of an athletic season or career.

With many of these issues, the real question is virtue. The primary purpose of participation in athletics is the cultivation of character, rather than points on a scoreboard. Stay the course. The outcome is incidental to excellence. If you take the attitude to do the right thing, simply because it is right, often the desired outcome will be there waiting for you as well.

0	Thursday	3/4-Effort, 2 x 600m at 800m Goal Pace
1	Friday	Active Recovery
2	Saturday	Time Trial, 3 x 150m with Accelerations
3	Sunday	Easy Effort, Long Run, 30-40 minutes
4	Monday	Day Before Race Routine
5	Tuesday	CONFERENCE PRELIM, Race 100m and 200m
6	Wednesday	Active Recovery
7	Thursday	CONFERENCE FINAL, Race 100m and 200m
8	Friday	Active Recovery
14/9	Saturday	Passive Recovery
13/10	Sunday	Easy Effort, Long Run, 30-40 minutes
12/11	Monday	Time Trial, 2 x 150m with Accelerations
11/12	Tuesday	3 x Starts and Handoffs
10	Wednesday	Day Before Race Routine
9	Thursday	REGION PRELIM, Race 400m
8	Friday	Active Recovery
7	Saturday	REGION FINAL, Race 400m
6	Sunday	Active Recovery
5	Monday	Passive Recovery
4	Tuesday	Time Trial, 2 x 150m with Accelerations
3	Wednesday	3 x Starts and Handoffs
2	Thursday	Day Before Race Routine
1	Friday	STATE PRELIM, Race 400m
0	Saturday	STATE FINAL, Race 400m

Regarding the high school 400 meters schedule, during the conference championship, specialists at 400 meters are well advised not to compete in the main race event. Since the athletes face two succeeding weeks of competition in the main race event and relays, it would be best to race under-distance or over-distance during the conference championship.

0	Thursday	Time Trial(s) 600m, full recovery, then 300m
1	Friday	Active Recovery
2	Saturday	1/2 Effort, Fartlek + 3 x 60m Starts
3	Sunday	Easy Recovery
4	Monday	Day Before Race Routine
5	Tuesday	CONFERENCE PRELIM, Race 400m
6	Wednesday	Active Recovery
7	Thursday	CONFERENCE FINAL, Race 2 x 400m
8	Friday	Active Recovery
14/9	Saturday	Easy Effort, Long Run, 40-60 minutes
13/10	Sunday	Passive Recovery
12/11	Monday	Time Trial 300m slow-fast, full recovery, then 3 x 150m with Accelerations, walk recovery
11/12	Tuesday	Active Recovery
10	Wednesday	Day Before Race Routine
9	Thursday	REGION PRELIM, Race 800m
8	Friday	Active Recovery
7	Saturday	REGION FINAL, Race 800m
6	Sunday	Easy Effort, Long Run, 40-60 minutes
5	Monday	Passive Recovery
4	Tuesday	Time Trial 300m slow-fast, full recovery, then 3 x 150m with Accelerations, walk recovery
3	Wednesday	Active Recovery
2	Thursday	Day Before Race Routine
1	Friday	STATE PRELIM, Race 800m
0	Saturday	STATE FINAL, Race 800m

Regarding the high school 800 meters schedule, during the conference championship, specialists at 800 meters are well advised to race under-distance, since they will run four competitions in the main event over the following two weeks.

0	Thursday	3/4-Effort, 4 x 1,000m at 3,000m Goal Pace
1	Friday	Active Recovery
2	Saturday	1/2-Effort Fartlek + 3 x 100m at Finishing Speed
3	Sunday	Easy Effort, Long Run, 40-60 minutes
4	Monday	Day Before Race Routine
5	Tuesday	CONFERENCE PRELIM, Race 800m
6	Wednesday	Active Recovery
7	Thursday	CONFERENCE FINAL, Race 800m and 400m
8	Friday	Active Recovery
14/9	Saturday	Easy Effort, Long Run, 60-80 minutes
13/10	Sunday	Passive Recovery
12/11	Monday	3/4-Effort, Time Trial 1,200m, then 300m slow-fast
11/12	Tuesday	Active Recovery
10	Wednesday	1/2-Effort, Fartlek + 3 x 100m at Finishing Speed
9	Thursday	Easy Recovery
8	Friday	Day Before Race Routine
7	Saturday	REGION FINAL, Race 1,500m
6	Sunday	Easy Effort, Long Run, 60-80 minutes
5	Monday	Passive Recovery
4	Tuesday	3/4-Effort, Time Trial 1,000m, then 300m slow-fast
3	Wednesday	Active Recovery + 3 x 100m at Finishing Speed
2	Thursday	Easy Recovery
1	Friday	Day Before Race Routine
0	Saturday	STATE FINAL, Race 1,500m

This 1,500-meter schedule is for an 800-meter sided specialist at 1,500 meters who would race 800 meters in the conference championship and 1,500 meters in the state championship. The time trials at 1,000 and 1,200 meters would normally be conducted at goal pace for 1,500 meters. After a full recovery, the slow-fast 300 meters would normally be run at 41-43 seconds (boys), and 48-51 seconds (girls). See Appendix I for alternate 1,500 and 3,000-meter schedules for an athlete who would compete in both events in the state championship.

0	Thursday	3/4-Effort, 4 x 1,000m at 3,000m Goal Pace
1	Friday	Easy Effort, Long Run, 60-80 minutes
2	Saturday	Easy Recovery
3	Sunday	Time Trial 1,200m, then 300m
4	Monday	Active Recovery + 3 x 150m at Finishing Speed
5	Tuesday	Easy Recovery
6	Wednesday	Day Before Race Routine
7	Thursday	CONFERENCE FINAL, Race 1,500m
8	Friday	Easy Effort, Long Run, 60-80 minutes
14/9	Saturday	Passive Recovery
13/10	Sunday	Time Trial 1,000m, then 300m
12/11	Monday	Active Recovery + 3 x 150m at Finishing Speed
11/12	Tuesday	Easy Recovery
10	Wednesday	Day Before Race Workout
9	Thursday	REGION FINAL, Race 3,000m
8	Friday	Active Recovery
7	Saturday	REGION FINAL, Race 1,500m
6	Sunday	Easy Effort, Long Run, 60-80 minutes
5	Monday	Passive Recovery
4	Tuesday	Time Trial 800m of 50-60 drill, then 300m
3	Wednesday	Active Recovery + 3 x 150m with Accelerations
2	Thursday	Day Before Race Routine
1	Friday	STATE FINAL, Race 3,000m
0	Saturday	STATE FINAL, Race 1,500m

This 3,000 meters schedule is for an athlete competing in the 1,500 meters during the conference championship, and both the 3,000 meters and 1,500 meters in the state championship. It is suited for more mature athletes who would advance and attempt to place in the top six in the state championship. The 3/4-effort time trials at 1,000 and 1,200 meters should be run at 1,500 meters goal pace. After a full recovery, the slow-fast 300 meters would normally be run at 41-43 seconds (boys), and 48-51 seconds (girls).

0	Tuesday	3/4 Effort, 4 x 1,200m at 5,000m Goal Pace
1	Wednesday	Active Recovery
2	Thursday	1/2-Effort, Fartlek + 3 x 200m at Finishing Speed
3	Friday	Active Recovery
4	Saturday	Time Trial, 1,600m
5	Sunday	Active Recovery + 4 x 150m with Accelerations
6	Monday	Easy Recovery
7	Tuesday	Day Before Race Routine
8	Wednesday	CONFERENCE FINAL, Race 5,000m
9	Thursday	Easy Effort, Long Run, 60-80 minutes
10	Friday	Passive Recovery
14/11	Saturday	Day Before Race Routine
13/12	Sunday	Time Trial 1,200m, then 300m
12/13	Monday	Active Recovery + 3 x 150m at Finishing Speed
11/14	Tuesday	Easy Recovery
10	Wednesday	Day Before Race Routine
9	Thursday	REGION FINAL, Race 5,000m
8	Friday	Easy Effort, Long Run, 60-80 minutes
7	Saturday	Passive Recovery
6	Sunday	Active Recovery + 6 x 200m at 1,500m Goal Pace
5	Monday	Day Before Race Routine
4	Tuesday	Time Trial 1,000m, then 300m
3	Wednesday	Active Recovery + 3 x 150m with Accelerations
2	Thursday	Easy Recovery
1	Friday	Day Before Race Routine
0	Saturday	STATE FINAL, Race 5,000m

This schedule for boys and girls cross-country is suited for mature high school athletes who would advance to the state championship.

Collegiate Track and Field / Cross-Country

The collegiate cross-country schedule is suited for athletes who must focus on peaking for the conference championship, and qualifying for the NCAA Regional Cross-Country Championships. The workout 8 days prior to the Regional Championships is therefore a stabilizing training effort. Mature athletes will be able to follow this schedule and successfully compete one week later in the National Championship. However, developing and 1,500-meter athletes should compete in their conference championships 5-7 days after the last sharpening workout, thus during the ascent or taper, and be held out of at least one of the two earlier contests.

COLLEGIATE CROSS-COUNTRY WOMEN'S 5,000 METERS AND MEN'S 10,000 METERS		
0	Thursday	3/4 Effort, 4-5 x 1,000m at 5,000m Goal Pace
1	Friday	Active Recovery
2	Saturday	1/2 Effort Fartlek + 3 x 200m at Finishing Speed
3	Sunday	Easy Effort, Long Run, 60-80 minutes
4	Monday	Passive Recovery
5	Tuesday	Time Trial, Men: 2,000m 30-40 drill Women: 1,200m 50-60 drill
6	Wednesday	Active Recovery + 3 x 150m at Finishing Speed
7	Thursday	Easy Recovery
8	Friday	Day Before Race Routine
14/9	Saturday	CONFERENCE FINALS
13/10	Sunday	Active Recovery
12/11	Monday	Passive Recovery
11/12	Tuesday	Easy Effort, Long Run, 70-90 minutes
10/13	Wednesday	1/2 Effort, 3(4 x 200m) at 1,500m Goal Pace
9	Thursday	Active Recovery
8	Friday	2/3 Effort, 4 x 1,000m at 10,000m Goal Pace
7	Saturday	Easy Effort, Long Run, 60-80 minutes
6	Sunday	Active Recovery + 3 x 150m at Finishing Speed
5	Monday	Passive Recovery
4	Tuesday	Time Trial, Men: 2,000m 30-40 drill, Women: 1,200m 50-60 drill
3	Wednesday	Active Recovery + 4 x 150m with Accelerations
2	Thursday	Easy Recovery
1	Friday	Day Before Race Routine
0	Saturday	NCAA REGIONAL FINALS

The reader should now be familiar enough with the vocabulary and notation in the training schedules to permit a comparative presentation with respect to the preparation of collegiate athletes in events ranging from 800-10,000 meters, prior to a conference championship. The schedule for a 10,000-meter specialist could be essentially the same as that for 5,000 meters. However, the time trial prior to the conference championship would then have to be moved back a day, as the 10,000 meters is normally contested the day before the 5,000 meters final.

Table 5.1 comprises an extended peak period that would allow an attempt at a personal best performance 10 days into the peak period, and thus maximize competitive productivity during the limited 14-to-21-day plateau of peak performance. An attempt at a personal best should normally be directed to an under-distance or over-distance performance, but could in some circumstances be directed towards the main race event in order to attain or improve a qualifying mark.

A brief discussion should help to clarify any ambiguities in the provided schedules. The last 3/4-effort sharpening workout falls approximately nine to 10 days prior to the first competition on the plateau of peak performance. After this last sharpening workout, the following training sessions can be conducted: a day of active recovery, a day of finishing speed work, an easy effort, a long run, and a day of passive recovery. This brings us to the time trial conducted four to five days before the first competition on the plateau. World-class athletes can sometimes conduct the time trial as close as three days before a major competition, whereas collegiate athletes normally catch the resulting wave of supercompensation by performing a time trial four days previous. However, when athletes are on the ascent, or have residual fatigue from sharpening efforts, they will sometimes need an additional day of recovery from the time trial. In this case, it can be advantageous to conduct a finishing speed session three days prior—in conjunction with a time trial performed five days before the competition, as shown in Table 5.1.

After the first competition, athletes will require four to five days to recover before assuming another demanding effort. The following training sessions could then be undertaken: a day of active recovery, an easy effort, a long run, and a day of passive recovery. Then, no closer than nine days prior to the conference championships, athletes should conduct a 2/3rds to 3/4-effort training session to stabilize their performance potential. An earlier acquisitive training session can then be repeated, but with suitable reduction in effort as to permit any resulting fatigue to be dissipated by the time of the conference championship.

Accordingly, between the first competition on the plateau and the conference championship, athletes ride the supercompensation waves generated by the demanding efforts that are all spaced four or five days apart:

- From the last sharpening workout to the first time trial
- From the first time trial to the first competition
- From the first competition to the stabilizing high quality training session
- From the stabilizing high quality training session to the second time trial
- From the second time trial to the conference championship prelim or final

Table 5.1 shows comparative schedules for collegiate track and field athletes for the 800–10,000-meter events.

Extended Peak Period for Collegiate Track And Field: 800-10,000 Meters

KEY TO ABBREVIATIONS

AR	Active Recovery	**MRE**	Main Race Event
FS	Finishing Speed	**DBR**	Day Before Race Session
ER	Easy Recovery	**ODE**	Over-Distance Event
PR	Passive Recovery	**UDE**	Under-Distance Event
LR	Long Run	**XUDE**	X Under-Distance Event
TT	Time Trial	**@ 1/4**	1/4 Effort
F	Fartlek	**@ 1/2**	1/2 Effort
FS	Finishing Speed	**@ 3/4**	3/4 Effort

	800m	1,500m	3,000m	5,000/10,000m
0	MRE 2 x 600m	ODE 5 x 1,000m	MRE 5 x 1,000m	AR
1	AR	AR	AR	MRE 4 x 1,600m
2	F+FS 4 x 100m	F+FS 4 x 150m	F+FS 3 x 200m	AR
3	LR	LR	LR	F+FS 4 x 200m
4	PR	PR	PR	LR
5	TT 1,200m, 300m	TT 400m, 400m	TT 800m, 400m	TT 1,000m, 300m
6	AR	AR	AR	AR
7	F+FS 3 x 100m	F+FS 3 x 150m	F+FS 3 x 200m	F+FS 4 x 200m
8	AR	AR	AR	ER
9	DBR	DBR	DBR	DBR
10	Race 1,500m	Race 800m, 400m	Race 1,500m	Race 3,000m
11	AR+FS 3 x 100m	AR+FS 3 x 150m	AR	AR
12	LR	LR	F+FS 4 x 150m	F+FS 4 x 150m
11	PR	PR	LR	LR
10	MRE 2 x 500m	ODE 4 x 1,000m	PR	PR
9	AR	AR	ODE 4 x 1,000m	ODE 5 x 1,000m
8	F+FS 3 x 60m Starts	F+FS 3 x 100m	AR	AR
7	AR	AR	F+FS 3 x 150m	F+FS 3 x 150m
6	LR	LR	LR	LR
5	TT 400m, 200m	TT 1,000m, 300m	PR	PR
4	AR 3 x 60m Starts	AR+FS 3 x 100m	TT 1,200m, 300m	TT 1,600m, 300m
3	ER	ER	AR+FS 3 x 150m	AR+FS 3 x 150m
2	DBR	DBR	ER	ER
1	800m Prelims	1,500m Prelims	DBR	DBR
0	800m Final	1,500m Final	3,000m Final	5,000m Final

TABLE 5.1

Elite Athletes: Track and Field

Table 5.2 provides illustrative schedules for elite athletes competing in the 800–10,000-meter events between the USATF National Championship and the World Championships.

Multiple Peak Period
USATF National Championships to the World Championships

KEY TO ABBREVIATIONS

AR	Active Recovery	**MRE**	Main Race Event
FS	Finishing Speed	**DBR**	Day Before Race Session
ER	Easy Recovery	**ODE**	Over-Distance Event
PR	Passive Recovery	**UDE**	Under-Distance Event
LR	Long Run	**XUDE**	X Under-Distance Event
TT	Time Trial	**@ 1/4**	1/4 Effort
F	Fartlek	**@ 1/2**	1/2 Effort
SS	Steady State	**@ 3/4**	3/4 Effort
ATSS	AT Steady State		

	800m	1,500m	5,000m	10,000m
14	ER	ER	5,000m Semis	DBR
15	DBR	DBR	AR	10,000m Final
16	800m Prelims	1,500m Prelims	5,000m Final	AR
17	800m Semis	AR	AR	PR
18	800m Final	1,500m Final	PR	PR
19	AR	AR	LR	LR
20	PR	PR	UDE 3(4 x 200m)	UDE 4(4 x 200m)
21	LR	LR	AR	AR
22	ODE 3(4 x 200m)	ODE 3(4 x 200m)	F @ 1/2	F @ 1/2
23	AR	AR	LR	LR
24	F @ 1/2	F @ 1/2	PR	PR
25	AR	AR	ATSS @ 3/4	ATSS @ 3/4
26	LR	LR	AR	AR
27	PR	PR	F @ 1/2	F @ 1/2
28	ATSS @ 3/4	ATSS @ 3/4	AR	AR
29	AR	AR	SS@ 3/4	SS @ 3/4
30	F @ 1/2	F @ 1/2	LR	LR
1	AR	AR	PR	PR
2	SS @ 3/4	SS @ 3/4	UDE 2(5 x 400m)	MRE 4 x 1,600m
3	LR	LR	AR	AR
4	PR	PR	F @ 1/4	F @ 1/4

TABLE 5.2

	800m	1,500m	5,000m	10,000m
5	MRE 3(3 x 300m)	MRE 2(4 x 400m)	AR	AR
6	AR	AR	MRE 5 x 1,000m	UDE 5 x 1,000m
7	F @ 1/4	F @ 1/4	AR	AR
8	AR	AR	PR TRAVEL	PR TRAVEL
9	MRE 3 x 500m	MRE 2 x 800m	F @ 1/4	F @ 1/4
10	LR	LR	ER	ER
11	PR TRAVEL	PR TRAVEL	DBR	DBR
12	F @ 1/4	F @ 1/4	TT 1,000m, 300m	TT 1,200m, 300m
13	AR + FS 4 x 150m	AR + FS 4 x 150m	AR + FS 4 x 200m	AR FS 4 x 200m
14	ER	ER	ER	ER
15	DBR	DBR	DBR	DBR
16	Race 400m	Race 800m	Race 1,500m	Race 3,000m
17	AR	AR	AR	AR
18	FS 3 x 100m	F+FS 3 x 150m	F+FS 3 x 200m	F+FS 3 x 200m
19	ER	ER	ER	ER
20	DBR	DBR	DBR	DBR
21	Race 800m	Race 1,500m	Race 3,000m	Race 5,000m
22	AR	AR	AR	AR
23	LR	LR	LR	LR
24	FS 3 x 100m	FS 3 x 150m	FS 3 x 200m	2UDE 12 x 200m
25	AR	AR	AR	AR
26	DBR	DBR	DBR	UDE 5 x 1,000m
27	Race 1,500m	Race 800m	Race 1,500m	LR
28	AR	AR	AR	PR
29	F+FS 3 x 60m	F+FS 3 x 150m	F+FS 3 x 150m	F+FS 3 x 150m
30	LR	LR	LR	ER
31	PR	PR	PR	DBR
1	TT 300m	ODE 4 x 1,000m	ODE 5 x 1,000m	TT 1,500m
2	AR Starts	LR	LR	AR+FS 3 x 150m
3	ER	AR+FS 4 x 150m	AR+FS 4 x 150m	ER
4	DBR	ER	ER	DBR
5	800m Prelims	DBR	DBR	10,000m Prelims
6	800m Semis	TT 600m, 300m	TT 1,000m, 300m	AR
7	AR	AR+FS 3 x 100m	AR+FS 3 x 150m	AR
8	800m Final	ER	ER	10,000m Final
9		DBR	DBR	
10		1,500m Prelims	5,000m Prelims	
11		1,500m Semis	5,000m Semis	
12		AR	AR	
13		1,500m Final	5,000m Final	

TABLE 5.2, continued

Mental Habits and Optimal Performance

There is a limit to how many outstanding performances athletes can deliver during an athletic season. Some individuals are incapable of getting it all from themselves in a supreme effort, while others seem to be able to do the impossible. Generally, when athletes receive gratification through training or any other avenue that leads to a state of satisfaction, they would dissipate an equal amount of mental energy, and sacrificed the gumption required for superior performance. To inwardly have a degree of contempt for flattery may be heterodox, but it is sound advice. That is one of the reasons why mature coaches and athletes are loath to make predictions, and as a rule, avoid pre-event interaction with the media: "It ain't over till it's over."

A host of physical and mental problems can arise from competing too frequently. Nothing exhausts peak condition faster than too frequently racing the main event. Moreover, the damage done to the competitive psyche of athletes could be permanent. For this reason, athletes should run the main race event infrequently, and only when physically and mentally prepared to deliver a supreme effort. When they do race the main event in a finals heat, it must be absolutely full out. To develop the conscious or unconscious habit of holding back in the main race event is self-defeating. This will happen if athletes are frequently being doubled, or running the main race event on a weekly basis. When an individual is not prepared to race as if it were a matter of life and death, then he or she can be beaten by someone who is.

It is important to protect those rare athletes who can give their all to the contest, from acquiring bad habits out of the need for self-preservation. Some big-meet personalities are born, and others self-made. Unfortunately, many are destroyed in their youth by the unenlightened expectations and demands of those on whom they depend for guidance. To compete well is an act. Habits are acquired by repeated acts. Right habits are virtues. This is the theory of disposition taught by Aristotle, Augustine, and Thomas Aquinas (Aristotle, in Thompson, 1946, Aquinas, in Pegis, 1948, Deane, 1963, and Lyden, 1986).

> *I believe that in any race you let a guy beat you—and you do let him beat you if you are not absolutely psychologically tuned up to winning at all costs—that creates a precedent that allows you to get beat in the race you care about... that was the sort of attitude that I had... But I had a dual goal in my running, that was to win and to achieve excellence, so I was never happy with a slow, tactical time.*
>
> —Herb Elliott

Fear of Failure

Fear of failure is commonly recognized and well understood. It often becomes most visible and acute during the peak period. Many athletes afflicted with a fear of failure actually suffer from a form of post-traumatic stress disorder. They often have prior learning experiences from a psychologically hostile environment in which failure at a task brought physical or psychological pain. These individuals are the walking wounded, and more vulnerable due to their psychological scar tissue. They might have dysfunctional or various levels of "dysfunctionally functional" emotional and behavior patterns. The forms of active aggression which they may have experienced as a child could have included physical abuse, confinement, hardships, or denial of privileges.

This can be a difficult and gray area for parent and coach alike. After all, a child disturbing others with a tantrum may require a time out. A child who takes the car without permission and hits a fire hydrant should perhaps be grounded. An athlete who breaks team rules could be benched. However, what perhaps matters most in matters of discipline are the actual and perceived intentions of the participants. Discipline with the emotional attachment of hate and rejection is destructive, but reasonable and appropriate discipline with a sense of fairness, and the emotional attachment of love is constructive. Parents, young children, even animals can discern one emotion from the other, and know whether or not they are loved.

Undoubtedly, with regard to fear of failure in sport, the most serious form of injury comes through the association of conditional love—with outcomes. Losing a game is no longer a matter of losing at play, but rather losing the love of one's parents, peers and the "tribe." Losing at play then means rejection and emotional death. Often associated with rejection are verbal attacks on the athlete's self-worth, such as, "you are no good—worthless," and so on. These forms of verbal abuse constitute active aggression. Passive aggression also qualifies as a form of abuse. It essentially communicates the same message of rejection and conditional love, but by acts of omission. When internalized, this negative self-image can be toxic and self-defeating, because the individual succumbs to believing what he or she hears. As a result, goal setting may not occur, or the goal may be set low. This negative self-fulfilling prophesy could also result in low levels of energy being directed toward a goal.

However, the more damaging aspect of internalization comes not only when individuals begin to believe the negative things they hear, but when, as a result of rejection and a loss of love, they blame themselves for it, and perhaps come to not love themselves. Thoughts such as, "damn, I missed the shot..." associated with self-disgust, are a symptom of this disease. The conditional attachment of love and self-worth to performing a successful outcome has then become internalized, and it is now the individual athlete who administers the abuse.

Coincidentally, this attachment constitutes a form of outcome orientation. Play and enjoyment are sacrificed for the desired end, or so-called success. Such attachment invariably results in numerous breaks in concentration. It diminishes the ability to focus on the task at hand, since attention is fixed on imagining a hypothetical outcome. In general, outcome orientation is also associated with an undue attachment to time, either the past or the future. Instead of focusing on the present, an individual may unduly cling to a positive or negative outcome that has just transpired. Similarly, an athlete might imagine a positive or negative future outcome. Wants, needs, and a variety of desires associated with the ego, can result in attachment to thoughts that do not relate to the here and now—the moment. These invariably result in numerous breaks in concentration and non-optimal levels of athletic performance. This phenomenon was well known to the Zen Masters (Suzuki, 1959, and Takuan Sōhō, in Wilson, 1987).

Fear of Success

Athletes who suffer a fear of success are less often recognized and understood. Those uninitiated to sport may find it surprising that athletes sometimes suffer an aversion to success. However, on any given day, the number of athletes suffering a fear of success generally equals the number suffering a fear of failure. The most common cure for both extremes is for athletes to transcend outcome orientation. This is simple to say, but can be difficult to accomplish. Years of errant thinking can result in deeply instilled beliefs and self-perceptions. For example, if a hundred negative thoughts have been registered, then it will generally take a hundred positive thoughts in order to have a 50/50 chance of breaking even. Further, when athletes face physical or mental stress, their old mental habits tend to dominate. Athletes afflicted with a fear of success generally have one of two basic problems:

- They are not prepared for the responsibilities, further demands or consequences associated with success.
- They suffer from a negative self-image, a lack of confidence, and feel unworthy or guilty about achieving success.

There can be many reasons why athletes might have an aversion to the responsibilities, further demands, or consequences associated with success. Sometimes, athletes face the pressure of little league parents, coaches, or their peers. In truth, pressure is something individuals put on themselves. Nevertheless, some athletes come to believe that failure provides the only avenue of escape. The "success monster" is never satisfied and only wants more. Sometimes the only way to escape from being consumed is to fail—and to do so in grand fashion in order to be left in peace.

Alternatively, it could be that athletes do not enjoy the activity for its own sake, but rather participate in athletics as a ticket to get something else. When they attain that something else, and extremely common and easy way to drop athletics is to fail. Sometimes athletes anticipate that they will face even greater responsibilities and demands if they attain a higher level of success. Consciously or not, they might judge the next level to be beyond their comfort zone. Failure can then provide an escape from the test. It can be easier to say, "I did not have the talent," than to admit, "I did not want to do it," (which may well be justified) or, "I did not have the guts to do it."

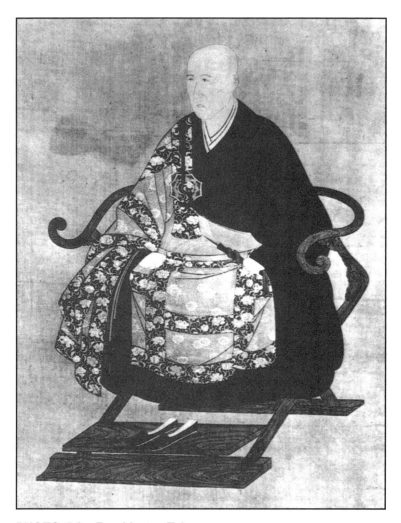

PHOTO 5.3—Zen Master Takuan. Plate 35, from Suzuki, Daisetz: *Zen and Japanese Culture*. Copyright © 1959, Princeton University Press. Reprinted by permission of Princeton University Press.

Those individual who suffer guilt over success are often the victims of abuse, and deserving of compassion. Something like the following can be said in such cases: It may be true that when an athlete competes to the best of his or her ability that some of the competitors will become psyched out. Consciously or not, these competitors might concede future contests and permit the athlete to dominate races from the start. While an individual can foreknow the probable effects of his or her superiority on the competition, this does not entail preordination. After all, the competitors can choose either to be intimidated or inspired.

A great performance, and the mark it establishes, contributes to excellence. The competitors, and those who come after, will be that much better for what an athlete achieves by honorable means—provided they have the strength of character to find that something extra within themselves and rise to the challenge. This is one of the reasons why the world loves a performer, whether in sport, or in any other realm.

Athletes who are afflicted with a fear of success due to a negative self-perception can sometimes be identified by their inability to verbalize in a strong voice, "I deserve to (whatever the goal happens to be)," in the presence of their coach and peers. Many find themselves completely tongue-tied or only capable of weak utterances. The Zen masters believed in the mutual interdependence and potency of thought, word and deed. If necessary, hold a private team meeting, and with the playful support of their teammates do not let any individual leave unless he or she can shout out, "the team deserves to..." but also, "I deserve to..." and most likely, the desired outcome will be achieved.

Whether the fear be of failure or success, athletes can become susceptible to illness or injury due to stress imposed by their mental state. One evening of anxiety can undo months of training. The adrenaline needed for the next day's competition can then go down the drain. Accordingly, the fittest athlete in the world will not be able to prove it unless he or she has trained for mental as well as physical fitness.

> *There's probably going to be a quantum leap forward when we understand our minds better. I believe that we just barely understand our physical capabilities at this stage of the game. There will come a time when knowledge of ourselves will enable us to tap that physical resource. At that time, we'll see a quantum leap in all sports.*
>
> —Herb Elliott

References

Aquinas, St. Thomas, *An Introduction to St. Thomas Aquinas: The Summa Contra Gentiles* (excerpts), Anton C. Pegis, Editor, New York: The Modern Library, Random House, Inc., 1948, pages 551-646.

Aristotle, *The Ethics of Aristotle: The Nichomachean Ethics*, Translated by J.A.K. Thompson, Introduction by Jonathan Barnes, London: Penguin Books, 1976.

Deane, Herbert, *The Political and Social Ideals of St. Augustine,* New York: Columbia University Press, 1963.

Liquori, Marty, and John L. Parker, *Marty Liquori's Guide for the Elite Runner,* Chicago, Illinois: Playboy Press Book, 1980, page 48.

Lyden, Robert M., *Ninety-Nine Questions: A Dialogue on the Nature of Just War with Francisco(s) De Vitoria and Suarez,* Plan B Paper for M.A. Degree, Hubert H. Humphrey Institute of Public Affairs, University of Minnesota, 1986.

Peters, Keith, "Conversation with Steve Scott and Herb Elliott," *Running*, May/June, 1981, pages 16-18.

Takuan Sōhō, *The Unfettered Mind,* Translated by William Wilson, New York: Kodasha International, 1987.

Suzuki, Daisetz, *Zen and Japanese Culture,* Princeton, New Jersey: Bollingen Foundation, Inc., Princeton University Press, 1959.

Will-Weber, Mark, Editor, *The Quotable Runner*, Halcottsville, New York: Breakaway Books, 2001.

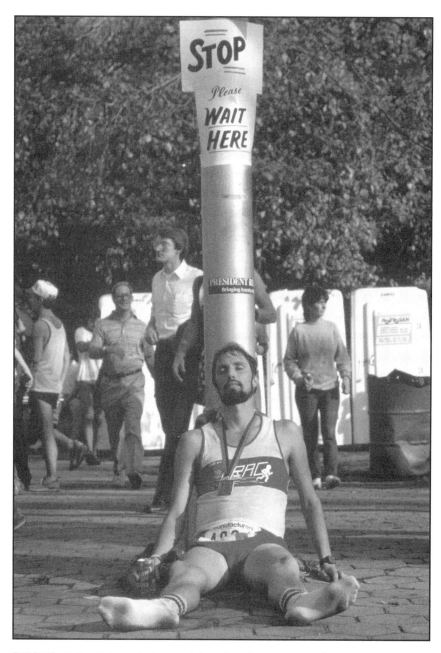

PHOTO 6.1—Exhausted... and leaning towards post-season recovery.
Copyright Owen Franklin / CORBIS, 1984. Reprinted with permission

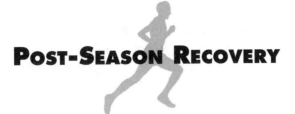

CHAPTER 6

POST-SEASON RECOVERY

The normal cycle of human existence over the millennia has included a period of diminished activity resembling a period of hibernation. In truth, the veneer of modern civilization has not gone far to supplant the handiwork of the ages. We need our vacations to get away from it all. Sometimes we need to do nothing. Doing nothing is sometimes doing something important. Sport is a highly compressed and intense form of life. Accordingly, athletes have great need for a period of post-season recovery following a competitive season.

Physical Aspects

Athletic development is characterized by three stages:

- Acquisition—hard training
- Consolidation—competition and performance
- Decline—post-season recovery

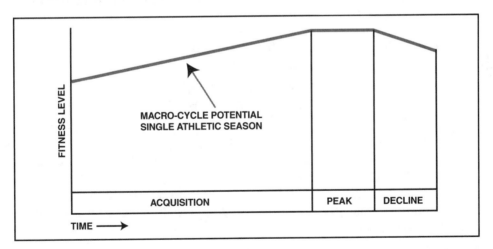

FIGURE 6.1

As discussed in Chapter 1, the effort of the training sessions vary within the weekly micro-cycle to permit adequate recovery from acute fatigue, and thereby facilitate super-compensation. However, after a more extended period of demanding work, an athlete needs a regenerative worthwhile break to consolidate the potential created by previous training efforts, and avoid the onset of residual or chronic fatigue. In brief, the more demanding the training, the greater the need for load-leaping and taking periodic worthwhile breaks. Accordingly, the training meso-cycles will be shorter and more frequent.

Nevertheless, even with the conduct of load-leaping and meso-cycles including worthwhile breaks, it is not possible to train and race indefinitely. Ten to fourteen weeks appears to be the limit of highly stressful work that distance runners can absorb before habituation or exhaustion sets in, and they cease to make substantial gains. In fact, athletes can become physically and mentally stale, and actually suffer a regression.

Aerobic work conducted well below the anaerobic threshold during the base and hill periods will not normally cause this regression. However, high quality aerobic work such as anaerobic threshold and steady state training, and also the anaerobic work performed during the sharpening period will do so. Symptoms of chronic fatigue and overstress commonly involve the disturbance of hormone and enzyme functions, and can include:

- Loss of appetite
- Insomnia
- Mental staleness
- Higher morning resting pulse rate
- Lower resistance to illness and injury

All demanding training approaches the threshold of imposing a chronic overload. The potential onset of debilitating fatigue and decline of an individual's athletic level makes it necessary to assume a period of post-season recovery. In the model shown in Figure 6.1, this corresponds to the period of decline, and serves as the prelude to the next athletic season.

Runner's High and Post-Race Recovery

The need for post-season recovery can be better understood by examining the various physical reactions that follow an athletic performance. A mental high that disguises the actual state of fatigue always follows in the wake of a full effort in athletic competition. The biochemical origin of this phenomenon is largely found in the central nervous system, and in particular, the midbrain, which triggers the release powerful natural drugs, such as cortisol, adrenaline and endorphins. If you know you have performed at full effort, then know you are tired and conduct yourself accordingly. You'll be glad that you did! For after the high comes the low, or crash, and the less you conserve of yourself, the more pronounced and prolonged the crash will be.

While still on their runner's high, athletes often become distracted and socialize immediately after a competition. But within an hour, the natural high will wear off, and their actual level of fatigue can hit them severely. Athletes can then go into mild shock, and become unable to ingest food for several hours. This mistake is fatal to a favorable result when preliminary heats of competition take place over several days. Instead, athletes should warm-down and immediately drink ample quantities of water after a performance. Additional electrolyte replacement drinks are also acceptable. When significant dehydration has occurred, and electrolyte replacement drinks are unavailable, sometimes a half-teaspoon of salt and/or baking soda (sodium bicarbonate) added to a quart of water can help. If possible, consume a natural pH buffer including a simple sugar—a citrus juice such as pineapple-grapefruit. Hard work tends to lower the blood pH, thus rendering it more acidic. The faster you can neutralize that acidity, the sooner and better you will recover. Why drink citrus juices containing citric acid? The simple answer is that within your body, citric acid acts as a natural buffer or base, thus neutralizing acidity. Generally, athletes can better ingest a blended citrus juice than straight orange or grapefruit juice. In addition, foods having a high glycemic index can facilitate recovery, and these include simple sugars such as glucose, fructose, sucrose, honey, and molasses—also present in various fruits and breads. However, athletes should follow up with foods having a moderate glycemic index such as corn, baked beans, grapes, oatmeal, oranges, rice, spaghetti, and yams (See Coyle, 1993, 1995, Podell and Proctor, 1993, and Brand-Miller, et al., 1999). What about the usual dorm food—greasy pizza and beer after the meet? The coach and athletes should stop and think about these.

Following the conduct of a 3/4-effort training session or a race, it is best to observe the above guidelines within 30 minutes—before the natural drugs wear off and the athletes begin to crash. Generally runners should not sunbathe, sightsee, or sit in hot tubs immediately before or after a competition, since these activities can drain them and retard recovery. And as much as they might want to celebrate a good performance with a party, what they really need to do is get some sleep. This description of proper conduct after a single race effort can be applied to all hard training efforts throughout the athletic season. It can also enhance our understanding concerning the need for post-season recovery. *The capacity to perform work ultimately depends on the ability to recover from it.*

Runner's High, and Post-Season Recovery

When early man had an unexpected encounter with a bear and had to fight or take flight, his central nervous system triggered the release of large doses of powerful natural drugs (including adrenaline, cortisol and endorphins). Think of these substances as roughly corresponding to the pharmaceutical drugs known as uppers, cortical steroids, and painkillers, but endorphins are many times more powerful than morphine. This alarm reaction made possible early man's survival. However, an alarm reaction of this magnitude was not part of his daily routine. Early man did not go out and wrestle with a bear every day, or even once a week.

Hence the problem, because modern training man commonly wants to wrestle a bear in the form of a training session that will provoke a substantial alarm reaction—several times a week. The central nervous system is not designed to sustain this constant high level of demand. The body's arsenal of natural drugs cannot respond indefinitely to alarm reactions of such great magnitude and frequency. Eventually, if training man persists, he will one day face the bear, and when the alarm reaction goes off, the body's pharmacy of natural drugs will be empty. As a result, the athlete's fitness will decline and possibly regress dramatically. This can happen through simple ignorance or technical error, such as believing that more training is always the answer.

Arousal Addiction

When athletes clearly know better, but cannot bring themselves to reduce their training, then they threaten to become arousal addicts. Arousal addicts need their daily runner's high or fix to feel good about themselves, which actually is the physical and mental state of not feeling bad due to the biochemistry of arousal. They are no longer in pursuit of excellence, but rather in need of counseling and professional help. The coach might hear rationalizations from an athlete such as: "Coach, I need to train harder to improve... I don't need or want to take that time off." However, the grim reality may be that the coach is listening to a running junkie pleading for his or her next fix.

In extreme cases, the functions of the central nervous system can collapse to such a degree as to result in death. What happens when you have not eaten for a while and you become hungry? At first you feel hungry and you want something to eat. Then after a while, if you still have not eaten, the feeling of hunger leaves you. In part, what happened is that your hunger induced an alarm reaction, which provided a fix of endorphins that dulled the pain associated with hunger. Excessive behavior associated with any of the following could indicate the presence of an arousal addiction:

fasting	alcohol	over-training
bingeing	sleep deprivation	pain
spicy food	sexual adventurism	tanning
chocolate	risk taking	danger
caffeine	attention seeking	gambling

Eating Disorders and Arousal Addiction

The preceding discussion concerning hunger illustrates what individuals with eating disorders are doing to themselves all the time. They are giving their central nervous system a punch to obtain a fix of natural drugs and escape or deny their personal suffering. Recognize that common sources of stress can include the individual's family, peers, coach, significant other(s), studies, and economic or environmental conditions. Further, these stressors can exert either a positive influence on the athlete (eustress) or a negative influence (distress). Now, take an individual with an eating disorder (punch one), and add the stress of training for distance running (punch two), a routine of coffee in the morning (stimulant, punch three), bits of sugar or pop during the day (a sugar high, punch four), social excitement and beer at night (stimulant and depressant, punch five), and you face an individual who has a good chance within two years of knocking out the life support function of their central nervous system. More likely, the athlete's running career will first come to an unfortunate end. Afterwards, the individual may continue to subsist as an arousal addict for decades at a subclinical level.

If this description fits the behavior of an athlete for whom you are responsible, seek out qualified professional help. Even a reasonably knowledgeable coach would be ill advised to take on the role of a clinical psychologist. Sports psychology is something well within the domain of the coach's responsibility and experience. However, the diagnosis, therapy and treatment of addictive disorders is out of bounds. For information on arousal addiction or eating disorders the reader may wish to contact clinical psychologist Scott Pengelly, Ph.D., who has the experience of working with many elite athletes: 1374 Willamette, Suite 6, Eugene, Oregon, 97401- 4075.

Eating disorders are generally found in women, but this is just one of a number of methods of provoking an alarm reaction from the central nervous system. Young men who stay out late (punch one), play video games with fantasy aggression or watch violent sports (punch two), have drinking binges (punch three), eat junk food loaded with excitotoxins such as MSG (punch four), pursue sexual adventures (punch five), and attempt competitive distance running (punch six) operate at nearly the same level. But not much is said

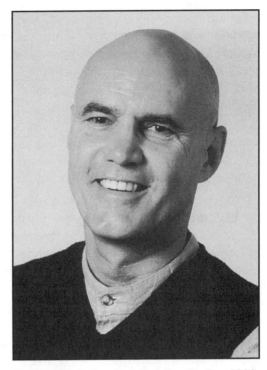

PHOTO 6.2 Scott Pengelly, Ph.D., 1999. (Photo courtesy of Scott Pengelly)

about this dysfunctional male behavior, perhaps due to a cultural blind spot. This behavior may not seem all that abnormal to many people. Such is the way of the world, but not the way of athletics.

Can an individual become a great athlete living this kind of life? Given enough talent, the answer is yes—but generally for less than two years. Alternatively, that individual might have an inconsistent career—with a good athletic season followed by several bad ones. Most natural substance abuse happens at a low enough level not to be life threatening, but it can impair an individual's quality of life. Obviously, an athlete's development can be severely affected, and there are periodic deaths that remind us of what can ultimately happen.

Properly conducted, athletic training comprises a delicate and prudent manipulation of an athlete's central nervous system, biochemistry, and in particular, a number of powerful natural drugs. If all the various stressors are handled just right, then an athlete will have the opportunity to peak at the right time and place. If not, any number of things can happen. The biggest potential stressor of all is the athlete's mind. One evening of toxic thinking can empty the natural drug pharmacy and wipe out a season of preparation as a match burning tinder.

Habituation and Stagnation

There is a limit to how much hard work the human body can tolerate, but also to what it can translate into positive adaptation and improvement. The need for variation cannot be overstressed, given its role in preventing habituation to the training, and resulting physical stagnation. Habituation is but another important reason for taking a period of post-season recovery. As the body becomes overly accustomed to training, less athletic development takes place. What the body once felt as a stressful training load will eventually come to resemble simple equilibrium. In some sense, the body numbs to the stimulus of the training program. Coincidentally, this condition is evidenced by mental staleness and boredom. An athlete needs to take time off to get a bit out of shape and off the natural drugs, so that when the training begins again, it will hurt! The body and mind then react with positive adaptations otherwise known as athletic development.

Unfortunately, many athletes attempt to train and race without a plan or a controlled respite. They end up training more and more to obtain less and less, and by pushing indefinitely, they eventually exceed the limit of their capacities and come down with a crash—the kind of crash an athletic career does not survive.

Resolution of Injuries

In the course of a given athletic season, most serious athletes come close to an injury that would prevent them from being in the best competitive shape of their lives. The best remedy for this is an ounce of prevention. Nevertheless, one day it can be one thing, and the next day another. To some degree we work around injuries during the competitive season, and in our own way, we then choose to ignore the message nature has been giving us. The problem is that in long ignoring nature, she begins to ignore herself. After a time, the body can become accustomed to the injury, and its healing powers begin to less actively focus on the injury in question. Imbalances and weaknesses can develop that could prove debilitating and become permanent. Quality performance in distance running is concerned with long-term processes and outcomes. So take care to remedy injuries during this time of rest and recuperation.

Momentum and Delayed Acquisitions

There is always a degree to which the hard training efforts devoted to acquiring a new athletic level actually suppress performance. Accordingly, athletes do not see all the improvement actually made during an athletic season. The momentum gathered might not become apparent until after the athletes have taken a period of post-season recovery and are well into the next training build-up. At that time, their enhanced athletic ability comes as something of a pleasant surprise. For this reason, the focus should be on quality and the refinement of athletic performance, rather than dramatic acquisitive efforts, during the desired peak athletic season in a multi-year developmental cycle.

De-Training

We are creatures of rhythms, cycles, and habits, and would do violence to nature by treating ourselves abruptly. An athlete's body becomes so accustomed to work that by the end of a season it can interpret the complete cessation of training as traumatic. Unless there is a pressing physical or psychological need, train down over a week's time to a period of post-season recovery.

How Much Time Off?

The phenomenon of delayed transformation also relates to the physical growth and development of young athletes. A growth spurt will suppress athletic development—thus performance—and vice-versa. Demanding training can suppress normal maturation. It is then extremely important to keep in mind the physical age of each athlete—the younger the athlete, the longer the post-season recovery. In the United States, the average high school freshman and sophomore participating in cross-country and track would do best to take off both the entire summer vacation and the winter sport season to obtain adequate post-season recovery. Juniors and seniors should take at least one full month off, and start around the first of July with easy base work to prepare for cross-country, and in late January or early February to prepare for the track season. Collegiate and national class athletes should take a minimum of two weeks of post-season recovery after the completion of an athletic season. More down time may be necessary depending on what physical injuries need to be resolved. And more may be desired, given the individual athlete's mental disposition. In the absence of a physical problem, the latter is the determining factor.

Post-season recovery should not include taxing physical or mental activities. Any recreational activities during this period should not exceed 1/2-effort. The danger here is that athletes flirting with an arousal addiction will simply substitute another activity for running to trigger the alarm reaction and obtain their fix, thereby defeating the entire purpose.

How Much Weight Gain?

Of course, metabolism will slow with diminished activity, especially if multiple training sessions have been the habit. The most noticeable result is a tendency to gain body weight, and sometimes nearly five pounds in two weeks for a 165-pound athlete. This is desirable and should not be discouraged. It is part of the body's way of recharging itself and restoring reserves. This is particularly important for female athletes given the degree to which their metabolism can be disturbed by athletic training. A failure to gain weight during the period of post-season recovery is a warning sign of a possible arousal addiction. However, a gain of over five percent of body weight is unwise for most individuals, as this would be counterproductive to the task of restoring the body's equilibrium. When in training or competition, female distance runners should not drop below eight percent body fat, and a healthy range would nine to 14%. Men should not drop lower than four percent body fat, and a healthy range would be five to 10% (Costill, 1986). Athletes are commonly near the lower limit of body fat during the peak period, and a five percent gain in weight during the post-season recovery period will herald a return to normalcy. For reasons both physical and mental, this practice will prevent a good many problems. No great athlete was ever made in a day, week, or month—but many have been undone in less time. Seek out therapy and appropriate measures for problems that arise. Never go into a new season with old problems. There will be enough new challenges in the coming season.

Psychological Aspects

Perhaps more important than the physical needs are the psychological and emotional needs for a period of post-season recovery. These vary considerably depending upon the maturity of the individual. The coach should normally observe the athlete from a distance at this time. Both the coach and athlete will need a hiatus. Nevertheless, this period can afford some insight into the athlete's personal development. For the sake of simplicity, the common needs and behavior of athletes during the period of post-season recovery can be characterized and divided into one of three levels of maturity:

- The Immature Athlete
- The Maturing Athlete
- The Mature Athlete, or Master

The Immature Athlete

Sports psychology is not the subject of this book, but it is appropriate to here make a few observations. Both coaches and athletes should guard against focusing on outcomes. Ron Clarke, an Australian World Record holder at 5,000 and 10,000 meters in the 1960's, observed that success is not all that rosy because an athlete then tends to become complacent, and failure is not all that bad since it leads an athlete to renewed reflection and determination. However, if a coach and athlete are to be extraordinarily successful and enjoy peace of mind, they need to transcend outcome orientation. That is, they must lose their attachment and desire for success, and their aversion to failure. The right reason for participation in athletics the pursuit of personal cultivation and excellence. Results are incidental to the process. This level of maturity is not often found in adults, and even less amongst young athletes. The young are generally handicapped by their social environment and relative lack of experience. And so the coach often encounters the immature athlete who regards the process as a personal sacrifice (See Percy Cerutty's chapter "On Sacrifice" found in *Success: In Sport and Life,* 1967). The immature athlete is quick to default from the straight and narrow during the athletic season and celebrate success with the usual worldly distractions, or go on a binge in lamenting over failure. Obviously, if still within the competitive season, the failure to maintain psychological integrity can have an adverse effect upon the remainder.

The immature athlete can sometimes be educated to defer the longed for gratifications, or hysterics as the case may be, until after the season. But then the immature athlete will proceed to do all those "sacrificed" things that generally run contrary to the purpose of post-season recovery—such as overexposure to the sun, parties, drinking, poor eating habits, and bad company. Clearly, the immature athlete is not practicing the way of athletics for the sake of the way. Instead, he or she is using athletics as a ticket to get something. That something might be love, attention, money, social esteem, a car, or the attention of the opposite sex.

If an athlete is not participating for the right reason, then it is the coach's job to point this out. The immature athlete should be advised with honesty and compassion to pursue what he or she really wants by a more direct route. If, after this the immature athlete still want to use athletics as a ticket to get something else, then he or she must search for another teacher. Why? Because the immature athlete is not sincere. The decision to become sincere transforms the immature athlete into a maturing athlete.

The Maturing Athlete

The maturing athlete is sincere and is searching for the way. The maturing athlete will show a readiness for enlightenment on a particular subject by asking appropriate questions. Then, the coach's role is to indicate the way—answer the question or direct the athlete to an environment or experience that holds the answer. When the maturing athlete finds the way, the coach's role is to nod and affirm the discovery. The maturing athlete still struggles with attachment to outcome orientation, and to various desires and aversions. But the maturing athlete is sincere in attempting to transcend these things and pursue personal cultivation.

The most common problem is the result of outcome orientation, whereby the maturing athlete focuses too greatly on becoming instead of being. Frequently, the maturing athlete views the way as a self-perfection project, ultimately defined by attachment of the ego to externalities. Moreover, the maturing athlete wants to complete the project NOW. The maturing athlete has a tendency to lose contact with the here and now and can miss enjoyment of the process. The maturing athlete has not yet "arrived" in life (as the outcome-orientated quest is sometimes called) and so lacks peace of mind. Obviously, we all fit the description of the maturing athlete during the larger part of our lives.

With the immature athlete, and to a lesser degree the maturing athlete, success and failure are like sticks of emotional dynamite. The coach sometimes then assumes the job of carefully measuring out small doses of each to use as carrots in order to maintain some kind of emotional equilibrium. Meanwhile, the coach attempts to wean the athlete away from outcome orientation and the quest for so-called success, towards process orientation and excellence.

Too much success too early can easily result in complacency. When it comes to the emotional gumption required for superior performance, this could mean that the immature or maturing athlete is finished—at least for that particular season. On the other hand, too much so-called failure can lead to despair, a crisis of confidence, and a premature end to participation.

Since the coach places a value on the activity and process, there is a natural desire to try to influence the situation to prevent either of these two extremes. Moreover, the unexamined assumption is that these unfortunate events are not supposed to happen. This assumption is not correct. In manipulating the carrots, a coach may be partly motivated by outcome orientation—the desire for a successful season. Moreover, the coach may also be acting out of compassion—a sincere desire to save athletes from the painful experiences associated with straying from the path. Regardless of the coach's intentions, manipulation of the carrots may come to be resented by the immature or maturing athlete as a form of mind game, and more so when the athlete's ultimate success has depended on the coach's management.

The problem is that society tells coaches they are expected to succeed and not to fail: winning is good, losing is bad. The unexamined assumption is that athletes under the coach must do the same. Athletics becomes a part of the entertainment industry as opposed to a vehicle of education. And so the coach acts to prevent the athletes from experiencing failure. Disaster occurs when the outward manifestation of success is out of step with their true level of maturity. This is a story with an unhappy ending. Sometimes athletes need to fail. Failure or temporary non-success is an essential part of the natural process. Coaches sometimes need to let athletes fail. Their response to non-success ultimately determines the course of their personal growth and character development.

The difficult question faced by every coach is—just where do actions taken as an educator end, and where do they threaten to interfere with the natural process? The line is not always easy to discern. As coaches mature and witness the destructive effects that so-called success can have, they often find themselves more reserved and much less inclined to mark and clear the minefield of athletic life.

Whereas the immature athlete may regard the period of post-season recovery as an opportunity to make up for lost sacrifices, the maturing athlete generally has a different perspective. Again, the maturing athlete is still not completely liberated from outcome orientation. Attaining an outcome at the end of the athletic season therefore impacts the maturing athlete. In the days following the mental high associated with the last event of the competitive season, regardless of its outcome, a maturing athlete generally experiences an emotional low, or mental state bordering depression. A pronounced feeling of relief, sometimes mixed with an inability to absorb it all, tends to leave the maturing athlete with an identity crisis.

Athletics is an intense and highly compressed form of life. The pressures, decisions and changes, which normally shape the personality over many months and years, come in the span of minutes, days and weeks. One moment, athletes aspire to become both within and without, what moments later they have become! Few things test the resiliency of the personality more severely. Sometimes, the personality cannot withstand the stress, and is harmed. Too much success can often be far more dangerous than failure. We have a natural inclination to overcome failure, but few guard themselves with respect to success.

In any case, the maturing athlete needs to assimilate and accommodate this experience and take stock of his or her new self. The maturing athlete will not be mentally refitted to pursue the question—where do I go from here—before having come to grips with the fundamental question—who am I? This may take but a few days.

A maturing athlete may be carried away by the feeling of the moment and be possessed to start training again in earnest. The maturing athlete is sincere about personal cultivation, but again, the common problem is he or she views the process with outcome orientation, and as a project to be completed now. This puts the maturing athlete in jeopardy of unwittingly becoming an arousal addict.

The coach and athlete must guard against this tendency, since subjective feelings are most deceptive—just as in the twilight of a superior performance, where mental excitement masks a state of exhaustion. This can be equally true in success or failure. The former can lead one on as an intoxicant, while the latter serves as a goad. And in an effort to prove himself or herself, the maturing athlete may be driven to an imprudent course of action.

In the event of success, the thinking often goes: if some was good, more is better. And with failure: if some was not enough, more is necessary. Neither may be true. Certainly neither is true at this time. If the maturing athlete has been truly serious about sport, it has been a long, hard season and the individual needs a rest. Returning directly to serious training will likely lead to a few days or weeks of largely misguided work, followed by a physical and mental letdown that could last indefinitely, thus impeding rather than enhancing further progress.

In purely rational terms, the maturing athlete's recent experience might be assimilated and accommodated directly. But it is the emotional and not the rational aspect of the personality that carries an athlete through the vicissitudes of an athletic season and life. Nothing great was ever accomplished without emotion. It is not a commodity an athlete would want to run out of halfway through an athletic season. There is a physical and a mental or emotional peak in athletics. They must both happen at the right time if a superior performance is to be possible.

In a short time, the feelings of the moment pass away and permit the athlete to see things objectively, with a certain detachment. There is a fine line between inspiration and obsession. The coach and athlete would do well to watch over themselves. In particular, when faced with adversity, the athlete should beware rationalizations or spin doctors, since words can deceive. Things are what they are. An old Chinese saying: Seek truth from facts.

During post-season recovery, the maturing athlete may alternate between states of unrest—even nervous irritability—and states of physical and mental fatigue brought on by no apparent reason. For the physical and psychological reasons above, it is not uncommon for an athlete to sleep and catnap more than usual. At this time, the subconscious faculty is working overtime to sort things out and perhaps even catch up. The expanded dream-life necessarily connected with expanded sleep time reflects this mental need. In waking life, the athlete may feel that they want to do something, and yet nothing in particular!

To some degree, these states give evidence that the maturing athlete is experiencing withdrawal symptoms from the aforementioned natural drugs. This is needed. A good indication of successful post-season recovery—is that the athlete does not feel the urge to run. An athlete will then do well to engage in some kind of activity, but not distance running. It is healthier to strike a balance and explore other areas of life. In a few weeks, the initial feelings of relief, and the question of whether one would ever do that again, will be answered. In sum, the sequence that a maturing athlete may experience following the seasonal high could include:

- Letdown and depression
- Fatigue alternating with energy, even irritability
- Restless desire to do things and yet nothing
- Boredom
- A certain self-awareness, determination and renewed enthusiasm to achieve new goals and purposes

At some point, an individual may become satisfied and will then have outgrown the vehicle of athletics as a means of achieving personal growth. In brief, the athlete has graduated, and it is time to move on to the next stage of life and other challenges. The coach's role is to then assist the individual, and facilitate his or her continued journey.

The Mature Athlete or Master

Living in the eternal present—the now—the mature athlete is not greatly affected by the outcome of the athletic season. Its conclusion is anticlimactic. No personal crises are evoked in its wake. Seeing no antics from a mature athlete who has just attained a great success, the immature or maturing athlete might think: "This person has no enthusiasm." Not so. The mature athlete was present, being there all along, and enjoyed the entire process, that is, each and every day. In contrast, the maturing athlete probably worked impatiently on an outcome-orientated quest, focused on becoming, and missed most of it. For the maturing athlete, the entire experience could well have ridden on the big race, or would-be payday—a single day. To miss so much life and to lack peace of mind for months or years, hoping to find it on one day in the externalities associated with success, seems an absurd proposition to the mature athlete.

Something should perhaps be said about the proper role of the coach regarding an individual who has progressed to the point of becoming a mature athlete or potential master: you have to let go. Sometimes coaches are people who like to control people. That is not healthy for either party. The external master of the coach, once having assisted in the process of cultivating the athlete's inner master to a critical mass of maturity, should then retreat to permit the natural process to complete itself (Dürckheim, 1989).

Often, athletes will suffer anxiety about having greater independence, and may even think the coach is no longer concerned about them. However, the external master can become a crutch, thus hindering athletes from truly exercising freedom of choice, and assuming responsibility for the consequences of their life decisions. This would prevent athletes from realizing their limitations—but also their ultimate potential. Sometimes athletes will take a fall from an established level and never return to it. Sometimes they will go onward and surpass their teacher. Either outcome can lead to personal growth, and simply reflects the natural order of things.

> *If the foundations we stand on in natural consciousness actually prevent us from experiencing Being, then the master who wants to lead us to experience must first do everything they can to knock them away. That is why their actions often startle like bolts from the blue, why they speak in riddles, why shock tactics are their tenderness, and nonsense their logic.*
>
> *The master of a skill has purged his technique of ego and is able to hand it over to a higher power and let that power act for him. No ordinary yardstick can be used to measure the result, since something more than visible achievement is at stake—namely, revelation of another dimension. When the student finally achieves mastery, this dimension reveals itself in five ways:*
>
> *In the basic attitude of the person performing the feat.*
>
> *In the perfection of the feat itself.*
>
> *In the power reflected in the feat.*
>
> *In what the person performing it experiences.*
>
> *In its numinous effect on those who witness it.*
>
> — Karlfied Graf Dürckheim

References

Brand-Miller, Jennie, and Kay Foster-Powell, Stephen Colagiuri, Thomas M.S. Wolever, Anthony Leeds, *The Glucose Revolution: The Authoritative Guide to the Glycaemic Index-The Groundbreaking Medical Discovery,* New York: Marlowe & Co., 1999.

Cerutty, Percy, *Success: In Sport and Life,* London: Pelham Books Ltd., 1967.

Costill, David L., *Inside Running: Basics of Sports Physiology,* Carmel, Indiana: Cooper Publishing Group, LLC, 1986.

Coyle, Edward F., "Substate Utilization During Exercise in Active People," *American Journal of Clinical Nutrition,* Volume 61, 4th Suppliment, 1995, pages 968S-979S.

Coyle, Edward F., and Effie Coyle, "Carbohydrates That Speed Recovery From Training," *The Physician and Sportsmedicine,* 1983, Volume 21, Number 2, pages 111-123.

Dürckheim, Karlfried Graf, *The Call For The Master*, New York: E.P. Dutton, 1989, pages 60, 61, and 64.

Pengelly, Scott, *Conversations on Arousal Addiction in Athletes,* Eugene, Oregon, 1988-1997.

Podell, Richard N., and William Proctor, *The G-Index Diet,* New York: Warner Books, Inc., 1993.

PART II

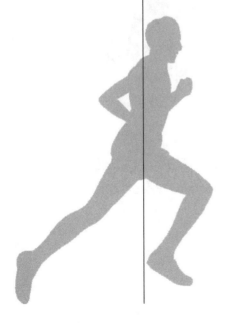

STRENGTH, FLEXIBILITY AND INJURY PREVENTION

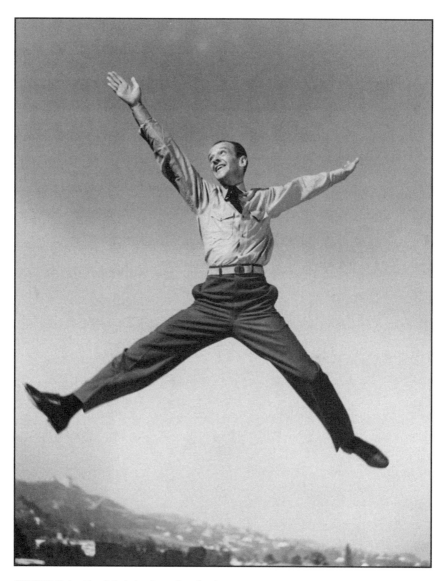

PHOTO 7.1—Fred Astaire jumping for joy. Copyright Otto Bettman / CORBIS, 1941. Reprinted with permission.

CHAPTER 7

Stretching, Flexibility and Movement

At the beginning of team practice, athletes commonly get together with their coach for a brief meeting. They then normally conduct a number of stretching exercises before running the day's primary workout. In the absence of sufficient discipline, young people will often turn this meeting, and the flexibility program, into a chitchat session. The resulting attention deficit is characterized by a lack of physical and mental awareness. Various stretching exercises are then performed imperfectly. In fact, the actual time spent on stretching might not be more than 25 percent of the time assigned to the task. Nevertheless, athletes will then conduct flexibility exercises to obtain full range of motion about their joints, and warm-up for at least a half-mile before performing a more thorough stretching routine. Generally, the athletes will assume a number of individual static stretching exercises, and perhaps even some contract-relax, or hold-relax Proprioceptive Neuromuscular Facilitation (PNF) stretching. The athletes then run the day's primary workout. Unfortunately, the training session will likely be conducted on a hard asphalt or artificial track surface. Afterwards, the athletes will perform another stretching session, but with the same lack of focus. Essentially, the same routine is repeated every day. As a result of common *unpractice* of the day, the athletes fail to enhance their flexibility and running technique.

Heredity, Education, and Experience

Our physical make-up and metabolism is largely determined by our genetic endowment. We are dealt our hand in life, and then do our best to play it. Human beings initially learn much through imitation. How we walk, talk, and even run can be the product of imitation. Individuals commonly have a cultural and personal blind spot to these largely unconscious, imitative habits. Some people walk with their toes pointed outwards, and others with their toes pointed inwards. And some athletes carry their arms high and close to the chest, whereas others carry them low and below the waist. Later in life, we may suddenly come to realize how much we speak and walk like one of our parents. Much of this behavior is self-taught and the product of informal education. Obviously, our technique can also stem from formal education, and how we were originally taught to perform an action. Experience is the product of action, and numerous repeated like actions create habits and neuromuscular stereotypes. In short, an individual's characteristic movements are a product of genetics, education, and experience. Unfortunately, part of this experience may include injury to the body and its movement patterns.

Neuromuscular Scar Tissue

An individual's biomechanics and running style sometimes reflects their history of injury. An adjustment once made to provide relief for an injury can replace an earlier and more desirable running technique. Robert Bly used the analogy of an invisible black bag to describe the subconscious psychological baggage that people often drag around behind them (Bly, 1988). Likewise, athletes sometimes drag behind them a black bag of physical and mental scar tissue from previous physical injuries. Unfortunately, after the injury has healed, the injured movement pattern can remain, and the affected athlete may have no kinesthetic awareness of this change. Athletes may believe they still move the same way, but in reality they do not.

Kinesthetic Sense, Lies and Video Tape

There can be a wide gap between what an athlete perceives concerning their running style, and what they are actually doing. An athlete's kinesthetic sense and mental image of their running style is generally a big lie. The fact that athletes run in protective footwear tends to decrease their kinesthetic sense of just where and what their feet are doing. Athletes commonly make biomechanical adjustments when running on various shoes and surfaces, and are not cognizant of these changes.

To remedy this situation, their level of awareness needs to be raised. They need to realize that there is a gap between their mental picture and reality. Given greater awareness, they can decide to do something about the discrepancy and close the gap. Athletes can stop themselves when they are about to make an error, and instead, make a conscious effort to perform the action correctly. Repeated actions form habits. Right habits of movement are biomechanical virtues. From a motor learning standpoint, this phenomenon is similar to the Pavlovian conditioned response, and the stimulus-response chains of the Behaviorist and Experimental psychologists (Pavlov, 1927).

This concept can also be found in the Alexander Technique, developed by F. M. Alexander in England (Alexander, 1995). Alexander found that the body's kinesthetic sense can indeed lie. He used the word "inhibition" to describe when an individual consciously stops and catches the body before it has a chance to commit another lie. Alexander used the phrase "directed activity" to describe the conscious performance of the activity in a proper manner.

Alexander realized that static positions and repetitive activities create strain on the body and cause it to become unbalanced. He understood that people use imitation in neuromuscular learning, and an individual's emotional distress can be imparted to the body and reflected in movement. Alexander taught the use of slow and reversible movements. When these were mastered, other actions could be performed with greater control, speed, and power. Alexander taught absence of effort—that is, only what needs to be done is done—and this was normally associated with slow and relaxed breathing. He recognized that end-gaining or outcome orientation could disturb the performance of an action. He then properly focused upon correct process—Alexander was an intelligent and progressive man.

The discoveries of Alexander came about due to his own inability to speak properly at a time when he was *desperately* trying to pursue an acting career on stage. In brief, he was outcome-oriented and literally choked. Like the ever-rational detective Sherlock Holmes, Alexander approached the problem or crime his body had committed by analytically observing the physical evidence. And in viewing the evidence, he recognized various physical phenomena and changed his bodily behavior. These changes in physical behavior brought changes to his basic mental outlook. Such was the nature of his path to enlightenment.

Today, someone like Alexander could seek the help of a good sports psychologist and focus on the primary problem, as opposed to the mere physical symptoms. Alexander would directly confront the problems associated with his outcome-oriented outlook. He would be instructed to recognize the physical and mental canaries. And he would be taught various methods of centering, relaxation, biofeedback, and how to successfully perform the desired activity in a manner not unlike what he eventually discovered for himself (For more on the Alexander Technique, see Alexander, 1995, and Drake, 1996).

Two things can be used to great advantage in wiping an athlete's slate clean of biomechanical faults and restoring sound running technique. One is the liberal use of videotape, which can prove invaluable for enhancing self-awareness. The other is walking and running barefoot on natural grass or sand surfaces. After starting to walk and run on grass, runners who have had injury problems for years and bounced from one doctor to the next without relief have come right in less than a month. There are many reasons why this works, but they largely boil down to one simple fact: walking and running barefoot on grass or sand is natural and normal. Asphalt and athletic shoes are relatively recent inventions, and they are not necessarily performance enhancing or healthy.

Faulty Surfaces Instill Faulty Technique

In the United States, athletes commonly run their primary training sessions on asphalt roads or the track. The road surfaces are normally hard, flat, and minimize turns or variations in elevation. Many roads incorporate transverse grades of five or more degrees to promote water run-off, and this can result in effective leg length differences. Athletes who run on asphalt tend to stagnate and habituate as a result of repeated motor actions. Instead of having to negotiate the nuances of surface variation, the body experiences sameness. Instead making frequent turns, the athletes might run in a straight line for miles. Instead of the challenge of rolling uphills and downhills, they experience the world as relatively flat.

Such extreme habituation and stagnation can develop into a certain stiffness and incompleteness in their movements. From the standpoint of motor learning, running on asphalt resembles what is referred to as blocked practice, as opposed to random practice—which takes place in a natural environment. Greater learning takes place when athletes experience random practice (Schmidt, 1988, and 1991). Further, when the body attempts to protect itself from shock loads, the biomechanical adjustments normally result in a shortening of the stride and less energetic application of force to the support surface. The athletes can become economic shufflers on the asphalt.

From the standpoint of mental concentration and focus, the continuity of the asphalt running surface and the monotony of the terrain can allow athletes to run without paying much attention to their biomechanics. They can, for the most part, run on automatic pilot. This can lead to muscular imbalances, injury and mental staleness. Athletes can't treat themselves like Pavlov's dog every day without starting to sniff, scratch, and bark at some point.

Running on natural terrain requires greater concentration, focus, and directed awareness. If athletes do not pay attention when running in a natural environment, they can easily trip or turn an ankle on a protruding obstacle. Running in a natural environment requires focus and one-pointed attention. The mind is absorbed in doing only what the body is doing. This oneness of mind and body is the *sine qua non* for physical and mental development.

Moreover, the enhanced cushioning effects of natural surfaces facilitate a fuller, more energetic stride, and higher oxygen demand, thus inducing a greater training effect. All things being equal, the better an athlete's running style, the less stretching and flexibility work he or she will have to do.

Proper Stretching and Flexibility

What constitutes correct stretching? Some might say to stretch like a cat and that is well. People do, in fact, stretch like a cat—that is, when they are not imitating a stretching activity they have seen or been taught. Think about how people stretch when they first awaken, as when lying on a couch. Their entire body moves in complete coordination. You cannot say there is a sequence of individual actions, rather, the entire activity happens together. Visualize how this happens:

Their feet alternately dorsiflex and plantarflex as they take a long deep breath. Then they subtly contract and relax the muscles of the lower leg, upper leg, buttocks, abdomen, back, shoulders and neck. Simultaneously, they raise their arms with the application of muscular contraction and relaxation, and move them asymmetrically as their head turns from side to side. And then they will slowly exhale with the sound of a yawn. It is as if their entire body responds to a continuous moving wave of muscular contraction and relaxation, just as a cat does when it first awakens. This is how human beings stretch naturally. Anything else is learned, and in that sense, contrived. Much of what is contrived is incorrect.

Conventional Stretching and Flexibility Exercises

How do conventional stretching and flexibility exercises rate? Is there a correct relationship or progression between different stretching and flexibility exercises? Ballistic stretching, that is, bobbing or forcing a muscle to stretch at a fast rate, is widely known to be ineffective and dangerous because it can induce injury (McAtee and Charland, 1993). However, this should not be confused with slow and deliberate stretching while moving the affected body part. Nor should it be confused with rapid actions that are the product of a progression of acquired skills.

Passive stretching, whereby the individual has a partner manipulate the body part to be stretched, also carries some of the injury risks found with ballistic stretch-

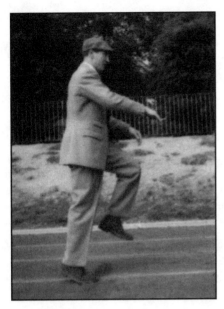 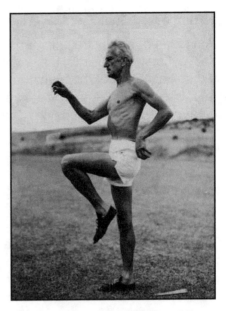

PHOTOS 7.2 & 7.3—The contrasting styles of rival coaches Franz Stampfl (left) and Percy Cerutty (right) are captured in these two photographs. The left photograph by Larry Burrows is from *Sports Illustrated*, November 26, 1956, page 84, courtesy of Russell Burrows; and the right photograph is from *Success: In Sport and Life*, London: Pelham Books, Ltd., 1967, and courtesy of Nancy Cerutty.

ing. These risks primarily stem from a possible communication gap between stretcher and stretchee. The presence of a partner can also result in numerous breaks in concentration. Given healthy individuals with full neuromuscular function, passive stretching is not advisable. However, if an individual has been incapacitated and cannot perform a stretching exercise, there is no other practical alternative.

Static stretching exercises are similar to learning the letters of the alphabet. They are a good place to start. Done properly, static stretching can accomplish basic stretching of targeted connective tissue including a muscle or muscle group. And static stretching can thereby enhance the athlete's flexibility consistent with the particular technique of a given static stretch. However, static stretching accomplishes little else. Muscles move in multiple planes, and one of the limitations of static stretching is that it tends to isolate only a single plane.

Proprioceptive Neuromuscular Facilitation (PNF) is more interesting since it uses what we understand to be natural stretching—that is, the kind of stretching that happens when we awaken from a nap. Hold Relax (HR), Contract Relax (CR) and Contract-Relax Antagonist-Contract (CRAC) more closely resemble how cats and humans stretch naturally. Single-muscle PNF stretching takes the letters of the alphabet—and is the first step towards forming individual words. When an individual applies muscular effort to affect the PNF single muscle stretch, a fuller stretch is possible. This is because of a greater recruitment of the affected muscle, due in part to subtle rotational movements. PNF stretching then becomes even more interesting when it turns to the use of spiral-diagonal patterns. Now an individual is forming words and even short sentences (Voss, et. al., 1985).

What Range And Quality of Movement Can The Unaided Individual Demonstrate?

The limitation of static stretching and PNF is that these activities are not sufficient to affect dynamic flexibility in the context of athletic performance. For example, in a seated static stretch of the hamstrings, athletes might be able to demonstrate an angle of less than 90 degrees between their torso and leg. But if they stand up and assume a normal vertical posture, then slowly raise their right leg as high as possible with their knee in a locked position, they may not be able to demonstrate even half of that range of motion.

When an individual maintains a normal posture of the head, neck and back, and conducts a slow, controlled movement of the limbs, pausing a moment to hold the maximum attainable position—that is their true range of motion and dynamic flexibility in the context of athletic performance. It certainly is not what they can attain during a static stretch with the assistance of a partner or a resisting surface. The range of dynamic flexibility that an individual can demonstrate in slow, smooth movements with proper posture, without any other means of support or application of force, approximates what they can exhibit when running.

For example, let's say that an individual stands up and assumes normal posture, then extends their right leg from the hip rearward with their knee nearly locked, and also moves their foot into plantar and dorsiflexed positions. Whatever they can exhibit when performing this movement slowly and deliberately approximates what they can exhibit when running. This is simple and fundamental, but unfortunately, sometimes not appreciated.

Dynamic stretching and flexibility movements are suggestive of the movements of great dancers. Arthur Lydiard and Percy Cerutty both held that distance runners could benefit by participating in dance at some point in their athletic development. The point is well taken.

Train the Whole and Get the Parts, Do Not Train the Parts and Miss the Whole

When athletes engage in dynamic stretching and flexibility exercises, many other aspects of fitness come into play. Their ability to balance, muscular strength, coordination, motor memory, learning, and neuromuscular inhibition all enter the picture. Some readers might have actually stood up and attempted to raise their leg in the positions described above and sensed that flexibility was not their limiting problem. They may have found themselves protesting that part of what the author suggested requires balance, part requires strength, and part requires coordination. And to hold the leg in a particular position for several seconds will require training in neuromuscular inhibition, and so on. That is right. That is precisely the point. The whole is larger than its parts. And unless you embrace the whole, the desired quality of flexibility will not be manifest during athletic performance. Our ego-conscious self prefers to slice reality up into many tiny pieces, but that is not the nature of reality.

If you cannot balance well enough to stand on the left leg and hold the right with almost a locked knee in various positions, then that is your limitation.

If you can balance well enough, but cannot hold your leg in a position for long due to a lack of strength, then that is your limitation.

If your agonist muscle sends a message to the antagonist to contract when a certain amount of tension or muscle fatigue sets in, then that is your limitation.

If your kinesthetic sense lies to you about your movements, then that is your limitation.

If you cannot perform multiple movements with grace due to a lack of coordination, then that is your limitation.

If you do not focus on an action, and perform it incompletely or badly, then that is your limitation.

Any number of possible combinations can determine an individual's range of motion and dynamic flexibility. The limitations of static and PNF stretching are that they do not address many of the above-mentioned phenomena.

> *All things and events of the universe originate, co-exist, and integrate simultaneously, being correlated not only in reference to space, but also time. Hence the fundamental idea is simultaneity*
>
> —Dōgen Kigen

Making Words into Sentences into Poetry

If static stretching is the alphabet, and aspects of PNF stretching are words and short sentences, then poetry is something resembling a hybrid of *T'ai Chi, Yoga*, and the *Kata* performed in Karate. Is the poem better than the sentence, or the sentence better than a single letter of the alphabet? This is a nonsensical question, because these things are mutually interdependent.

T'ai Chi as a meditative movement teaches mental concentration and personal cultivation. The relatively vertical relationship maintained between the head, neck, and back while performing the movement is also consistent with the Alexander Technique. Some of the individual forms are appropriate for distance runners, but the historical evolution of T'ai Chi was heavily influenced by the martial arts, and so many of its forms are best suited to those activities. Further, T'ai Chi is not a stretching or flexibility exercise, at least not in the conventional sense.

The student of Karate often performs the Kata. The Kata is an exhibition of correct technique performed in a continuous manner so as to resemble dance. Sometimes the Kata is practiced at full speed and with considerable exhibition of power. However, the specific forms practiced in Karate are far removed from distance running.

The strongest teachings regarding stretching and flexibility are in the Yogic tradition. However, the Yogic forms and poses are seldom taught to comprise one continuous flowing movement as found in T'ai Chi or the Kata. The Yogic *Soorya Namaskar*, or Sun Exercise, perhaps comes closest to the type of sequencing, dynamic stretching and flexibility that would prove advantageous for distance runners. There is an outstanding need to identify Yogic forms suitable for distance runners, and to choreograph them into a sequence that enables them to be performed in a continuous, flowing manner, as in T'ai Chi and the Kata—to comprise a suitable dynamic stretching and flexibility routine.

All three of the aforementioned disciplines teach essentially compatible and desirable breathing techniques. The following dynamic stretching and flexibility routine integrates all three traditions.

Dynamic Stretching and Flexibility Routine

The following dynamic stretching and flexibility routine includes numerous individual poses conducted in a sequence as part of one continuous exercise. While many might find this particular form suitable for themselves in daily practice, it reflects the author's own physique, age, experience and particular areas of weakness. Athletes are encouraged to try this particular routine for themselves, but also to create their own. In the light of circumstances, they might want to adapt their routine on a daily basis. The essential part lies in the principles and manner in which the routine is practiced, and not in a particular set of poses or sequence. However, in order to grasp the principles and basic technique, athletes can begin with the following routine:

Start by standing with your feet spaced normally, with correct posture (Photo 7.4). Take a relaxed, deep breath. Then slowly bend forward from the waist towards the floor with outstretched arms, and slowly exhale. Time your exhale to end at the lowest portion of the movement. Pause and retain your diaphragm in the contracted position for several seconds as you briefly hold the lowest portion of the movement, while still maintaining the integrity between the alignment of the head, neck and back. During this movement, slowly contract and relax the muscles of the toes, then legs, and so on up to the head and fingers, as when waking from sleep. This directed awareness and contract-relax activity should take place as you reach the maximum stretch in each and every individual movement within the routine (Photo 7.5).

Then inhale as you straighten up at a rate twice as fast as when descending. This should provide a ratio with respect to the duration of inhalation, retention, and exhalation approximating 1:4:2 (Swami Vishnu-devananda, 1988). Then, with a full breath in the up position, and no break in movement, bend from the waist backwards, gradually thrusting the hips forward and exhaling (Photo 7.6).

Recover to the upright position while inhaling, and then bend from the hip to the right while exhaling (Photo 7.7).

Then, recover to the upright position while inhaling, and do the same routine to the left (Photo 7.8). Then step into a wider figure "X" stance with the arms and legs outstretched, and repeat the above-mentioned forward, backward, and side-to-side movements (Photos 7.9—7.13).

Then, from the standing position, bend at the right knee and lower the torso over the right foot, leaving the left leg in the extended position and thereby stretch the adductors of the left leg (Photo 7.14).

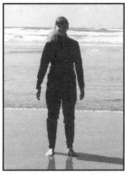 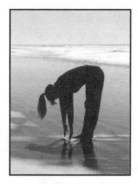 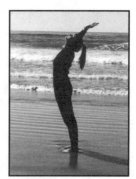

PHOTO 7.4   **PHOTO 7.5**   **PHOTO 7.6**

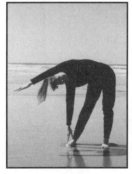 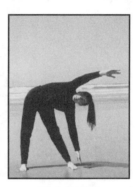

PHOTO 7.7   **PHOTO 7.8**

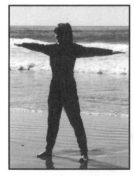 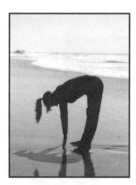 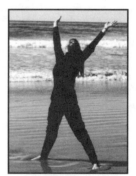

PHOTO 7.9   **PHOTO 7.10**   **PHOTO 7.11**

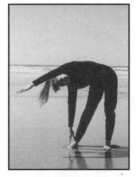 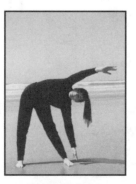

PHOTO 7.12   **PHOTO 7.13**

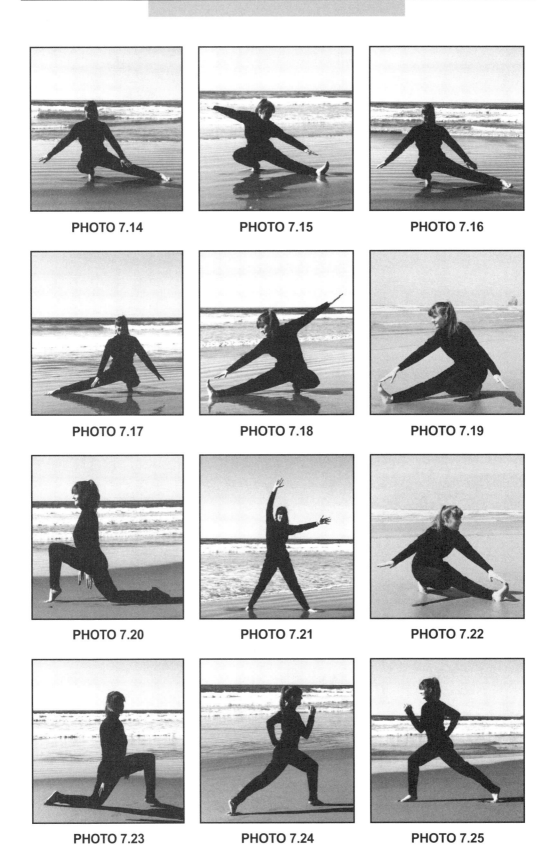

PHOTO 7.14

PHOTO 7.15

PHOTO 7.16

PHOTO 7.17

PHOTO 7.18

PHOTO 7.19

PHOTO 7.20

PHOTO 7.21

PHOTO 7.22

PHOTO 7.23

PHOTO 7.24

PHOTO 7.25

In all of these movements, exhale during the stretch. Then, as you achieve the maximum stretch, pause, holding the diaphragm in the contracted position, and inhale during the release. Conduct the muscular contraction and relaxation from toes to head (including the primary target group) in unison with the movement. Your arms can be raised to the sides and extended overhead so that the fingers of your hands touch at the maximum position.

Inhale while rotating the extended leg so that the foot points upward. Then exhale while bringing your arms towards the leg, and perhaps grasp the toes of the extended foot to stretch the hamstrings of the left leg (Photo 7.15). Next, inhale as you rotate your extended leg downward to again bear weight on the support surface (Photo 7.16).

Exhale while ascending from the weight-bearing right leg, switch over to the left, and exhale while lowering the torso in a similar manner over the left leg. Again, for balance and to help maintain a vertical alignment, your arms can be raised, extended, and the fingers of your hands can be locked over your head while completing the lowering motion. This will stretch the adductors of the extended right leg (Photo 7.17).

Then, inhale while rotating the extended right leg so that your right foot points upward, and exhale while extending your arms toward it, and perhaps grasp the toes of the extended foot to stretch the hamstrings of the right leg (Photo 7.18).

Then, inhale while rotating your left thigh from its perpendicular position (in relation to the extended right leg) to a position parallel and adjacent to the right leg. The ball of the left foot and the heel of the extended right foot remain planted during this movement (Photo 7.19).

Then, as you begin to exhale, shift forward on the extended right foot, which will then flatten on the support surface while the right knee rises. At the same time, lower the left knee to the support surface, and continue the forward movement until the left thigh extends rearward from the hip, and the right knee is slightly forward of the ball of the right foot (Photo 7.20).

Again, this is done in one continuous movement, and the position resembles a fully extended stride. For runners, this is a functional version of the splits, and it stretches the quads of the leg that has its knee bearing upon the support surface. You should exhale as you assume the forward extended position, and then simultaneously attempt to flex forward the rearward extended upper leg, which should nevertheless remain in the planted and fixed position. While executing this movement, you can raise both arms over your head and join the fingers of your hands.

Next, rise up on both feet enough to disengage the planted left knee, and then, while evenly bearing weight on the balls of both feet, rotate 180° (Photo 7.21). Then descend, bending the right knee, and sit over the right foot with your left leg in the extended position. This duplicates the position in Photo 7.19, but now for the opposite side (Photo 7.22).

Then descend on the right knee to conduct the same movement for that side, as described earlier. While attaining and retaining the forward extended position, exhale and hold the diaphragm briefly in the contracted position (Photo 7.23). Then inhale while elevating the torso, and in so doing, raise the weight-bearing knee from the support surface so that the weight rests on the balls of both feet, thus moving into the position of a fully developed running stride. Then, as you move the knee of the rearward extending right leg to an almost locked position, exhale, and contract and relax the flexors of the rearward-extended leg (Photo 7.24). Next, pivoting on the balls of the feet, rotate 180° and reverse the relative position of both legs (Photo 7.25).

Then, perform the same dynamic stretching and flexibility movement for that side, as just described, with the breathing pattern coordinated with the movements. As you complete some of the individual dynamic stretching and flexibility movements, you might do the contract-relax stretch that happens when awaking from sleep, which travels in a continuous wave from toes to head and outstretched arms.

Having completed this progression in a slow, deliberate manner, athletes are usually quite flexible. While saving time is not a goal, this routine actually takes far less time than most athletes often spend doing disassociated static and PNF stretching exercises.

In order to enhance the effect of the dynamic flexibility exercise: Both before and after the above routine, the athletes should visualize the entire conduct of the routine. In particular, the athletes should imagine the external and internal movements of the body, and in particular, mentally project the desired practical effects. This is in contrast with the athletes' focus during the physical performance of the routine, when their attention should be directed to actual performance of the movements. One simple way to recall the sequence of movements in the larger routine is to visualize while mimicking the breathing pattern. This makes recollection easy.

There are a number of reasons for using visualization or imagery techniques both before and after physical exercise. The visualization exercise before the routine turns on the key—effectively starting and warming up the body. It is then possible to conduct the physical aspects of the routine more effectively. As athletes prepare to take strenuous exercise, they also warm up mentally and emotionally. The memories and emotions from previous experiences, step up the nervous system to an increased "tone." Done correctly, this helps to prepare the body for the demands soon to be placed upon it.

After the dynamic stretching and flexibility routine, athletes should again conduct the visualization routine because, as those familiar with the Feldenkrais method are aware, actual improvement is greater through visualization than through action (Feldenkrais, 1990). However, note that in the Feldenkrais teachings, so-called visualization is not merely visual. Rather, individuals are directed to imagine the sensory feelings and input associated with the actions, and to focus on the kinesthetic sense. Imagining what the action will *feel* like and noticing these subtle differences is more effective than visualizing the action, that is, merely seeing it.

Conducting the imagery routine after a dynamic stretching and flexibility session also serves to turn the key off—and quiet the mind and body. Otherwise, even after the workout, the athlete's mind and body might remain in a state of heightened readiness and activity. This phenomenon is well understood in Yogic teachings.

> *More of our energy is spent keeping the muscles in continual readiness for work than in actual useful work done. To regulate and balance the work of the body and mind, you need to learn to economize the energy produced by our body, which is the main purpose of learning how to relax.*
>
> —Swami Vishnu-devananda

To turn off and cool down the body after exercise, athletes should lie in the Yogic corpse pose, flat on their back upon a supporting surface with arms slightly outstretched. They should then engage in relaxed breathing, and imagine their internal body parts and the intended action, while sequentially contracting and relaxing the primary target muscles of the body, starting with the toes and working up towards the head and arms. This completes the dynamic stretching and flexibility routine. When athletes observe this practice, they will find that their muscles do not tighten up so greatly in the hours following exercise. Otherwise, only a few hours later, they might find themselves less flexible than they were shortly after exercise. At a subliminal level, this can easily interfere with their ability to get to sleep.

Yoga

Almost every stretching pose imaginable is a part of the Yogic tradition and has therein been given a name. The previous dynamic stretching and flexibility routine can be considered a hybrid form of Yoga. A serious student of yoga will recognize that it begins with meditation, then flows to *pratikriya*, then to goal-oriented *asana* practice, then back to *pratikriya* and to meditation. However, many other Yogic poses and routines can be advantageous for distance runners. In this regard, the reader may see two fine books: *The Runner's Yoga Book*, by Jean Couch, 1990, and *Yoga For Wellness*, by Gary Kraftsow, 1999, which contains an excellent discussion of sequencing.

Distance runners should occasionally practice at least the following yogic forms: the cobra, dog, superman or locust, bow, triangle, Lord Nataraja, ankle-knee, open angle, head-knee, reclining hero, wheel, wind relieving, supine hand to foot, shoulder-stand, plough, and corpse poses. When performing a sequencing routine, it is relatively easy to transition from the cobra pose to the dog pose to the superman or locust pose, and then to the bow pose. Likewise, it is easy to transition from the wind-relieving pose to the supine hand to foot pose, to the shoulder-stand pose,

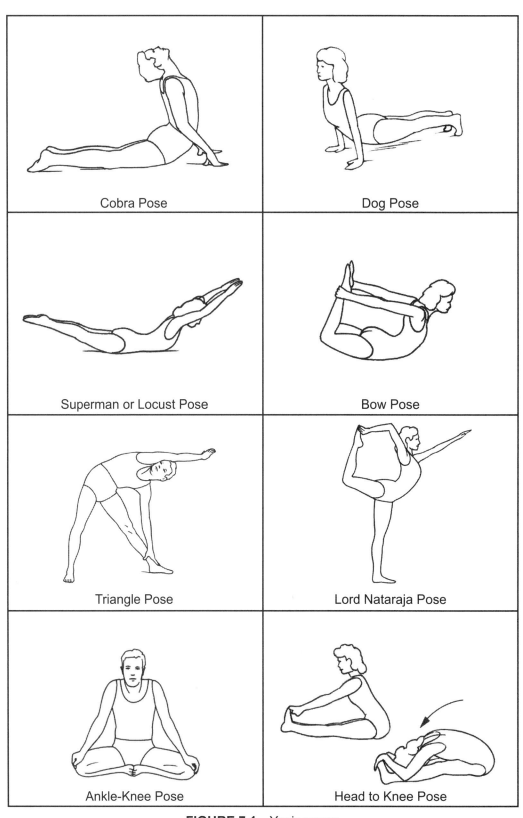

Cobra Pose

Dog Pose

Superman or Locust Pose

Bow Pose

Triangle Pose

Lord Nataraja Pose

Ankle-Knee Pose

Head to Knee Pose

FIGURE 7.1—Yogic poses

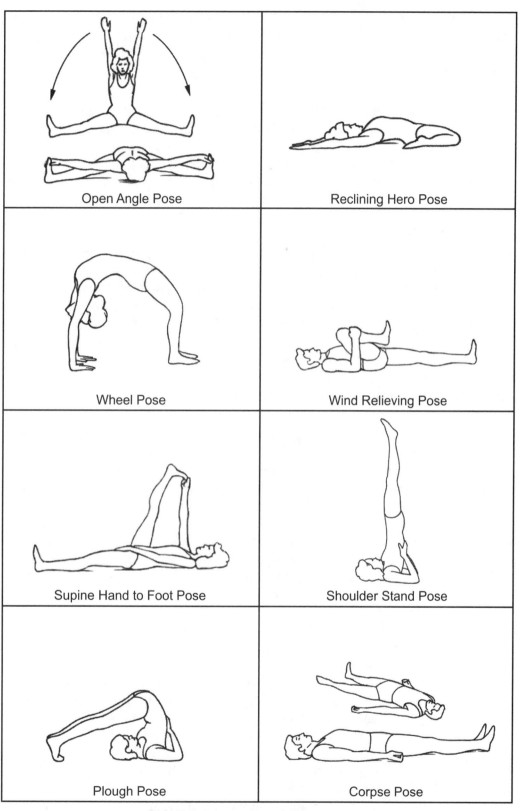

Open Angle Pose	Reclining Hero Pose
Wheel Pose	Wind Relieving Pose
Supine Hand to Foot Pose	Shoulder Stand Pose
Plough Pose	Corpse Pose

FIGURE 7.1 continued—Yogic poses

and then to the plough pose. To help clear the legs of the by-products of a hard workout or race, distance runners might wish to perform the shoulder-stand pose. Athletes should normally end a dynamic stretching and flexibility session in the corpse pose, lying flat on their back with arms slightly outstretched (See Swami Vishnu-devananda, 1988, Couch, 1990, and Kraftsow, 1999).

However, it is inadvisable for distance runners to perform extremely pretzel-like Yogic forms. They should not over-do things and stretch ligaments or tendons to such a degree as to cause injury. There is such a thing as being too tight, but also being too loose. Somewhere in between lies the golden mean. Athletes should progress so as to be capable of performing a series of Yogic forms in a continuous flowing manner.

Rehabilitation and Acquisition

Nevertheless, static stretching, PNF stretching, and the dynamic stretching and flexibility routine are not sufficient to fully rehabilitate an individual. Muscles are educated by movement, and repetition is the mother of learning. Rehabilitation of a movement pattern requires recreating a neuromuscular stereotype, and that entails a high number of repetitions. The process of rehabilitation therefore closely resembles the original *habilitation* process, and also acquisitive efforts directed to achieving higher levels of performance. Running faster or jumping higher also requires the creation of new neuromuscular stereotypes. And it demands a considerable investment of time and effort directed towards the repetition of a movement pattern.

Athletes generally have tight muscles and limited flexibility for a reason. Their inflexibility is normally the direct result of how they use a particular muscle group or limb. And all the conventional stretching and flexibility work in the world will not necessarily change their movement pattern. For example, athletes having tight quads are generally over-using that muscle group and under-utilizing their hamstrings. If they want to increase the flexibility of their quads, then they might need to do exercises such as walking squats to increase the strength of their hamstrings. Athletes also differ greatly in their ability to perform movements while in a state of fatigue. And during athletic performance they must manage not only high loads and rates of movement, but also the presence of fatigue.

Fatigue and Inhibition

If the coach instructs a group of athletes to stand on one leg and simply perform leg raises (that is, bend at the knee and raise the thigh parallel to the support surface), then return the foot while not quite touching the ground, some interesting things will be seen. When athletes are properly trained they can perform 100 reps, or so-called 100-ups. But what happens when a group of athletes have not been trained in this form drill? The first 10-20 reps are easy—but wait—by 30 reps it becomes difficult, and by 50 reps some athletes become bound up and incapable of maintaining anything resembling correct form. By the time they reach 60 reps some will drop out, and only a few will manage 100 reps. For some, the limitation is balance, for others it is coordination, and for still others strength. But something else is going on here as well.

Athletes vary greatly in their neuromuscular coordination, and also their relative inhibition between agonist and protagonist muscle groups. As athletes fatigue, the effort taken to recruit the agonist muscle can sometimes engage the antagonist as well. The muscle spindles and golgi tendon organs have their role to play in protecting connective tissue and facilitating movement. Nevertheless, the threshold of engagement for neuromuscular inhibition can be trained and elevated to enhance performance.

Further, when extreme fatigue is present, the neuromuscular system does not respond in the same way, nor do athletes accurately perceive their movements. For example, when finishing the last 100 meters of the 400 meters, their legs might feel heavy, sluggish, and not moving properly. Sometimes this is precisely what is happening, but sometimes that is only the way their legs feel. When properly trained, athletes might still feel their form breaking down, but they will correctly respond to that feedback and largely prevent it from happening. Learning how to interpret feedback and move with proper technique while in a state of fatigue is something of a whole new bag of tricks. In some sense, it is as if the athletes need to learn how to walk or run all over again. The possible gap between perception and reality needs to be made apparent so that they can close the gap in a constructive manner.

Stationary Form Drills

The medicine usually required is what some coaches refer to as form drills. The so-called "100-up" drill discussed previously is one example (See Figures 7.2 and 7.3). When it is conducted in front of a mirror, athletes can have immediate feedback regarding their movements.

The late University of Oregon Coach Bill Bowerman used to teach a running form drill in which athletes stood on one leg while alternately raising and extending the opposite leg in a natural running motion, in synchronization with the opposing arm. Essentially, athletes perform the running motion while stationary on one leg. To steady themselves, they can initially stand with one shoulder against a wall, but should later perform the exercise in a freestanding position. Athletes should also progress to a point where their elevated foot only barely touches the ground, thus the muscles of the leg are not permitted to rest. Athletes can eventually progress so they can perform 100 repetitions non-stop before changing over to conduct 100 reps with their opposite arm and leg. In no instance should an athlete proceed if they cannot perform a form drill with complete control and perfect form (See Figures 7.4 and 7.5).

Again, when performing form drills, athletes need feedback, and in particular visual feedback. Their untrained kinesthetic sense can, and generally will, lie. What their body is doing, and what athletes think it is doing can be two very different things, but they may not be able to sense it. Athletes need to develop an accurate kinesthetic sense through repeated practice and observation.

Another common stationary form drill includes arm swings—that is, holding light free weights in one's hands and practicing proper arm movement for the duration of a middle distance race. This exercise should also include the transition in running form and arm action that takes place during the kick (See Figures 7.6 and 7.7).

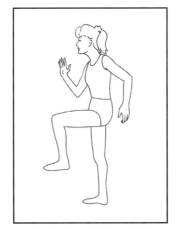
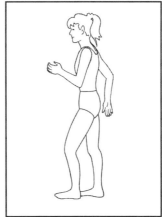

FIGURES 7.2 and 7.3—up and down positions of the 100-up drill

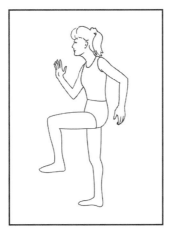
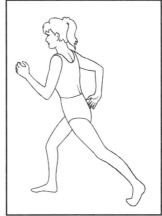

FIGURES 7.4 and 7.5—up and down positions of the running form drill

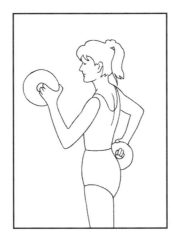
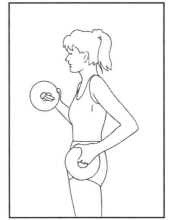

FIGURES 7.6 and 7.7—up and down positions of arm swings

Another form drill is especially suitable for hurdlers and the steeplechaser. The athletes stand and raise their thigh parallel to the support surface directly to the side, imitating the up position when hurdling the barrier, and perform 50-100 reps. Hurdlers commonly practice several other different types of stationary form drills. For example, they will often stand beside a hurdle and repeatedly move their trail leg over the hurdle in a continuous circular action. If athletes do not perform a movement correctly and commit it to motor memory so that it becomes automatic during competition when they are in a state of fatigue, their performances will suffer. Errors would then occur, such as hitting a hurdle or steeplechase barrier. Stationary form drills focus on key specific movements that can improve an athlete's coordination, balance, strength, endurance, and ability to perform—even when highly fatigued.

Plyometric Form Drills

If an athlete cannot perform static stretching, PNF stretching, a dynamic stretching and flexibility routine, and simple stationary form drills proficiently, then they should not engage in more demanding plyometric form drills. Examples of plyometric drills are also provided in Chapter 8, and illustrated in Figure 8.1. Some of the drills used in circuit training by the Kenyan runners also comprise plyometric form drills (Abmayr and Kosgei, 1991). The only limit to the various possibilities is one's imagination. It can be advantageous for athletes to include specific plyometric form drills during their warm-down. For example, athletes can perform relaxed high-knee, alternating leg butt-kick, locked-knee, and also skip-bounding, as shown in Figure 7.8.

The introduction of music can solicit flowing movements and positive energy, as opposed to robotic movements (Matesic and Cromartie, 2002). Aerobics demonstrates the power of music in this connection. In truth, many aerobics classes include stationary and plyometric form drills. Movements having a desired training effect can also be conducted in the form of dance.

A Practical Stretching and Flexibility Program

What would constitute a sound daily training practice with regards to stretching and flexibility? Unless the temperature is over 60°, the athletes should be fully clothed. In order to attain a full range of motion, they should silently conduct a dynamic stretching and flexibility routine of their own design. This can normally be completed in five to 10 minutes. Thereafter, they should warm-up by running moderately for five to 20 minutes so as to break a sweat and attain a pulse of 120 beats per minute. Unfortunately, many athletes will have to wear athletic shoes and run a large portion of their training on asphalt roads. However, it is often possible to run the daily warm-up and warm-down barefoot on the infield grass of a track and field facility, or the soccer fields found at most high school and college facilities. The warm-up should then finish with a series of 100-meter accelerations, with a short continuous jogging recovery. This can be accomplished by running diagonals on the infield grass and jogging to the opposite corners. However, the coach and athletes should first carefully inspect the area for any debris that could possibly

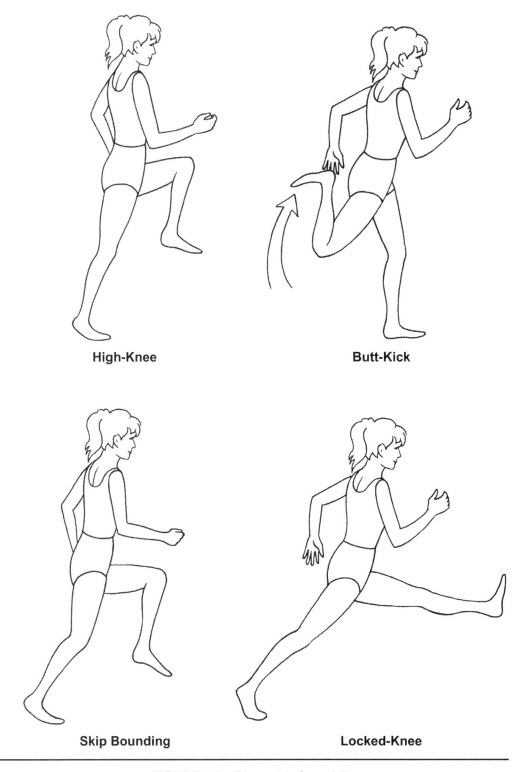

High-Knee

Butt-Kick

Skip Bounding

Locked-Knee

FIGURE 7.8—Plyometric form drills

result in injury. Even a relatively small amount of barefoot running can result in a visible improvement of an athlete's running style, and will often provide one second/400 meters improvement in athletic performance.

The athletes should then engage in whatever focused static, PNF, or other dynamic stretching and flexibility routines are deemed necessary to properly prepare themselves for the primary training session. Depending on the athlete's physical condition, and the nature of the training session, this second round of stretching and flexibility work is sometimes unnecessary. If a high quality workout is to be conducted, then the athletes should change into appropriate footwear and run at least three to six accelerations in the range between 50 and 200 meters. These accelerations or strides should gradually build up to, and slightly exceed the prescribed pace that will be undertaken. Athletes will then be ready to conduct the primary training session.

After completing the primary training session, whenever possible, athletes should run barefoot on a natural surface. Towards the end of their warm-down, they should conduct plyometric form drills such as high knee, locked knee, butt kicks, and skip-bounding. They should then put on warm clothes, drink water, and ingest a citrus juice or electrolyte replacement drink including a source of simple carbohydrates. Athletes should then perform a 20 to 30 minute 1/4-effort strength training session to restore equilibrium and facilitate recovery (as discussed in Chapter 8). On some days, athletes might even play a fifteen-to thirty-minute game of barefoot, non-contact soccer using a tennis ball. Alternately, they could play a few sets of tennis. These activities require brief accelerations and use the balancing muscle groups in lateral movements. All of the aforementioned post-exercise activities will restore equilibrium and speed recovery. They induce a shift in metabolism from catabolic processes associated with distance running towards anabolic processes and neuromuscular recovery. The athletes should then conduct various static, PNF, and dynamic stretching and flexibility exercises, including yogic forms, and finish in the corpse pose. They will then walk away from practice feeling pleasantly tired, in search of a good meal and rest, but not suffering from severe physical or mental exhaustion.

Running is the Ultimate Form Drill

The ultimate form drill is running on undulating natural terrain. The best movers are, in some sense, practicing flexibility with every stride they take. And the better their technique, the less remedial stretching and flexibility work will be required. The importance of cultivating good running technique becomes apparent when it is remembered that each day's running workout typically involves several thousand repetitions—as opposed to the relatively small number of repetitions associated with conventional strength training and flexibility exercises. The Australian coach Percy Cerutty wrote several books that address running technique and the importance of training in a natural physical environment (1961, 1964, and 1967). While difficult to locate, these books are highly recommended reading.

Cerutty sometimes worked an evening job that required little of his mental faculties. He then surrounded himself with his books, music, and barbells in order to make use of the hours. Likewise, Arthur Lydiard of New Zealand was a foreman in a shoe factory by trade, and sometimes also a milkman. These two individuals, who probably contributed as much as anyone over the last century to our understanding of training distance runners, were men of humble origins. They were largely self-educated and "the salt of the earth," rather than products of a celebrated university. Accordingly, they *earned* their knowledge through experience and reflection, allowing nature to be their guide.

> *Grace does not abolish Nature but perfects it.*
>
> — Thomas Aquinas

References

Abmayer, Walter, and Mike Kosgei, "Kenya Cross-Country Training," *Track & Field Quarterly Review*, Volume 91, Number 2, 1991, pages 43-44.

Alexander, F. Matthias, *The Alexander Technique: The Essential Writings of F. Matthias Alexander*, Edward Maisel, Editor, New York: Carol Publishing Group, 1995.

Aquinas, St. Thomas, *An Introduction to St. Thomas Aquinas: The Summa Contra Gentiles* (excerpts), Anthony C. Pegis, Editor, New York: The Modern Library, Random House, Inc., 1948.

Bly, Robert, *A Little Book on the Human Shadow*, William Booth, Editor, San Francisco, California: HarperCollins Publishers, 1988.

Cerutty, Percy, *Athletics*, London: The Sportsman's Book Club, 1961.

Cerutty, Percy, *Middle Distance Running*, Great Britain: Pelham Books, Ltd., 1964.

Cerutty, Percy, *Success: In Sport and Life*, London: Pelham Books, 1967.

Couch, Jean, *The Runner's Yoga Book*, Berkeley, California: Rodmell Press, 1990.

Cowan, James, *Mysteries of the Dream-Time*, Dorset, England: Prism Press, 1989.

Drake, Jonathan, *The Alexander Technique In Everyday Life*, Musselburgh, Scotland: Scotprint Ltd., 1996.

Fagan, J., and I.L. Shepherd, Editors, *Gestalt Therapy Now*, Palo Alto, California: Science and Behavior Books, 1970, Harper Colophon, 1971.

Feldenkrais, Moshe, *Awareness Through Movement*, San Francisco, California: HarperCollins Publishers, 1990, page 137.

Hatcher, Chris, and Philip Himelstein, *The Handbook of Gestalt Therapy*, Northvale, New Jersey: Jason Aronson Inc., 1995.

Hyams, Joe, *Zen in the Martial Arts*, Los Angeles: J.P. Tarcher, Inc., distributed by St. Martin's Press, 1979.

Kim, Hee-Jin, *Dōgen Kigen: Mystical Realist*, Tuscon, Arizona: University of Arizona Press, 1987, page 152.

Kraftsow, Gary, *Yoga For Wellness*, New York: Penguin Group, 1999.

Liao, Waysun, *T'ai Chi Classics*, Boston, Massachusetts: Shambhala, 1990.

Maier, Hanns, "Seko," *Runner's World*, June, 1981.

Man-ch'ing, Cheng, and Robert W. Smith, *T'ai-Chi, The "Supreme Ultimate" Exercise for Health, Sport, and Self-Defense*, Rutland, Vermont: Charles E. Tuttle Co., 1994.

Matesic, Brian C., and Fred Cromartie, "Effects Music Has on Lap Pace, Heart Rate, and Perceived Exertion Rate During a 20-Minute Self-Paced Run," *The Sport Journal*, Daphne, Alabama: The United States Sport Academy, February, 2002, http://www.thesportjournal.org/2002Journal/Vol5-No1/music.htm

McAtee, Robert E., and Jeff Charland, *Facilitated Stretching*, Champaign, Illinois: Human Kinetics Publishers, 1993, page 6.

Pavlov, Ivan P., *Conditioned Reflexes: An Investigation of the Physiological*, New York: Dover Publications Inc., 1927.

Schmidt, R.A., *Motor Control and Learning: A Behavioral Emphasis*, 2nd Edition, Champaign, Illinois: Human Kinetics Publishers, Inc., 1988.

Schmidt, R.A., "Motor Learning Principles for Physical Therapy," in M.J. Lister, Editor, *II Step Contemporary Management of Motor Control Problems*, Alexandria, Virginia: Foundation for Physical Therapy, Inc., 1991, pages 49-63.

Swami Vishnu-devananda, *The Complete illustrated Book of Yoga*, New York: Crown Trade Paperbacks, 1988, pages 49, 201 and 239.

Voss, Dorothy, and M.K. Ionta, B. Myers, *Proprioceptive Neuromuscular Facilitation*, 3rd Edition, Philadelphia, Pennsylvania: Harper & Row, 1985.

Westmoreland, Barbara, and Jeff Charland, *Facilitated Stretching*, Champaign, Illinois: Human Kinetics Publishers, 1993, page 6.

Westmoreland, Barbara, et al., *Medical Neurosciences*, Third Edition, New York: Little, Brown and Company, 1994.

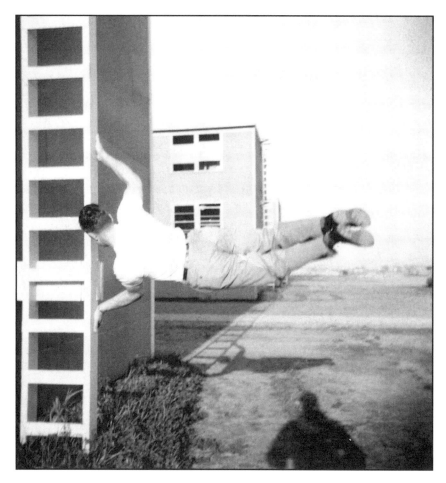

PHOTO 8.1—The author's father, Bob Lyden, demonstrating the benefits of strength training, Camp Parks Air Force Base, Pleasanton, CA, 1953.

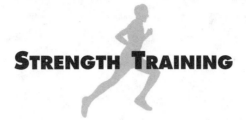

CHAPTER 8

STRENGTH TRAINING

Only the complete athlete finds success at the national and international levels. In championship competition few athletes can expect to be aerobically superior enough to sustain a pace none can follow. And in a race where the stakes are high, a front-runner cannot expect to drop all competitors with only surge and breakaway tactics. An athlete must be prepared for all this as a matter of course. The race goes to the complete athlete who can survive a testing pace, including surge and breakaway attempts, and still execute a winning drive to the tape. World class men in the 5,000 and 10,000 meters will commonly run the last 400 meters in under 56 seconds, and in the 1,500 meters nearer 52 seconds, with the final 200 meters in less than 25 seconds. That kind of anaerobic power and speed flows from strength.

Many of the training principles advocated by Arthur Lydiard of New Zealand have proven to be correct (Lydiard and Gilmour, 1962, and 1978). Nevertheless, there has been ongoing debate over the relevance of strength training to performance in middle distance and distance events. Lydiard is correct to stress that the number one limiting factor to performance in distance running is aerobic ability. However, some might mistakenly believe that the athletes who won fame under Lydiard were not exceptionally powerful men. The intensive hill phase that Lydiard advocates involves demanding resistance work, as does any running over the testing New Zealand terrain. Have a look at photos and film dating from the 1960's showing the build of Peter Snell. Americans watched Snell some years ago in the Superstars competition, and as his rowing demonstrated, he was still an extremely powerful man. So do not let the slender build of some distance runners fool you. Appearances can be deceiving. All things being equal, the race goes to the strong.

Distance running is a skill consisting of many components, and is not an activity sufficient unto itself for athletic development. Proper strength training can facilitate recovery from demanding endurance and sharpening work. It can enhance cardiovascular endurance, speed, and flexibility. Strength training can provide the durability and resistance to injury that figures so prominently in the longevity of an athletic career.

Exercise Physiology

A brief discussion of relevant exercise physiology will make it possible to later address a number of important questions relating to strength training and athletic performance. Strength is perhaps the most acquirable component of athletic fitness. Few possess the genetic gift, even allowing for an enhancement of 35% over their natural endowment, to permit them to become world-class distance run-

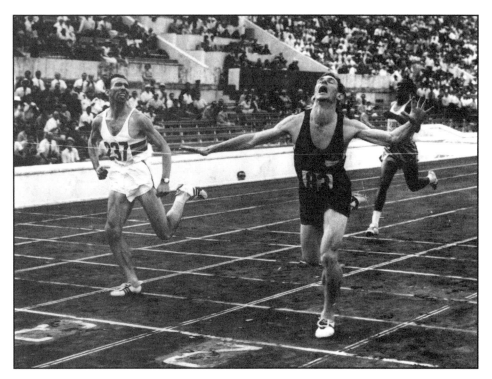

PHOTO 8.2—Peter Snell of New Zealand winning the 800 meters over Roger Moens, 1960 Olympic Games. Photo from AP/ Wide World Photos.

ners. And few possess the neuromuscular innervation and predominant muscle fiber type to become elite sprinters. But athletes can be stronger for the task of distance running than they ever need to be. Distance runners are not interested in muscular hypertrophy, but rather packing the highest level of strength and power into their competitive body weight. Many runners avoid strength training altogether, fearing cumbersome muscular development that would compromise their aerobic ability. However, this need not be a concern, given a properly constructed weight-training program.

Muscle Fiber Type

Muscle fiber has two predominant types:

- Slow-twitch (Type I)   associated with endurance
- Fast-twitch (Type II)   associated with explosive strength and power

Although some exercise physiologists suggest the possibility of muscle fibers splitting and replicating themselves as to type, our ratio of Type I and Type II muscle fibers is substantially fixed and genetically determined. At least three general subtypes exist within the fast-twitch muscle fiber type. These classifications between Type II muscle fiber types are based largely on biochemical rather than structural differences (Åstrand, 1986).

- Type IIa associated with ATP-Lactic Acid energy utilization
- Type IIb associated with the ATP-PC system
- Type IIc exhibits the ability to cross-train and assume many characteristics of the slow-twitch (Type I) muscle fiber

What does this imply for the training of distance runners? The genetic endowment as between the Type I and various Type II fibers does establish ultimate limitations. Some athletes are born for a given event. Certainly, this is true at the extreme ends of the spectrum, that is, the marathoner versus the sprinter, but things become much grayer as we move towards the middle distance events. In fact, by continually stressing a particular energy system and fiber sub-type amongst the Type I and Type II fibers, that particular type will develop and hypertrophy, whereas the other fibers types will remain the same or perhaps atrophy. The same number of fibers of the various muscle types still remain, but their relative development and proportional space utilization would change dramatically (Åstrand, 1986). Today, we can appreciate that the best performers at 800 meters are former specialists at 400 meters who have conducted the stamina work required to more fully develop their Type I, IIa and IIc muscle fiber metabolism. Table 2.1 (page 58) provides an estimate of the predominant energy system used in different events. The ratio of anaerobic to aerobic work would differ considerably between a mile run in 5:00 versus 3:45. The greater the speed, and the shorter the duration of the performance, the more anaerobic the event. And the more anaerobic the event, the more will Type II muscle fibers be utilized.

What are the wider implications of Type I and Type II fiber adaptation for distance runners? Athletes must train specifically for the duration and speed projected for the goal performance in the main race event. That is why Lydiard found it was not possible to simply train a 10,000 meters specialist for the 1,500 meters and thereby produce a high quality performance at 5,000 meters. The date pace and goal pace work done during the season educates the twitch to the proper tune.

With regard to muscle fiber composition, the natural athlete has an edge over the made athlete, since the latter must spend more time educating their metabolism to perform at a comparable level. This has more serious implications: When athletes cease their acquisition efforts, their muscle fiber type and metabolism detrains—that is, it heads back towards their natural endowment (Åstrand, 1986). For example, after the end of a season, an athlete genetically disposed to be a specialist at 800 meters will lose little form compared to another athlete genetically inclined to be a specialist at 3,000 meters, but who had nevertheless trained in order to achieve the same level of performance at 800 meters. The less specifically gifted need to train longer and harder to fool Mother Nature. That is one of the reasons why athletes need to recognize early and develop from the under-distance side towards their best racing distance.

The initial investment of time and energy in strength training can be substantial. However, athletes will find returning to a previously attained level of fitness far less expensive, and characterized by faster progression on succeeding attempts. And when out of form, they will also find a higher base level of fitness has been established. The higher the level of fitness the athletes attain, and the more extensive their training background, the higher the base level of fitness that will be naturally maintained with less further investment. This is an important factor when it comes time to back off of strength training and concentrate on performance at the end of an athletic season. It is also important when developing to peak in a multiple year cycle such as one culminating in the Olympic Games. In this case, during the first years of acquisitive developmental work, athletes should engage in relatively energy-inefficient efforts directed towards their areas of weakness. In some sense, the athletes must fight Mother Nature to bring their apparent deficiencies up to certain minimums. This will later permit their natural line of strength to be fully exploited without the relative areas of weakness unduly restraining their ultimate performance potential. In an athletic season when optimal performances are desired, athletes should then train towards their natural strengths, and place special emphasis on quality in order to refine previously acquired powers. This will minimize any counterproductive macro-cycle (seasonal) and mega-cycle (multi seasonal) suppression of performance and permit optimal competitive results.

Strength and Muscular Endurance

Muscular endurance should not be confused with cardiovascular endurance. In the context of muscular endurance, an athlete who exhibits greater strength in a maximum lift will also normally exhibit greater muscular endurance in that exercise. For example, all things being equal, an athlete who can bench press 200 pounds will exhibit greater muscular endurance in reps with 100 pounds than another athlete whose maximum bench press is only 150 pounds. Of course, this assumes both individuals have comparable backgrounds with respect to training volume (the number of sets and reps being performed), since this would substantially determine the magnitude of local stores of muscle glycogen.

The popular notion that distance runners should do endless repetitions with light weights to improve their endurance is a lot of nonsense. Serious distance runners will be spending untold hours swinging their arms and legs in hundreds of thousands of endurance reps during weeks and months of training. They do not need to spend several hours a week flapping paperweights around. In any case, the maximum duration of an endurance weight training set would be the duration of the main race event.

In brief, distance runners should not cower away from high quality strength training or would-be impossible tasks simply because they may resemble the proverbial 138-pound weakling. And athletes should not lift light weights for fifteen minutes and fool themselves that they are doing something constructive. Distance runners should strive to become as strong as possible, but without inducing significant muscular hypertrophy or increasing their competitive body weight. Given their natural body chemistry, women need not be concerned about the development of unusual muscle definition or a resultant loss of sex appeal. In fact, the consensus among men is that just the opposite is true, and in this regard, female distance runners have the better deal over their male counterparts. For even after years of training, by all outward appearances, male distance runners might still beg having sand kicked in their faces—the bully making a big mistake!

Strength and Cardiovascular Endurance

The relationship between strength and cardiovascular endurance has not been fully explored by exercise physiologists. One effect of weight training is an increase in blood pressure to help perfuse working muscles, but this normally has little or no chronic effect upon the resting blood pressure. This temporary increase in blood pressure is largely caused by vasoconstriction, that is, by partially turning off the blood supply to relatively inactive tissues. The blood pressure is then raised so as to increase the perfusion pressure and blood flow through active tissues. This offsets the occlusion pressure and resulting impedance of blood flow caused by muscular contractions in the active tissues. The increased afterload on the heart from weight training (caused by resistance to pumping blood through working muscle tissue) induces concentric and ventricular hypertrophy, but without significantly increasing stroke volume or the ejection fraction. In short, the heart muscle becomes bigger and stronger.

In contrast, interval training increases the preload of venous return on the heart. This induces an enlargement of the heart and a corresponding increase in stroke volume (NSCA Journal, 1987). The heart then becomes more efficient, since it can pump more blood with fewer beats per minute (bpm). The practical result is bradycardia, or a slowing of the rest pulse rate—commonly observed in endurance athletes. Cardiac output figures largely in the formula of aerobic ability and the performance of distance runners (See Chapter 2, page 72).

Weight training can increase local stores of energy in the form of muscle glycogen, but if muscular hypertrophy results, the relative density of mitochondria (the powerhouse of the cell) could actually decrease due to a dilution effect. That could possibly compromise the aerobic ability of the athletes. In sum, weight training per se has little impact on the gross structure of the cardiovascular system. However, it has been determined that strength training can dramatically affect cardiovascular endurance by other means (Hickson, et al., 1988, Marcinik et al., 1991, Houmard, et al., 1991, Paavolainen et al., 1999). Strength training causes the body to generate higher levels of anabolic hormones, such as testosterone, which can generally promote acquisition and even increase the number of red blood cells. Further, if two athletes are placed on a treadmill, but one is much stronger than the other, the stronger athlete will demonstrate a less dramatic fatigue curve and will outlast the weaker. Generally speaking, stronger muscles fatigue slower than weaker muscles. The reasons for this defy an easy explanation, but they largely concern the so-called anaerobic threshold. In this regard, the higher level of fatigue in the nervous system caused by the weaker athlete's effort to manage the workload can be a contributor to early exhaustion. Further, the more forceful contraction of the weaker athlete's muscles to accomplish the same amount of work can result in greater occlusion, thus less adequate blood perfusion. The latter would result in a mechanical lowering of the anaerobic threshold. Less clear is how higher strength levels contribute at the cellular level to the use of fatty acids, carbohydrates and the removal of blood lactate. However, it has been found that some athletes learn to distribute the work load spatially, and then use more muscle mass while performing a task, thereby reducing the load on individual muscles (Coyle, 1995).

Strength training can significantly improve the technique and efficiency of distance runners. This ultimately determines just how much of their aerobic ability is ultimately translated into performance. The running economy of individual athletes can be tested on a treadmill and expressed as a percentage of their VO_2 maximums. If runners use a significant portion of their limited oxygen uptake on incidental movements (induced by muscle imbalances or weakness), the practical effect will be diminished performance. For example, athletes having weak plantar flexion at the ankle will tend to strike more heavily on their rearfoot. This often shifts their pelvis and center of gravity out of place, that is, substantially behind the point of footstrike. Thus the athletes must pull themselves forward, lift themselves up and across, and then push themselves forward from their center of gravity. That will use the larger muscle groups and incur a higher oxygen demand. By comparison, smaller and stronger calf muscles could have provided superior plantar flexion, and so would have consumed much less oxygen. This biomechanical adaptation would permit athletes to continually fall forward from their center of gravity and catch themselves with their next footplant. Athletes can have a deficient way of moving for any number of reasons, but when the problem stems from muscle imbalances or weakness, all the thinking or visualizing in the world will not remedy the situation. They have to do something about it, and that entails some form of strength training. Moreover, athletes should identify and eliminate their possible wobbles and whips in order to avoid injury.

Due to a combination of the above mechanisms as well as others, weaker athletes will cross their anaerobic threshold earlier (and possibly at a lower percentage of maximal oxygen uptake) than stronger counterparts. In practice, stronger athletes clearly demonstrate a marked advantage in arduous conditions. This becomes apparent when cross-country championships are held on demanding courses, and also when athletes confront headwinds or other adverse environmental conditions.

Speed and Strength

Speed flows from strength. The shorter the main race event, the stronger an athlete must be to compete at the highest levels. In this regard, there is need for greater force and power to be applied over time and space. In the middle distance events athletes require considerable anaerobic power, since the ATP-PC and ATP-Lactic Acid Systems provide the predominant energy source. This suggests the necessity for considerable strength training.

Athletes having greater strength in the appropriate muscle groups will demonstrate a longer stride, but will also be able to maintain more of their stride length during competition. A gradual shortening of stride length normally takes place during competition as athletes fatigue—this prevents an exorbitant slowing of cadence or stride frequency. The act of running can be divided for analytical purposes into a flight phase, and a support phase. Increases in speed are largely correlated with a decrease in the duration of the support phase. And a shorter support phase means that athletes must perform more work in less time, that is, they must demonstrate greater power. The significance of the support phase for speed can be seen in the finish of many distance events. Some athletes invariably tighten up in the last straight and then seem to spend an eternity on the ground, thereby permitting their relatively light-footed adversaries to pull away.

The proper cue for athletes attempting a strong finish is to drop and quicken by slightly increasing their forward body lean while simultaneously lowering their hips. However, the actual increase in stride frequency and acceleration is initiated in the forefingers and is directed by the hands. Accordingly, the hands of the athletes should drop and drive below hip level as the change in posture is initiated, and then drive in a flurry with short, fast strokes relatively close to the torso, and reach nearly to chin level. Athletes never need think about their legs, since all else will follow the rhythm dictated by their hands (Cerutty, 1964).

All things being equal, stronger muscles are also more capable of rapid movement. Superior spatial and temporal neuromuscular recruitment and coordination (induced by strength training) plays an important role. If an athlete cannot perform a movement requiring maximal exertion slowly, then imagine how much less efficient the movement will be when performed quickly. Moreover, the stronger a set of muscles and connective tissues are throughout a requisite range of motion, the less inhibitory feedback will proprioceptors and protective sensors such as the golgi tendon apparatus send to turn off muscle groups via the reflex arcs. In brief, the body attempts to protect areas of weakness in a way that prohibits maximal exertion, thus resulting in a loss of power and speed.

Strength and Skill Levels

In order to maintain skill levels, stretching and flexibility work is always advisable following a strength-training session. However, activities including fine motor skills should also be undertaken. Otherwise, the skill level of the athletes could regress whenever rapid adaptation takes place. The same phenomenon can be seen when young athletes undergo a growth spurt—their skill levels drop. Because of this, including a skilled activity in the warm down is doubly important in those activities which require higher skill levels. For example, athletes can practice form drills, or jump rope after a weight training session. Free throw shooting can also help the athletes' arms to recover. Their skill levels will then be considerably impaired, and not just because of fatigue. In short, athletes need to engage in a warm-down including a skilled activity—otherwise their strength training efforts could prove counterproductive to maintaining desired skill levels.

Often, if young athletes appear slow, they are labeled as such and made distance runners. Too often these athletes will thereafter compete only in the distance events. Many are naturally reluctant to venture into events where they have less proficiency. Moreover, their coach may see ten points stamped on the shorts of the athletes with respect to the distance events in every dual meet, and so little or nothing is done to develop their basic speed ability. A self-fulfilling prophecy! Some individuals do have less athletic ability, but this should not confuse the issue, as talented distance runners are not slow by layman's standards. They do not have the speed to become world-class sprinters, but that does not preclude, for example, male middle distance runners from running 100 meters under 11 seconds, and 400 meters in under 47 seconds.

Some athletes are naturally faster or slower in terms of their neuromuscular function and coordination, but that does not mean nature cannot be taught. Slow is sometimes a state of mind, and may reflect an individual's level of excitement. In a life-threatening situation, self-preservation can override learned inhibitions. Take a so-called slow athlete, and also a fast athlete, and sit them down on a piano bench. Observe how well they can perform the scale or a trill. If the slow athlete has years of piano over the fast athlete you could be in for a surprise! And so an athlete's speed ability is in part an acquired skill. It can be learned through repetition and practice. Just as in playing the piano, it requires an investment of time. Not many are Mozarts. Athletes must train speed to have speed, or they will be overtaken by someone more talented, or perhaps more diligent.

Again, speed flows from strength. The great mistake middle and distance runners can make is to neglect strength training because of the degree it can suppress performance when they are in the midst of hard training. Seeing the immediate effect on performance, coaches and athletes might think it bad (just as they might think more and more sharpening work is good). Granted, strength training must be done prudently to avoid adverse effects on the larger training program and performance. Hill work can normally suppress performance by two seconds/400 meters, and adding weight training can put it closer to three full seconds. However, given a properly constructed training program, this two-to-three-second deficit can be translated into a rebound and substantial improvement in performance at the right time and place.

Strength, Durability and Flexibility

Many athletes fear that strength training will hurt their flexibility. It can, when conducted improperly. Anything done improperly can cause problems. But performed correctly, strength training can actually enhance the flexibility of athletes and even reduce their need for stretching. Within certain limitations, stronger muscles have the capacity to be more durable. As a result, athletes will not become as stiff and sore from a given training activity. They will recover faster and require less stretching or therapy to get the kinks out. Strength work can help to restore equilibrium, thus accelerate recovery after a demanding training effort or performance. In short, when it comes to durability the key concept is—*strength saves*.

Flexibility is therefore vitally important to strength and demonstrable speed. Inflexibility is associated with diminished range of motion, and slower performance. Again, tight tendons and muscles send inhibitory messages back through the reflex arcs to protect themselves from overextension and overuse, due to their being under-conditioned. Those messages turn off motor units, resulting in a loss of strength and speed. Moreover, weak muscles in specific regions of an otherwise outstanding range of motion produce muscle imbalances and a condition of dynamic inflexibility. Again, it is one thing to static stretch, but quite another to demonstrate the same range of motion in the practical application. We are concerned about the running technique of the athletes, not what they look like sprawled out on a gym floor. So an important component of athletic ability is the possession of adequate strength throughout a required range of motion. If athletes have weaknesses or muscle imbalances, then they will normally be more beat-up as the result of distance running. All things being equal, the more efficient their running technique, the less damage will be done. As discussed in Chapter 7, the better movers are dynamically stretching by virtue of superior technique with every stride they take.

Neuromuscular Stereotypes or Habits of Movement

An established, dominant pattern of neuromuscular function is commonly called a neuromuscular stereotype, or habit of movement. We all have them. Try to change the way you walk for just one day and you will appreciate how difficult these habits are to break. It takes time and endless repetition to instill a new neuromuscular stereotype. Every time athletes seek to attain a new level they must break the old habits and build the new. This requires patience and consistency. Take the hurdle event for example. It requires considerable repetition to change some aspect of their technique. And initially, the attempt to instill a new stereotype will likely decrease their skill levels. Later, the athletes will be able to demonstrate the new technique so long as their higher consciousness holds sway. But put them into a competition and often half way through the contest (as conscious control gives way to instinctive and unconscious automatism) the athletes will revert back to their old technique, which at a deeper level is still the dominant neuromuscular stereotype.

Some are able to learn and unlearn neuromuscular stereotypes more readily than others, but expect no miracles. Accurate and immediate feedback provided by video can greatly accelerate the process. Athletes must be careful when engaging in numerous repetitions and sessions, as fatigue can cause them to deviate from the desired technique. Again, there are no practice heats, nor do we ever do anything twice. The competition will be what the training has been. Every time an athlete performs an action, that act is a brick in the wall forming a dominant neuromuscular stereotype. So each and every time you do something, do it with proper technique. That goes for weight training, hurdle drills, or anything else in life. In the realm of philosophy and theology, the analogous concept is known as disposition (as taught by Aristotle, Augustine, and Thomas Aquinas).

To a great degree, an athlete's running technique can reveal self-perception, attitude, mood and the like. It is sometimes necessary to work with an individual at a subconscious level in order to change their technique (Cerutty, 1961). In truth, the coach merely serves as a catalyst, and athletes change themselves. As everywhere else, body language can be important. Consciously or not, experienced athletes can acquire an ability to read the physical and mental status of their competitors. This ability can entail the telegraphing phenomenon well understood in the martial arts (Hyams, 1979). Emil Zatopek, the only man to win the 5,000 meters, 10,000 meters, and marathon events in a single Olympic Games made the following observation (Spear, 1982):

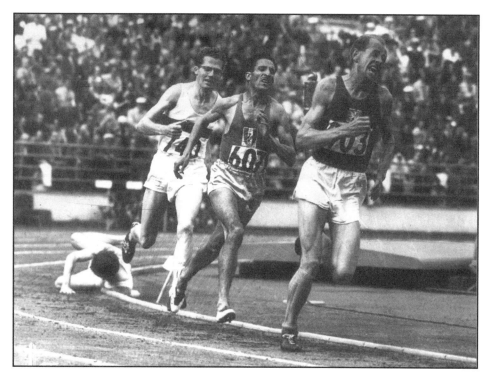

PHOTO 8.3—Emil Zatopek attacks the final straightaway of the 5,000 meters, 1952 Olympic Games. Photo from Hulton / Getty Images.

Question: How do you explain someone like Miruts Yifter of Ethiopia who won the 5,000 and 10,000 at Moscow (1980 Olympic Games) and who may be well over 40?

Zatopek: He is a very nice exception. Not only are his legs an exception, but his brain also. He has a very high intelligence quotient. After the last Olympics he said, "For me it is not so difficult. After five or six laps I have read everyone like a newspaper, and I know who is able to do this or that. And I know what I am able to do." He was able to play with them like a cat with a mouse.

Physical Age, Sex and Level of Development

The body protects itself by conspiracy of nature. It does not acquire much capacity for strength training or respond to it until the growth process has nearly completed. By then the body has sufficiently matured to withstand the stress. Pay attention to nature, since mere chronological age means nothing. It is best to use strength training exercises that employ the athlete's own body weight until the epiphyseal growth plates have settled down and early adult maturity been reached. The years of puberty and rapid skeletal growth should then be limited to introducing proper methods, habits and attitudes relating to strength training.

Pay close attention to nature, since some athletes might be ready at age 16, but others not until age 21. There is no virtue in hurrying things on the creative plane. More athletes have been destroyed by attempting too much too early, than by erring on the side of leniency. Exercise caution in strength training activities, because athletes are especially vulnerable to injury when going through a growth spurt. Note that taller and slighter builds (ectomorphs) tend to mature later than the other body types. Most distance runners roughly fit this description, and as a rule they are later in maturing. It is prudent to record the height, weight and relevant measurements of young athletes and to monitor their physical development quarterly. In this regard, young people are a lot like puppies. Foot size usually arrives before height—so do not use unchanging foot size as an indicator and try to beat the gun. Moreover, adult height arrives before mature body chemistry and physique—thus recognize and respect the sign of the times. When male athletes have nearly reached their adult height (that is, after their growth plates settle down), then they are ready to engage in more demanding weight training.

The same guidelines hold true for female athletes, but their development and maturation is more complicated. With a young man, the maturation process results in a more or less continual improvement in performance. When the maturation process absorbs physical energies, there can be some delays or short-lived plateaus in an athlete's progress. The young woman faces a more trying experience. Initially, she may gain height, strength, and maturity earlier than her male counterpart, and realize radical improvements in performance, perhaps from ages 12 to 15. But then she becomes a woman. Most of the changes that occur are, for the first time, detrimental to her running performance. Indeed, some of the changes could prove to be permanent liabilities, since nature does not intend for many women to become elite distance runners. Do not despair—there *are* other things in life more rewarding!

In any case, the female maturation process typically results in at least a temporary decline in a woman's aerobic ability and athletic performance. Many young women experience metabolic changes that can make weight gain a so-called problem. Women are not ready for serious weight training or otherwise demanding work involving the legs until their hips have fully arrived. Do not push things in this regard, since maturation of the pelvic girdle can result in biomechanical changes that place additional stress on their legs at this time. So perhaps from ages 16 to 18 a young woman will be doing all that she can to hold her ground. The training effort she is putting forth is being absorbed, suppressed or counteracted by the changes occurring in her body. Young women may then encounter a plateau or setback for several years, despite their honest efforts. It can be a tough time for women, emotionally and otherwise. It is important that they clearly understand what is happening, and that expectations are not placed upon them that do not take into account the relevant facts of life. The key is to channel emotional and physical energy in a positive direction. Provided that nature has permitted, after these changes run their course, often a startling leap in performance can follow. Some men might have a hard time understanding why such a fuss is being made. But realize how you might react if for a number of years the changes in your physique seemed detrimental to your athletic performance. And at the same time, society and most eligible women would be telling you rather loudly and clearly that without those changes you are nobody.

Female structural differences do exist that call for some limitation of intensity and variation in technique with respect to certain weight training exercises. As a rule, women have 30% less strength than men. However, there is little or no difference between the training of men and women at the same athletic level. For example, there is negligible difference in the strength training of a male or female athlete for a 5:00 mile. The training prescriptions would vary more out of individual differences than as a consequence of gender. Simply focus on the athlete and projected goal performance, and work to eliminate areas of weakness.

The years 18 through 25 normally represent the time for optimal strength development. Once attained, athletes can maintain acquired powers with relatively less investment of time and energy, and then concentrate on other tasks. Obviously, athletes can greatly improve their strength levels in later years, especially if they have previously neglected strength development. But in that case, they will have to work a bit harder to achieve the same result. It is important to be as efficient as possible in athletic development, since there is only so much energy and so much time.

Cross-Training

Cross-training is not an extra or alternative activity, but rather a vital component to the athletic skill that distance runners need to acquire. Athletes are not likely to achieve balanced physical development without engaging in some form of cross-training. However, runners should exercise moderation when participating in cross-training activities. The balance of primary to secondary activity and suitability of cross-training activities is of primary importance. It has been suggested that the ratio of primary to secondary athletic activity be on the order: 30/70 for the sprinter, 60/40 for the middle distance athlete, and 80/20 for the marathoner (Cerutty, 1961). That could be pushing things a bit, but the point is well taken. Distance runners should be conducting more cross-training than is common practice today.

Barefoot Running On Natural Surfaces

If athletes have access to a stretch of sand and a dune suitable for training purposes, they should consider themselves lucky and take advantage of it. However, avoid running on a beach with a marked grade or deep sand, and always use moderation when beginning this activity. Unfortunately, sand training and naturalistic technique have been largely ignored in the United States in recent years. Bill Dellinger related that his quantum leap to international caliber came after an extended period of training on the beach (Dellinger and Beres, 1978). This was no mere coincidence. Sand running has figured into the training regime of too many world-class athletes to be ignored. Percy Cerutty's athletes incorporated a great deal of barefoot running in the sand dunes surrounding Portsea, Australia (Cerutty, 1961, 1964, and 1967). Accordingly, this activity figured in the training background of Herb Elliott, former World Record holder in the mile and 1,500 meters, and 1960 Olympic Champion. An article in *Runner's World* similarly revealed another former World Record holder at 1,500 meters, Steve Ovett, running barefoot up a sand dune (Schneider, 1979). And you can bet that most of the African runners did not sport sneakers on their first training runs. So if you have wondered about sand training, stop wondering about it and start doing it. And if the circumstances and your structure permit, do so barefoot.

Again, begin slowly, and gradually introduce the activity by merely walking in sand for several days—even a few weeks. Athletes can later build up from five to 20 minutes of easy jogging (perhaps during the warm-up and warm-down). Although noticeable positive adaptations can be seen in days, skeletal adaptation alone requires a minimum of five to six weeks before more taxing efforts should be done. So do not think of sand training as a short-term gimmick. As with everything else in distance running, athletes need to make a long-term commitment.

What does sand training do for distance running athletes? For one thing, they can simultaneously stress their cardiovascular and muscular systems to the point of exhaustion at greatly reduced speeds. That cannot be done with such specificity by many other means. It is therefore possible to assume less quantity at lower levels of speed and experience a supra-normal training effect. Running in such an environment also conditions an elusive aspect of an athlete's aerobic ability and anaerobic threshold. Sand training can also enable many forms of work to be performed with less resultant wear and tear on the body. The shock loads associated with running on pavement—and in particular, the punishment normally inflicted by uphills and downhills—is not present. It would actually be difficult for athletes to hurt themselves by running uphill or downhill on sand, whereas the risk of doing so on hard surfaces is high.

The athletes will become stronger and enjoy better muscle balance with naturalistic technique. Many athletes have a tendency to prove themselves to themselves in training, and that often translates into running at high speeds on paved roads. The hardness of the surface returns much of the energy associated with the athletes' footstrike, and the evenness of the surface makes for high levels of efficiency. However, running on grass or other natural terrain can be relatively costly from the standpoint of energy demand, and in this sense, it is uncomfortable. On a natural surface, athletes will often have to work harder, using more of their balancing muscle groups at reduced speeds and with greater mental concentration. That can be beneficial depending on which aspect of aerobic ability is targeted for improvement.

There is also a degree to which conventional athletic shoes inhibit dorsiflexion and plantarflexion of an athlete's foot and toes. The relatively weak plantarflexion and restricted range of motion that many American athletes exhibit relative to the Kenyan distance runners is largely the direct result of Americans pounding their natural technique flat on the asphalt, rather than genetics. If you would like to see how weak your feet are, find two five-gallon buckets and fill them partially with water so they are an effort to handle. Then put on training shoes and climb up 10 steps on stadium bleachers, and return by the same route, carefully stepping down backwards. Repeat this several times, as necessary, while maintaining good form and without spilling anything. Allow a complete recovery. Now remove your shoes and repeat the above process. You might find yourself straining, wobbling and with

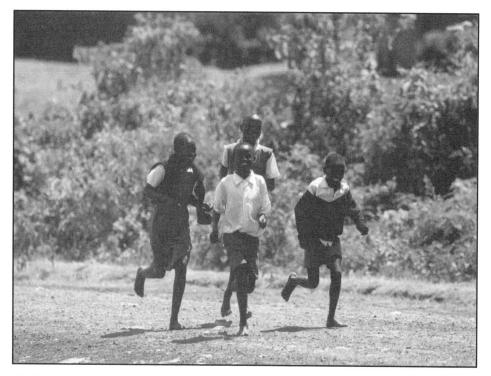

PHOTO 8.4—Kenyan children running barefoot to school. Photo from Victah Sailer/Photorun.

an empty bucket before you are finished. Why? Because conventional shoes more widely distribute the forces generated by contact with the underlying support surface, and that is not how it works in nature. Some researchers even argue that the lack of stimuli to proprioceptors in the foot and shoe-shielding from these stressors, can reduce the body's adaptation and level of resistance to injury (Robbins and Gouw, 1990).

Does that mean you should throw your shoes away? No, but it does mean that athletes who condition their feet are wise. Some barefoot jogging on a natural surface in the warm-up and warm-down, whenever circumstances permit, is extremely important. The human body was not made for athletic shoes or asphalt. Those are relatively recent inventions, and the adaptations from these stimuli are not necessarily performance-enhancing. The human body by contrast is a product of the millennia. The most elementary piece of equipment or facility for training purposes would then be a grass track with a two-lane sandbox around the perimeter. The artificial track is an ideal venue for athletic performance, but it is no place for the larger part of training conducted by distance runners.

Cross-Country Skiing

For athletes living in northern latitudes, cross-country skiing can provide a beneficial supplement to running during the winter months. An immediate danger for a runner who is just learning to cross-country ski is a groin pull, and also running into trees! So take precautions and do some flexibility work beforehand in order to avoid the necessity of remedial work later. When athletes resume training for distance running, another danger is straining their calf muscles. Cross-country skiers are well known to develop the highest aerobic ability of any athletes as a result of the stress placed on their entire body. If athletes think they're fit, they might be shocked by their first experience with cross-country skiing. Even when they do acquire the technique, finding their upper body fatigued and failing could be a new and callusing experience. Nevertheless, the neuromuscular development associated with extensive cross-country skiing is not conducive to performance on the track. The specificity is not there. However, taken in moderate amounts, the strength and power which cross-country skiers develop does translate reasonably well into performance in the 3,000 meters steeplechase.

Indoor use of cross-country skiing equipment can also be helpful—when used in moderation as a supplement, and in particular, to restore equilibrium after demanding running workouts. But beware of extensive use, which might affect your running technique. The posture of the cross-country skier generally has a more pronounced forward lean than that of a runner. Their hands pass more widely at the hip and there is relatively little knee lift. These neuromuscular habits should not supplant those associated with optimal running technique. Accordingly, cross-country skiing can be used as a supplement, but never as a complete substitute for running.

Biking and Swimming

One might think the Almighty intended the bicycle and swimming pool for injured runners—at least this is the conclusion that might be drawn from how runners most often use them! These exercises are sometimes viewed by athletes as activities to keep busy with until they can run again. The time devoted to running is primary, but again, we need to look at running as a skill, and consider how to better integrate various components that contribute to that skill. It is far better to do some supplemental bike or pool training on a regular basis than to become seriously injured—that is to do some "prehabilitation." Biking and swimming can aid in recovery from the demanding running sessions, help to develop strength, and serve to restore balance and equilibrium to the training program. Athletes would do well to conduct some form of alternative exercise such as biking or swimming in one of the two training sessions during active recovery days.

Too much concentration on endurance, like excessive sharpening work, presents a danger, because requisite levels of strength may not be maintained. When athletes conduct a quality endurance or sharpening effort, they expend some measure of their muscular strength and resiliency. Prudent athletes can be found instinctively assuming a bit of strength work after a hard training session or competition. Demanding training sessions or competitions deplete muscular strength and resilience. When athletes make too many withdrawals, they might end up bankrupt, injured, and doing all those so-called "little things" anyway, but now with the possible loss of a season or athletic career. It is a "pay now or pay later" proposition.

If an athlete is incapacitated and requires an extended layoff from running, then pool workouts having the same duration and format as the running sessions can help to maintain aerobic fitness. It is difficult for athletes to get their pulse rate above 160 bpm in a pool session, but since this approaches their anaerobic threshold, a remarkable degree of the aerobic fitness acquired via their base and strength work can be maintained. However, their local stores of muscle glycogen will normally be depleted when they finally resume running. They will suffer local fatigue and low energy levels for several weeks. When on a time line, athletes might first think the situation hopeless. Do not despair. Keep a cool head and do not attempt too much in trying to get back. The legs will arrive, having had a chance to catch up. Again, all those "little extra" things are not little, nor are they extra. They are a necessary and vital part of the larger skill distance runners need to acquire.

Plyometrics and Circuit Training

The hill bounding advocated by Arthur Lydiard comprises a form of plyometrics. Again, it is best to conduct this bounding technique on forgiving natural surfaces. Figures 8.1 and 8.2 show common examples of bounding and circuit training drills. The substance of plyometrics and circuit training sessions can be easily varied. For other potentially useful plyometric and circuit training programs, see Abmayer and Kosgei, 1992, and Martin and Coe, 1992.

Unfortunately, the potential benefits of plyometrics and circuit training can be easily compromised. Athletes having little or no foundation in strength training should not be introduced to explosive jumping or bounding activities. Runners should not undertake such activities unless they are physically mature young adults who have completed at least two years of consistent strength training. Further, the training loads must be reasonable, and the support surfaces should be forgiving. It is generally better for distance runners to conduct various plyometric drills upon a grass infield, instead of a relatively hard artificial track surface. Moreover, these exercises are best not performed as regimented drills. This method can be appropriate for use with sprinters, or large groups, but it is generally not suitable for use with distance runners. Regimented plyometric exercises can be far removed both physiologically and psychologically—from Herb Elliott leaping with exhilaration in the sand dunes and swimming in the ocean near Portsea. Given a choice, more can be gained by running barefoot on grass during the warm-up and warm-down, than by thirty minutes of bounding in shoes on a mat in a gymnasium. In warm weather conditions, it can be advantageous to play a controlled game of ultimate Frisbee—or non-contact soccer, utilizing a soft ball while running barefoot on grass. When faced with cold winter conditions, athletes can sometimes run barefoot and perform these activities upon an indoor artificial grass surface.

When attempting to restore equilibrium, the goal is to accomplish the required training task while permitting the athletes to physically and mentally recover from the preceding high quality training session. And the best way to do that is to adopt the naturalistic approach and play ethic.

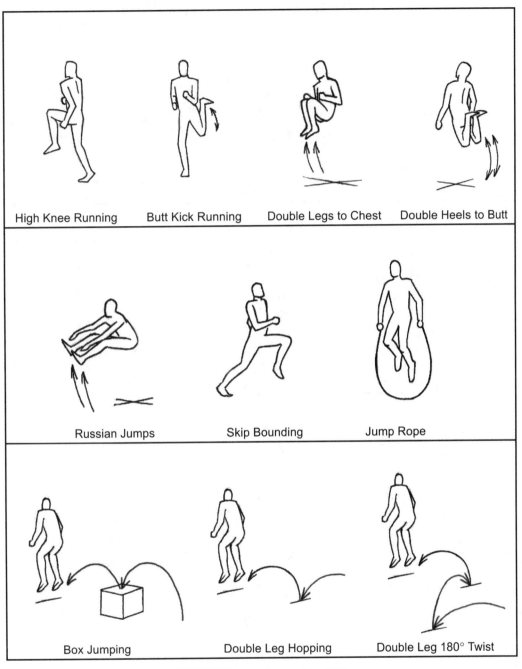

FIGURE 8.1—Plyometric Drills

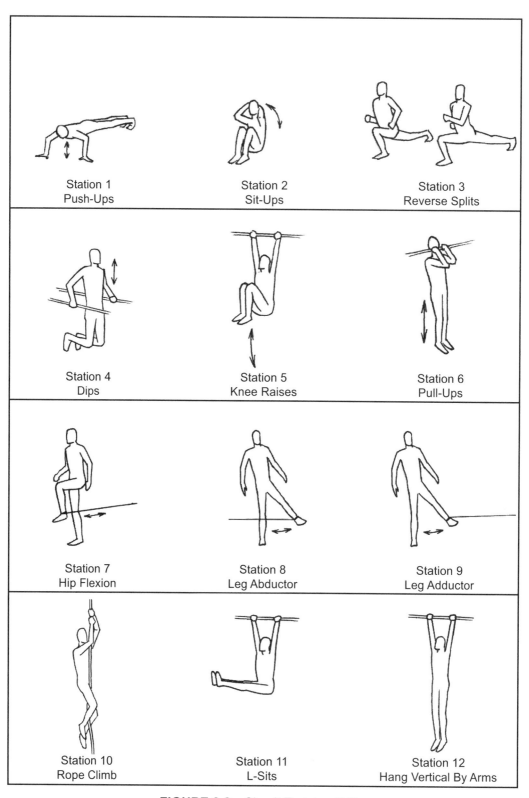

FIGURE 8.2—Circuit Training Drills

Dance, Rhythm, and Coordination

It would be difficult to find a sub 46-second specialist at 400 meters who would not be a superb dancer. The reason being that such performance requires superior neuromuscular control, balance, and coordination. Music and dance are perhaps the best activities for enhancing these qualities. Athletes are advised to participate in dance at some point, since it would both strengthen their feet and enhance flexibility. When athletes appear to be forcing or wrestling with their running technique, the coach might create an opportunity to observe them dancing. The coach may discover that the problem stems from an undeveloped sense of rhythm. However, it could also stem from an effort to maintain full conscious control of their movements—blocking the natural flow of the activity. Miyamoto Musashi, revered by the Japanese as *kensei* or swordsaint, wrote on these matters shortly before passing beyond in the year 1645. It should be noted that Musashi, besides killing over 60 men in individual combat, produced masterpieces of ink painting that are perhaps more highly valued by the Japanese than any other.

> *Whatever the Way, the master of strategy does not appear fast... skillful people never get out of time, and are always deliberate, and never appear busy. From this example the principle can be seen.*
>
> —Miyamoto Musashi

Job and Work Activity

The late University of Oregon coach Bill Bowerman made a practice of having some of his athletes employed in the sawmills of Eugene, Oregon (Moore, 1992). And under coach Bill Dellinger, the late Steve Prefontaine spent his summers working the docks in Coos Bay. Obviously an individual's employment, whether it be seasonal or year round, should not be such as to impair athletic development. But what Bowerman's athletes did certainly did not hurt them—quite the contrary. One school of thought would suggest that athletes must devote 24 hours of the day to athletics, and have the finest facilities, regimented training, and so on—*ad infinitum*.

However, there is no better way to develop strength than physical work that employs the entire body. Much can be said for a few summer months applied to the well-rounded approach to strength development found in the honest farm-boy or farm-girl ethic. So do not avoid the opportunity if it presents itself. If an athlete has a choice between two to three weight-training sessions a week, or helping someone build a house, well, help build the house! In so doing, you will spend more time engaged in countless reps that will be more beneficial all around. Murray Halberg of New Zealand, the 1960 Olympic Champion at 5,000 meters, once worked during the summer installing fence posts as a way of strengthening himself, despite having a crippled left arm.

Some coaches openly question whether athletes drawn from middle class suburbia possess the mettle required for world-class achievement. And it is easy for athletes on a scholarship stipend to think they are hard working, dedicated individuals on a holy quest for athletic excellence. An occasional eight-hour day of boring work is a good antidote for that attitude. Moreover, it will provide them with perspective, and keep their will to excel in athletics and future career high. It is easy for Americans to become runaholics, because we tend to worship number one and then wrongly equate the measure of an individual with their athletic performance on a given day. That is a lot of nonsense. Most of those who want to accomplish something in this world work hard at thankless tasks and enjoy no fanfare for their toil. On occasion, young people should be reminded of this.

The Principle of Equilibrium

Speed, strength and endurance are as three corners of a triangle that must be balanced upon a central point of equilibrium. To maximize performance on a given day, it is most productive to emphasize one or another of the above aspects at various times in training. Nevertheless, equilibrium between these components must be continually maintained. Again, imagine the athletes' endurance, speed, and strength as three corners of a triangle with the center being balanced on the head of a pin. When they try to raise one corner of the triangle, the other two will be lowered. When they raise two corners of the triangle together, one corner is lowered. In short, it is difficult to raise all three corners simultaneously (Bompa, 1994).

Another way of explaining this phenomenon is by using the analogy of a bank. If athletes attempt to purchase Endurance X, they pay for it in terms of a direct cost, but also an opportunity cost associated with the commodities, Speed Y and Strength Z. For example, when athletes run an endurance training session (such as a steady state run), making a deposit into the endurance bank account, they simultaneously make a withdrawal from their speed and strength bank accounts. A speed training session will normally cause a withdrawal from their strength and endurance accounts. And strength training normally results in a withdrawal from their endurance and speed accounts. Obviously, the various training effects of most activities do not fall neatly into a single category. Nevertheless, this analogy illustrates the interrelationship of the major assets in the "Bank of Athletic Fitness."

When athletes do not observe and implement the principle of equilibrium, they risk unbalanced development, illness, and injury. Repeated withdrawals from the strength account due to demanding running workouts, can easily lead to bankruptcy in the form of an injury. There is also a real danger of developing muscle imbalances when athletes conduct a great deal of endurance work on paved roads. The smooth and rigid nature of the surface provides a level of efficiency not found when running on a natural surface. And the paved surfaces do not permit the athletes to extensively work their balancing muscle groups. They can run faster workouts on paved surfaces, but if the object of the training is to cultivate endurance, it makes more sense to seek out natural grass, sand, or dirt roads. Athletes can then place a higher training load on their cardiovascular system at lower speeds, saving themselves wear and tear. In addition, natural surfaces impart less shock loading than paved surfaces. Moreover, the inherent strength demanded for running on natural surfaces permits athletes to maintain equilibrium without needing as much supplementary strength work.

When athletes finish a demanding aerobic effort (such as an anaerobic threshold or steady state session), the last thing they will want to do, given the feelings of the moment, is to engage in a 1/4-effort strength training session. But subjective feelings are deceiving, and *this* is precisely what they *will* need to do in order to restore equilibrium. What this entails is first conducting a warm-up set, then a second set with a training load no greater than the first set commonly used in the acquisitive strength training session. Half way through this recovery strength training session, athletes commonly feel unusually refreshed, and the fatigue which normally lingers after a demanding running workout will dissipate.

It is well known that distance running tends to shift an athlete's biochemistry towards catabolism, as opposed to anabolism. An athlete's metabolism should not continue in a catabolic mode long after a run. This would undermine the process of adaptation and acquisition. After a hard training session, it will help to stop further catabolism and promote anabolism if athletes ingest water, but also a citrus juice including a simple sugar such as pineapple-grapefruit. Carrot juice also works well. Alternatively, other forms of sugar also have this effect, such as glucose, sucrose, maltodextrin, honey or foods having a high glycemic index. Getting adequate rest and sleep also promotes anabolism and acquisition, thus athletes would be prudent to take an afternoon siesta, and get to bed at a reasonable hour. However, the important point here is that strength training can dramatically shift the metabolism of athletes from catabolism to anabolism.

Let's return to the earlier analogy in which the triangle of athletic fitness (endurance, speed, and strength) lies balanced on the head of a pin. When athletes first raise the corner of endurance, this causes the strength and speed corners to lower. Then, by conducting a recovery strength training session, the athletes can elevate the corner of strength to an equal position relative to endurance. Nevertheless, this still leaves the speed corner flagging. One of the most noticeable and potentially dangerous characteristics can be a loss of elasticity in connective tissue. After a demanding running workout, athletes can experience tightness, weakness, and a brittle feeling in connective tissues—particularly in their tendons. In short, the snap has substantially gone out of their legs. Accordingly, after a demanding running workout and before the next, it is prudent to solicit the return of elasticity to their connective tissue.

During the warm-down, when conditions permit, barefoot walking and jogging on a natural grass or sand surface can go far to restore the flagging speed corner and equilibrium. Obviously, the surface must be free of glass or other possible hazards. Swimming can also be especially effective. Both of these activities permit athletes to be grounded. A trampoline, or alternatively, a miniature trampoline or so-called rebounder can also be used to good effect. Music and aerobics, or dance activities associated with lateral movements can also facilitate recovery. Depend-

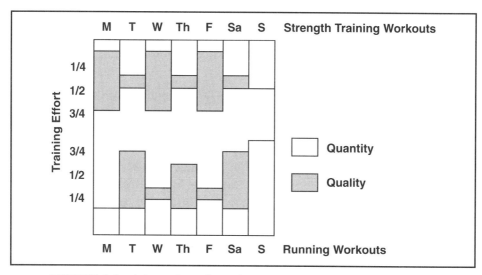

FIGURE 8.3—Integration of running and strength training workouts

ing upon which corner of the triangle had been stressed, other activities might be done in order to restore equilibrium. However, these activities should be as natural, spontaneous, and rhythmic as possible. Psychologically, this means they should correspond to active play.

Strength Training Schedules

Strength exercises often place training loads on multiple parts of the body, but here these exercises will be divided by their primary focus into upper body, abdominal, and lower body groups. In addition, these sessions will be further characterized by their express training purpose:

- Acquisitive efforts—increase strength levels
- Consolidative efforts—stabilize the gains made by acquisitive efforts
- Maintenance efforts—hold on to acquired strength levels
- Recovery efforts—use strength training to restore equilibrium

In no way should weight training compromise the running workouts—which are of primary importance. This means that adequate separation between succeeding weight training and running sessions should be provided to eliminate any counterproductive interaction. Thus, the structure of the weekly running program largely dictates the frequency and magnitude of the weight training sessions that will be assumed. The micro-cycle or weekly training schedule provided in Chapter 1 has been adapted for present use and shown in Figure 8.3.

The timing and interaction between the quality weight training and running sessions is critical, given:

- The positive role of strength training in restoring equilibrium and enhancing recovery
- The negative effects that would attend an improper integration of weight training and the running sessions

Base Period Strength Training Schedule For Workweeks

Monday: Acquisitive upper and lower body strength training session before the passive recovery running workout

Tuesday: Recovery upper and lower body strength training session after the 3/4-effort running workout

Wednesday: Acquisitive upper and lower body strength training session before the active recovery running workout

Thursday: Recovery upper and lower body strength training session after the 1/2-effort running workout

Friday: Acquisitive upper and lower body strength session before the active recovery running workout

Saturday: Recovery upper and lower body strength training session after the 3/4-effort running workout

Sunday: Recovery upper and lower body strength training session after the easy long run

This schedule would provide ample opportunity to conduct three acquisitive weight training sessions, as well as three to four recovery efforts during each workweek. The *early-cycle* and *mid-cycle* weight training progressions would then be used (See Table 8.3). The schedule provided below corresponds to worthwhile breaks during the base period.

Base Period Strength Training Schedule For Worthwhile Breaks

Monday: Upper and lower body strength training performance evaluation before the passive recovery running workout

Tuesday: Recovery upper and lower body strength training session after the time trial or date pace running workout

Wednesday: Recovery lower body strength training session after active recovery running workout

Thursday: No strength training, easy recovery running workout

Friday: No strength training, Day Before Race running workout

Saturday: Recovery upper and lower body strength training session after the control run, time trial, or race

Sunday: No strength training, easy long run

This schedule includes a strength training performance evaluation on Monday, that is, five days prior to a control run, time trial or race. In this way, no counterproductive interactive effects will be experienced. As shown in Table 8.3, the *late cycle* weight training progression would be conducted during this strength training performance evaluation. Throughout the base period, the strength training undertaken largely comprises general conditioning exercises.

After completing the base period, athletes will begin the hill period, which is characterized by more extensive anaerobic work and specific conditioning exercises, both on and off the track. The acquisitive strength training session is then dropped from the schedule, since at least one running workout normally entails strength conditioning during the hill period.

Hill Period Strength Training Schedule For Workweeks

Monday: Acquisitive upper and lower body strength training session before the passive recovery running workout

Tuesday: Recovery upper and lower body strength training session after the 3/4-effort running workout

Wednesday: Maintenance upper and lower body strength training session, body weight exercises being preferred, before the active recovery running workout

Thursday: Recovery upper and lower body strength training session after the 1/2-effort running workout

Friday: Acquisitive upper and lower body strength training session before the active recovery running workout

Saturday: Recovery upper and lower body strength training session after the 3/4-effort running workout

Sunday: Recovery upper and lower body strength training session after the easy long run

This schedule would provide ample opportunity to conduct two acquisitive weight training sessions, one maintenance effort using body weight exercises, and three to four recovery efforts during each workweek. The *early-cycle* and *mid-cycle* weight training progression would then be used (See Table 8.3).

Hill Period Strength Training Schedule For Worthwhile Breaks

Monday: Upper and lower body strength training performance evaluation before the passive recovery running workout

Tuesday: Recovery upper and lower body strength training session after the time trial or date pace running workout

Wednesday: Recovery lower body strength training session after the active recovery running workout

Thursday: No strength training, easy recovery running workout

Friday: No strength training, Day Before Race running workout

Saturday: Recovery upper and lower body strength training session after the control run, time trial, or race

Sunday: No strength training, easy long run

Once again, this schedule includes a strength training performance evaluation on Monday, that is, five days prior to a control run or race. The *late-cycle* weight training progression would be conducted during this strength training performance evaluation (See Table 8.3).

Sharpening Period Strength Training Schedule For Workweeks

Monday: Acquisitive upper and lower body strength training session before the passive recovery running workout

Tuesday: Recovery upper and lower body strength training session, recreational swimming preferred after the 3/4-effort running workout

Wednesday: Recovery upper and lower body strength training session after the active recovery running workout

Thursday: Recovery upper and lower body strength training session, recreational swimming preferred after the 1/2-effort running workout

Friday: Acquisitive upper and lower body strength training session before the active recovery running workout

Saturday: Recovery upper and lower body strength training session, recreational swimming preferred after the acquisitive running workout

Sunday: No strength training, easy long run

This schedule would permit two acquisitive upper and lower body weight-training sessions, conducted on Monday and Friday during the sharpening period, thus alternating three to four days apart. The *mid-cycle* weight training progression would be used during the Monday acquisitive strength training session, and the *late-cycle* progression would be used during the Friday session (See Table 8.3). The practical effect is to permit some strength acquisition, but at a reduced rate and with considerably less investment of time and energy. This will enable athletes to focus on the demanding sharpening work during this time.

Once again, the strength training sessions during the sharpening period are placed to minimize suppression of the quality running sessions normally run on Tuesday (3/4-effort), Thursday (1/2-effort) and Saturday (3/4-effort). The preferred mode of active recovery after the running workouts of Tuesday, Thursday and Saturday would be recreational swimming. In addition, the recovery upper and lower body sessions on Wednesday would focus on body weight exercises. Sunday would then essentially be a day off with regard to strength training, but whenever possible the long aerobic effort should be run on natural surfaces. Obviously, assigning particular tasks to various days of the week is only intended to serve as an illustration, since it is the pattern and integration of activities that is most important.

Sharpening Period Strength Training Schedule For Worthwhile Break

Monday: Upper and lower body strength maintenance session before the passive recovery running workout

Tuesday: Recovery upper and lower body strength training session, recreational swimming preferred, after the time trial

Wednesday: Recovery upper and lower body strength training session after the active recovery running workout

Thursday: No strength training, easy recovery running workout

Friday: No strength training, Day Before Race running workout

Saturday: Recovery upper and lower body strength training session, recreational swimming preferred after the competition

Sunday: No strength training, easy long run

During the worthwhile break in the middle of the sharpening period, a single strength maintenance session comes on Monday, that is, five days prior to a Saturday competition. The *peak period* weight training progression would be used in the Monday maintenance session (See Table 8.3). The recovery upper and lower body session on Wednesday would consist of body weight exercises. Recreational swimming is the preferred mode for recovery after the Tuesday time trial and the Saturday competition.

Peak Period Strength Training Schedule

For The 9-to-10-Day Ascent to the Plateau of Peak Performance

9 Thursday: Recovery upper and lower body strength training session, recreational swimming preferred, after the last 3/4-effort running workout

8 Friday: Upper and lower body strength maintenance training session before the active recovery running workout

7 Saturday: Recovery upper and lower body strength training session, recreational swimming preferred, after the finishing speed running workout

6 Sunday: No strength training, easy long easy run

5 Monday: Upper and lower body strength maintenance training session before the passive recovery running workout

4 Tuesday: Recovery upper and lower body strength training session, recreational swimming preferred, after the time trial

3 Wednesday: Recovery upper and lower body strength training session, body weight exercises preferred, after active recovery workout

2 Thursday: No strength training, easy recovery running workout

1 Friday: No strength training, Day Before Race running workout

0 Saturday: Recovery upper and lower body strength training session, recreational swimming preferred, after the competition

TABLE 8.1—Overview of Athletic Season Strength Training Schedules

No acquisitive strength training sessions are conducted once the athletes begin the peak period. Table 8.1 summarizes this discussion.

Format Considerations for the Individual Strength Training Sessions

Again, the progression of primary weight training sessions during the base, hill and sharpening periods must follow the structure of the meso-cycles adopted in the competitive racing schedule. As a result, distance runners have more frequent cycles and rapid weight training progressions, compared to those of athletes in other sports, such as American football.

An effective means of inducing muscular hypertrophy would be to direct exercises towards a particular muscle group with numerous sets and reps in the range of 80% maximal effort, and take brief recovery periods to keep the muscles hot and pumped. However, runners desire to pack the highest possible level of muscular strength into their competitive body weight. Unlike football players or throwers, they are not interested in muscular hypertrophy or gains in competitive body weight, because normally this would lower their aerobic ability and be counterproductive to performance.

The distance runner must then take a more intensive, quality-oriented approach to strength training. As a result, the number of sets in a distance runner's weight training program will be limited, and the progressions will also include fewer reps. The weight training progression is also faster, given the brevity of the meso-cycles dictated by the racing schedule. Also, the sets and reps within a given training session (and in the larger progression) will normally reduce in volume, and progress in intensity. This process will possibly culminate in maximum lifts at the end of each worthwhile break prior to the next training meso-cycle (See the *late cycle* training session in Table 8.3).

The limited number of sets and reps tends to offset the fact that distance runners generally lift intensively—that is, above 80% maximal effort, which could otherwise induce muscular hypertrophy. Distance runners should also take care to widely separate exercises that would cumulatively load-up specific muscle groups. For this reason, they might conduct roaming sets, proceeding from station to station in a series, as opposed to doing three straight sets of a given exercise. Some call this super-setting, whereas others use the same term to describe just the opposite practice. Distance runners might be advised to conduct three sets by doing three passes at a larger series of exercises that do not cumulatively load a specific muscle group.

In contrast with the arm exercises, athletes should not attempt a maximum in any of the primary or secondary leg exercises. And because of the greater strength of the primary leg muscles relative to the joints being stressed, athletes should not exceed 20 reps. Moreover, with reference to the legs, a maximum lift should not be characterized by fewer than six reps. The primary requirement is complete control. If this cannot be demonstrated, regardless of the weight involved, the activity should not proceed!

The *late cycle* or *peak cycle* training sessions in Table 8.3 would be conducted after the time trial or competition. At that time, the primary goal would be to maintain acquired strength levels and facilitate recovery. In order to maintain acquired powers with a minimal risk of injury and without introducing high fatigue levels, athletes should first conduct a warm-up set, and then a second set with the quality reduced to between 80 and 90% of the repetition maximum. This normally translates into a second set of four or five reps.

There is a practical limit to how much positive adaptation can be elicited by the combined running and strength training work loads. Accordingly, the risk of introducing high levels of fatigue or incurring injury can be a concern. However, by well structuring the strength training program, athletes can be in and out of the weight room within an hour. One-hour Maximum! In this way, high school athletes might be able to catch the early activity bus, and collegiate athletes can make supper at the dorms and be able to complete their studies.

The primary weight training progressions being provided are developmental in nature. As a result, they incorporate more volume than would be assumed by athletes who have already arrived, whose primary task is to maintain strength levels. Moreover, the progressions represent something near the developmental end point for mature specialists at 1,500 and 3,000 meters. Thus, the percent body weight (% BW) and repetition maximum (% RM) correspond to the desired performance guidelines (See Table 8.2). Obviously, athletes competing in 400 or 800 meters might increase their strength-training program approximately 15% over this example. On the other hand, those competing in 5,000 or 10,000 meters might decrease their program by the same amount. A truly comprehensive treatment would progress the schedules by physical age and athletic level, but that is beyond the scope of this book.

Acquisitive Upper Body Session

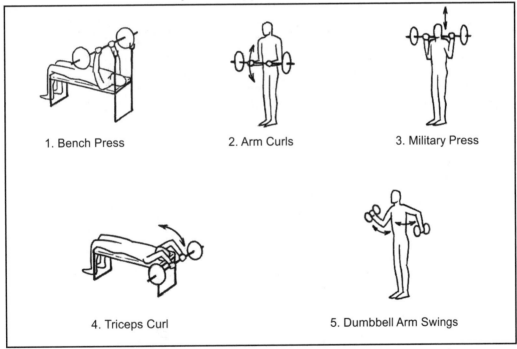

1. Bench Press   2. Arm Curls   3. Military Press

4. Triceps Curl   5. Dumbbell Arm Swings

FIGURE 8.4—Strength Training Sessions

Acquisitive Lower Body Session

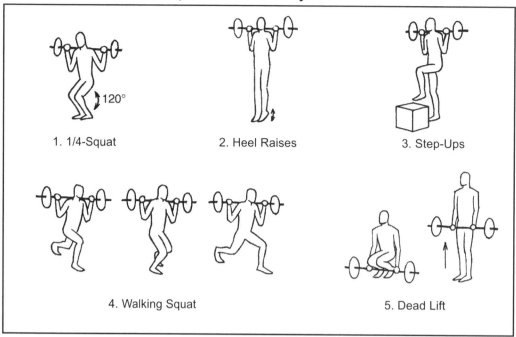

Recovery Upper Body Session

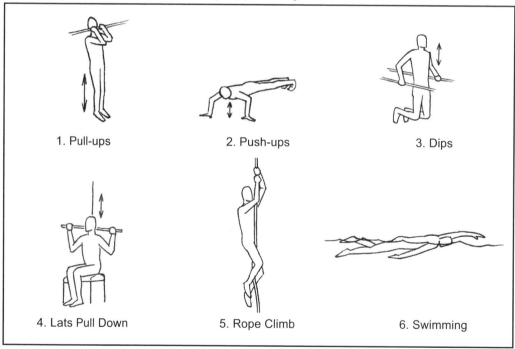

FIGURE 8.4 (continued)—Strength Training Sessions

Recovery Lower Body Session

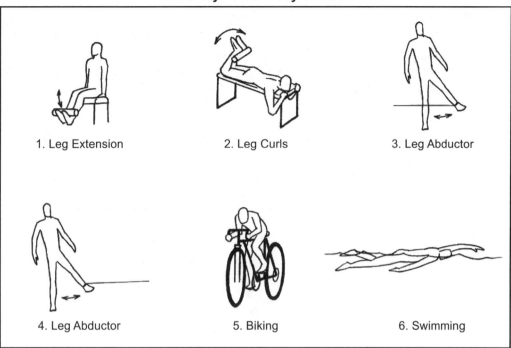

1. Leg Extension   2. Leg Curls   3. Leg Abductor

4. Leg Abductor   5. Biking   6. Swimming

Daily Abdominal Session

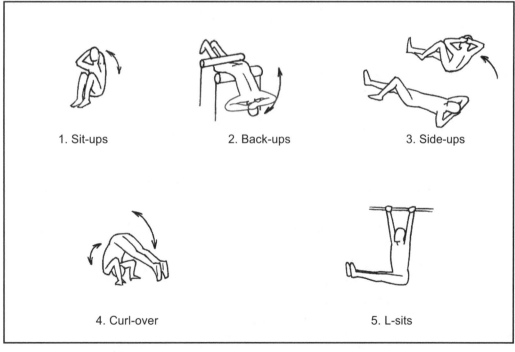

1. Sit-ups   2. Back-ups   3. Side-ups

4. Curl-over   5. L-sits

FIGURE 8.4 (continued)—Strength Training Sessions

Strength Training Performance Guidelines

Table 8.2 provides abstract strength training guidelines that are not specific by event. Athletes competing in the middle distance events should assume more extensive and higher quality strength training than those in the long distance events. These exercises do not exhaust the possibilities, but rather provide an appropriate indication of required strength levels.

Weight Training Progressions

Table 8.3 provides weight-training progressions for both the men's and women's primary upper body, and lower body exercises. Table 8.4 is based on Table 8.3, and can serve as a weight training workout card.

Male and Female
Free Body Weight Exercises

Pull-ups	Men	15 routine, 20 possible
	Women	10 routine, 15 possible
Push-ups	Men	50 routine, 75 possible
	Women	35 routine, 50 possible
Dips	Men	20 routine, 30 possible
	Women	10 routine, 20 possible
Sit-ups	Men	50 routine, 100 possible
	Women	50 routine, 100 possible
Back-ups	Men	25 routine
	Women	25 routine
Side-ups	Men	25 routine
	Women	25 routine
Curl over	Men	25 routine
	Women	15 routine
L-Sits	Men	20 routine
	Women	15 routine
Jumping Jacks	Men	100 routine
	Women	100 routine
Mountain Climb	Men	25 routine
	Women	25 routine
Reverse Splits	Men	25 routine
	Women	25 routine
Rope Climb	Men	1 Climb without using Legs
	Women	1 Climb using Legs

TABLE 8.2—Strength Training Performance Guidelines

Male and Female
Upper Body Free Weight Exercises

RM = Repetition Maximum = 1 Repetition at 100% Effort
BW = Quality Expressed as Percentage (%) of Body Weight

Bench Press	Men	1 x 150% BW
	Women	1 x 105% BW
Incline	Men	10 x 110% BW
	Women	10 x 75% BW
Military	Men	10 x 100% BW Standing
		10 x 75% Behind Head
	Women	10 x 70% BW Standing
		10 x 50% Behind Head
Flat Flies	Men	10 x 50% BW
	Women	10 x 35% BW
Arm Curls	Men	10 x 55% BW Normal
		10 x 50% Reverse
	Women	10 x 45% BW Normal
		10 x 40% Reverse
Triceps Curls	Men	10 x 50% BW
	Women	10 x 35% BW
Bent Rows	Men	10 x 75% BW
	Women	10 x 50% BW
Hang Cleans	Men	10 x 125% BW
	Women	10 x 75% BW

Male and Female
Lower Body Free Weight Exercises

Heel Raises	Men	10 x 125% BW
	Women	10 x 90% BW
Step-ups	Men	10 x 80% BW
	Women	10 x 55% BW
Walking Squats	Men	10 x 50% BW
	Women	10 x 35% BW
Dead Lift	Men	1 x 225% BW
	Women	1 x 150% BW
1/4 Squats	Men	6 x 225% BW
	Women	6 x 150% BW

TABLE 8.2 (continued)—Strength Training Performance Guidelines

Male Athletes
Upper Body Weight Training Progression

RM = 1 Repetition Maximum   BW = Body Weight
RV = Reverse Curls   BH = Military Behind Head
FR = Military Free Standing   WK = Walking Squats

Early-Cycle	Set 1	Set 2	Set 3
1) Bench Press	20 x 50% RM	15 x 60% RM	10 x 70% RM
2) Arm Curls	15 x 40% BW	15 x 40% BW RV	10 x 50% BW
3) Military BH	20 x 40% BW	15 x 50% BW	10 x 60% BW
4) Triceps Curl	20 x 30% BW	15 x 40% BW	10 x 50% BW

Mid-Cycle	Set 1	Set 2	Set 3
1) Bench Press	10 x 70% RM	6 x 80% RM	3 x 90% RM
2) Arm Curls	10 x 50% BW	10 x 50% BW RV	6 x 60% BW
3) Military BH	10 x 60% BW	6 x 80% BW	3 x 90% BW
4) Triceps Curl	10 x 50% BW	6 x 55% BW	3 x 60% BW

Late-Cycle (MAX)	Set 1	Set 2	Set 3
1) Bench Press	10 x 65% RM	3 x 90% RM	1 x 100% RM
2) Arm Curls	10 x 40% BW	6 x 60% RV	3 x 70% BW
3) Military FR	10 x 60% RM	3 x 90% RM	1 x 100% RM
4) Triceps Curl	10 x 55% BW	3 x 60% BW	3 x 65% BW

Peak Period	Set 1	Set 2	Set 3
1) Bench Press	10 x 65% RM	3 x 90% RM	—
2) Arm Curls	10 x 40% BW	6 x 60% BW	—
3) Military	10 x 60% BW BH	3 x 90% RM FR	—
4) Triceps Curl	10 x 40% BW	3 x 60% BW	—

TABLE 8.3

Male Athletes
Lower Body Weight Training Progression

RM = 1 Repetition Maximum	BW = Body Weight
RV = Reverse Curls	BH = Military Behind Head
FR = Military Free Standing	WK = Walking Squats

Early-Cycle	Set 1	Set 2	Set 3
1) 1/4 Squat	10 x 100% BW	10 x 125% BW	10 x 150% BW
2) Heel Raises	20 x 50% BW	10 x 80% BW	10 x 100% BW
3) Step Ups	10 x 45% BW	10 x 60% BW	10 x 70% BW
4) WK Squats	10 x 30% BW	10 x 40% BW	10 x 45% BW

Mid-Cycle	Set 1	Set 2	Set 3
1) 1/4 Squat	10 x 125% BW	8 x 175% BW	6 x 200% BW
2) Heel Raises	10 x 80% BW	10 x 100% BW	6 x 110% BW
3) Step Ups	10 x 60% BW	10 x 70% BW	10 x 75% BW
4) WK Squats	10 x 40% BW	10 x 45% BW	10 x 50% BW

Late-Cycle (MAX)	Set 1	Set 2	Set 3
1) 1/4 Squat	10 x 125% BW	6 x 175% BW	6 x 225% BW
2) Heel Raises	10 x 80% BW	6 x 100% BW	6 x 125% BW
3) Step Ups	10 x 60% BW	6 x 70% BW	6 x 80% BW
4) WK Squats	10 x 40% BW	6 x 45% BW	6 x 55% BW

Peak Period	Set 1	Set 2	Set 3
1) 1/4 Squat	10 x 125% BW	6 x 175% BW	—
2) Heel Raises	10 x 80% BW	6 x 100% BW	—
3) Step Ups	10 x 60% BW	6 x 70% BW	—
4) WK Squats	10 x 40% BW	6 x 45% BW	—

TABLE 8.3 (continued)

Female Athletes
Upper Body Weight Training Progression

RM = 1 Repetition Maximum	BW = Body Weight
RV = Reverse Curls	BH = Military Behind Head
FR = Military Free Standing	WK = Walking Squats

Early-Cycle	Set 1	Set 2	Set 3
1) Bench Press	20 x 50% RM	15 x 60% RM	10 x 70% RM
2) Arm Curls	15 x 30% BW	15 x 30% BW RV	10 x 40% BW
3) Military BH	20 x 30% BW	15 x 35% BW	10 x 40% BW
4) Triceps Curl	20 x 20% BW	15 x 25% BW	10 x 30% BW

Mid-Cycle	Set 1	Set 2	Set 3
1) Bench Press	10 x 70% RM	6 x 80% RM	3 x 90% RM
2) Arm Curls	10 x 40% BW	10 x 40% BW RV	6 x 50% BW
3) Military BH	10 x 40% BW	6 x 45% BW	3 x 55% BW
4) Triceps Curl	10 x 30% BW	6 x 35% BW	3 x 40% BW

Late-Cycle (MAX)	Set 1	Set 2	Set 3
1) Bench Press	10 x 65% RM	3 x 90% RM	1 x 100% RM
2) Arm Curls	10 x 30% BW	6 x 50% BW	3 x 60% BW
3) Military FR	10 x 60% RM	3 x 90% RM	1 x 100% RM
4) Triceps Curl	10 x 35% BW	3 x 45% BW	3 x 55% BW

Peak Period	Set 1	Set 2	Set 3
1) Bench Press	10 x 65% RM	3 x 90% RM	—
2) Arm Curls	10 x 30% BW	6 x 50% BW	—
3) Military	10 x 40% BW BH	3 x 90% RM FR	—
4) Triceps Curl	10 x 25% BW	3 x 45% BW	—

TABLE 8.3 (continued)

Female Athletes
Lower Body Weight Training Progression

RM = 1 Repetition Maximum   BW = Body Weight
RV = Reverse Curls   BH = Military Behind Head
FR = Military Free Standing   WK = Walking Squats

Early-Cycle	Set 1	Set 2	Set 3
1) 1/4 Squats	10 x 100% BW	10 x 125% BW	10 x 135% BW
2) Heel Raises	20 x 50% BW	10 x 70% BW	10 x 90% BW
3) Step Ups	10 x 25% BW	10 x 35% BW	10 x 45% BW
4) WK Squats	10 x 20% BW	10 x 25% BW	10 x 30% BW

Mid-Cycle	Set 1	Set 2	Set 3
1) 1/4 Squats	10 x 125% BW	8 x 135% BW	6 x 145% BW
2) Heel Raises	10 x 70% BW	10 x 80% BW	6 x 100% BW
3) Step Ups	10 x 35% BW	10 x 45% BW	10 x 55% BW
4) WK Squats	10 x 25% BW	10 x 30% BW	10 x 35% BW

Late-Cycle (MAX)	Set 1	Set 2	Set 3
1) 1/4 Squats	10 x 100% BW	6 x 130% BW	6 x 150% BW
2) Heel Raises	10 x 80% BW	6 x 100% BW	6 x 110% BW
3) Step Ups	10 x 35% BW	6 x 45% BW	6 x 55% BW
4) WK Squats	10 x 25% BW	6 x 30% BW	6 x 40% BW

Peak Period	Set 1	Set 2	Set 3
1) 1/4 Squat	10 x 125% BW	6 x 130% BW	—
2) Heel Raises	10 x 80% BW	6 x 90% BW	—
3) Step Ups	10 x 35% BW	6 x 45% BW	—
4) WK Squats	10 x 25% BW	6 x 30% BW	—

TABLE 8.3 (continued)

Workout Card
Male and Female Athletes
Upper Body Weight Training Progression

RM = 1 Repetition Maximum	BW = Body Weight
RV = Reverse Curls	BH = Military Behind Head
FR = Military Free Standing	WK = Walking Squats

Early-Cycle	Set 1	Set 2	Set 3
1) Bench Press	20 x	15 x	10 x
2) Arm Curls	15 x	15 x RV	10 x
3) Military BH	20 x	15 x	10 x
4) Triceps Curl	20 x	15 x	10 x

Mid-Cycle	Set 1	Set 2	Set 3
1) Bench Press	10 x	6 x	3 x
2) Arm Curls	10 x	10 x RV	6 x
3) Military BH	10 x	6 x	3 x
4) Triceps Curl	10 x	6 x	3 x

Late-Cycle (MAX)	Set 1	Set 2	Set 3
1) Bench Press	10 x	3 x	1 x
2) Arm Curls	10 x	6 x	3 x
3) Military FR	10 x	3 x	1 x
4) Triceps Curl	10 x	3 x	3 x

Peak Period	Set 1	Set 2	Set 3
1) Bench Press	10 x	3 x	
2) Arm Curls	10 x	6 x	
3) Military	10 x BH	3 x FR	
4) Triceps Curl	10 x	3 x	

NAME: _____

DATE: _____

TABLE 8.4

Workout Card
Male and Female Athletes
Lower Body Weight Training Progression

RM = 1 Repetition Maximum	BW = Body Weight
RV = Reverse Curls	BH = Military Behind Head
FR = Military Free Standing	WK = Walking Squats

Early-Cycle	Set 1	Set 2	Set 3
1) 1/4 Squat	10 x	10 x	10 x
2) Heel Raises	20 x	10 x	10 x
3) Step Ups	10 x	10 x	10 x
4) WK Squats	10 x	10 x	10 x

Mid-Cycle	Set 1	Set 2	Set 3
1) 1/4 Squat	10 x	8 x	6 x
2) Heel Raises	10 x	10 x	6 x
3) Step Ups	10 x	10 x	10 x
4) WK Squats	10 x	10 x	10 x

Late-Cycle (MAX)	Set 1	Set 2	Set 3
1) 1/4 Squat	10 x	6 x	6 x
2) Heel Raises	10 x	6 x	6 x
3) Step Ups	10 x	6 x	6 x
4) WK Squats	10 x	6 x	6 x

Peak Period	Set 1	Set 2	Set 3
1) 1/4 Squat	10 x	6 x	
2) Heel Raises	10 x	6 x	
3) Step Ups	10 x	6 x	
4) WK Squats	10 x	6 x	

NAME:_____

DATE:_____

TABLE 8.4 (continued)

Beyond the Physical Aspects of Strength Training

This chapter has been largely devoted to physical aspects of strength training and athletic performance. However, the mental or spiritual contribution is equally important. It has been said that everything lies in the execution, and this requires an integration of concentration, timing, and focus. These qualities and abilities derive from a wider process of personal cultivation.

> *Mind and body are but two aspects of the one reality: energy. One informs the other. The "informing" is found in the combined exercise of meditation flowing into concentration flowing into focus.*
>
> *When an individual converts concentration into action, the movement is called focus. A vitalized mental image becomes a physical reality. The combination of concentration and focus intensifies power two-, four-, ten-fold.*
>
> —Sang Kyu Shim

When teaching any physical activity, at some point, athletes can be enlightened to mentally project in time and space the desired physical action and result. This important subject falls into the realm of sports psychology, and lies beyond the scope of this book. In brief, the optimal performance state transcends a superficial causal explanation. Athletics at the highest level is ultimately an art form. In this regard, the role of the deeper personality cannot be overstressed.

> *For the superlative athletic performances of the future, a contemplation of, and some understanding of, the highest forms of art, music and philosophy can be seen as a sine qua non of the era of new world records...*
>
> *A superlative performance does not merely require a few grimaces in the last stages of a race, but the capacity of the athlete to fully express himself—in every way open to him, through his strength, stamina and technique; his spirituality, which will supply the inner strengths: and his artistic response, which will make his physical movements more efficient and successful.*
>
> —Percy Cerutty

References

Abmayer, Walter, and Mike Kosgei, "Kenya Cross-Country Training," *Track & Field Quarterly Review*, Volume 91, Number 2, 1991, pages 43-44.

Åstrand, Olaf, and Kaare Rodahl, *Textbook of Work Physiology*, 3rd edition, New York: McGraw-Hill, 1986, pages 33-39.

Bompa, Tudor O., *Theory and Methodology of Training*, Dubuque, Iowa: Kendall/Hunt Publishing Company, 1994.

Bowerman, William J., *Coaching Track & Field*, William H. Freeman, Editor, Boston, Massachusetts: Houghton Mifflin Co., 1974.

Cerutty, Percy, *Athletics*, London: The Sportsmans Book Club, 1961, pages 60, and 151.

Cerutty, Percy, *Middle Distance Running*, London: Pelham Books, 1964, page 57.

Cerutty, Percy, *Success: In Sport and Life*, London: Pelham Books, 1967, pages 54 and 134.

Coyle, Edward F., "Integration of the Physiological Factors Determining Endurance Performance Ability," *Exercise Sport Science Review*, 1995, Volume 23, pages 25-63.

Dellinger, Bill, and George Beres, *Winning Running*, Chicago, Illinois: Contemporary Books, Inc., 1978.

Fox, Edward, Donald Mathews, *The Physiological Basis of Physical Education and Athletics*, 3rd Edition, New York: Saunders College Publishing, 1981, page 313.

Hickson, R.C., and B.A. Dvorak, E.M. Gorostiaga, T.T. Kurowski, C. Foster, "Potential for Strength and Endurance Training to Amplify Endurance Performance," *Journal of Applied Physiology*, Volume 65, 1988, pages 2285-2290.

Houmard, J.A., and D.L. Costill, J.B. Mitchell, S.H. Park, T.C. Chenier, "The Role of Anaerobic Ability in Middle Distance Running Performance," *European Journal of Applied Physiology*, Volume 62, 1991, pages 40-43.

Hyams, Joe, *Zen in the Martial Arts*, Los Angeles, California: J.P. Tarcher, Inc., 1979.

Lydiard, Arthur, and Garth Gilmour, *Running the Lydiard Way*, Mountain View, California: World Publications, Inc., 1978.

Lydiard, Arthur, and Garth Gilmour, *Run to the Top*, Auckland, New Zealand: Minerva, 1962.

Marcinik, E.J., and G. Potts, S. Schlaback, P. Will, P. Dawson, B.F. Hurley, "Effects of Strength Training on Lactate Threshold and Endurance Performance," *Medicine and Science in Sports and Exercise*, Volume 23, 1991, pages 739-743.

Martin, David, and Peter Coe, "Training Distance Runners," *Track & Field Quarterly Review*, Volume 91, Number 2, 1992.

Moore, Kenny, *Best Efforts*, Florida: Cedarwinds Press, 1992.

Musashi, Miyamoto, *A Book of Five Rings*, Translated by Victor Harris, New York: Overlook Press, 1982, pages 49, and 91.

Paavolainen, L., and K. Hakkinen, I. Hamalainen, A. Nummela, H. Rusko, "Explosive-Strength Training Improves 5-Km Running Time by Improving Running Economy and Muscle Power," *Journal of Applied Physiology*, Volume 86, Issue 5, May, 1999, pages 1527-1533.

Robbins, Steven E., and Gerard J. Gouw, "Athletic Footwear and Chronic Overloading," *Sports Medicine*, Volume 9, Number 2, 1990, pages 76-85.

"Roundtable: Cardiovascular Effects of Weight Training," *NSCA Journal*, Volume 2, April/May, 1987, pages 10-20.

Schneider, Howard, "Steve Ovett," *Runner's World*, 1979.

Shim, Sang Kyu, *The Making of a Martial Artist*, 1st Edition, Published Privately in the United States, 1980, pages 13, 91, and 93.

Sparks, Ken, and Garry Bjorklund, *Long Distance Runner's Guide to Training and Racing*, New Jersey: Prentice-Hall, 1984.

Spear, Mike, "Emil Zatopek gives Modern Day Runners the Truth Behind the Myth," *Runner's World*, 1982 Annual, page 11.

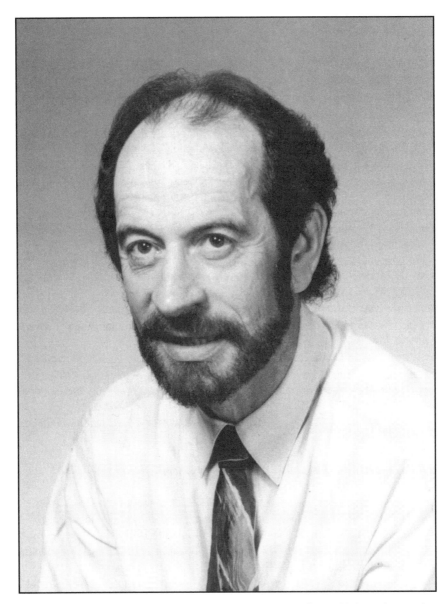

PHOTO 9.1—Peter Cavanagh, educator at Penn State University, and a pioneer of modern footwear research. Photo courtesy of Peter Cavanagh.

CHAPTER 9

INJURIES AND ATHLETIC SHOES

When you have questions about your health or that of someone for whom you are responsible, always consult a qualified medical professional such as a doctor, podiatrist, or physical therapist. Consider the following suggestions about the possible origin, rehabilitation and prevention of athletic injuries. Share whatever information you feel may be of interest or assistance with a health professional. Because this chapter deals with athletic shoes, you should know that the author has a connection with the athletic footwear industry as a former employee of Nike, Inc., but also as an independent consultant and inventor. However, the beliefs and opinions expressed herein are the author's, and do not reflect those of any other individual or company.

Functional Footwear Versus the Consumer Feeding Frenzy

Military and safety footwear have specifications, and there are industry standards for certain footwear materials and components, but there is no government or private agency regulating the footwear industry. Footwear designers and companies are relatively free to do as they wish. Practically speaking, the only real check upon the footwear industry is the footwear industry. Between the companies there is some level of scrutiny regarding the claims of competitor products concerning their performance. Occasionally, if one company makes a blatantly false statement, or grossly misrepresents another competitor's product, then the irritated party will let the other know by taking legal action.

However, the great and final arbiter of what the footwear industry does or doesn't do is the consumer, and general public. Unfortunately, the public often lacks sufficient information to make prudent decisions when selecting athletic footwear. It can be difficult for consumers to separate reality from the nonsense often present in the marketing blurbs provided by major manufacturers. Further, most researchers who are well educated on the subject are gainfully employed by the footwear manufacturers. Moreover, their published works are steeped in scientific jargon, and not well known to the public. Coaches, who might have valid insights and contributions, generally do not have a mastery of the scientific literature, neither do they often publish their observations and conclusions.

The consumer looking for an article of footwear needs to have answers to some basic questions: Does the shoe fit foot properly? Is it comfortable? Does it provide adequate cushioning? Does it provide stability? Does it provide good traction? What is the shoe's expected service life? These questions are increasingly becoming difficult if not impossible to answer, given the accelerating rate at which new products are being introduced.

This constitutes the second major problem facing those searching for functional athletic footwear. In the past, new footwear designs were introduced relatively infrequently, thus a particular model would be available for several years. Presently, new products are being launched three to five times a year. If an individual manages to find a good product, they are unlikely to find it again. Instead, when they next go shopping for footwear, they must once again take their chance at the roulette wheel and make their best guess.

Is there someone to blame? Everybody and nobody, since there are some large, impersonal, amoral forces at work. Consumer goods, such as a pair of athletic shoes, can be viewed as an essential tool. However, they can also constitute symbols with secondary meanings. "Goods carry meanings, and consumers buy goods to get hold of those meanings and use them to construct the self" (McCraken, 1988). In other words, the herd instinct is alive and well. People sometimes judge themselves and others by the external symbols they accumulate to communicate who they are—or at least, who they want to be. In this respect, how different are humans from bower birds that collect all sorts of interesting, shiny stuff to attain social status and attract a mate? Obviously, the mentality of our culture of consumption is a trap and an illusion. Individuals who literally buy into it are living in denial. In particular, relatively insecure young people, who have not yet matured and discovered their true self, often use external symbols and their stereotypical meanings as a substitute.

> *Symbols are transitory—they come and go. Chasing symbols is like settling for the map instead of the territory. It creates anxiety. It ends up making you feel hollow and empty inside, because you exchange your Self for symbols of your Self.*
>
> —Deepak Chopra

The so-called "consumer" may not be a fit athlete, rather, a so-called "ordinary" person. In truth, we are all unique, extra-ordinary people. To have dignity or worth, we do not need to be anyone else, or collect symbols to fool ourselves or others about who we are. The letterhead of Hee-Jin Kim, an expert on Zen Master Dōgen, bears the following quote from Abraham Heschel: "Just to be is a blessing. "Just to live is holy" (Kim, 1987). What is the driving force behind the appeals made to sex, youth, and rebellion so often seen in modern advertising? Denial of mortality—denial of death. More importantly—denial of the true Self. Yes, denial of that which is truly unique and individual, and replacing it with a branded stereotype or caricature of "the individual." The truth is, we all die. As my father once said, "Armageddon, or the end of the world, comes for many people every day." No one survives life. And we can take no material thing with us. Embrace the fact. Transcend it. It may transform the nature of your life.

At the present time, consumers have an insatiable thirst for the new—for change—and corporations are responding with more numerous and faster product introductions. And corporations, in the business of making profits for shareholders, fan the feeding frenzy, thereby pursuing the best interest of the amoral corporation, since its primary guiding principle is the dollar. The result of this escalation is a consumption monster that neither party really controls. Those consumers looking for functional footwear will have to look long and hard, and perhaps without success. Those wanting to make a good product within a corporation will have an uphill battle in making corporate "cents," when it is much easier to feed the frenzy and enjoy so-called success. Athletes may have to spend quite some time to actually identify those functional footwear presently being made by various manufacturers. Three months from now most of those shoes will likely be gone, and there may be little or no continuity with what comes next. The baby is often thrown out with the bath water.

Realize that you are the consumer, and the consumer is still king. If you want to continue to buy shoes that are pretty, cool, or have gizmos, then go ahead and do it. This is a free country and people are permitted life, liberty and the pursuit of happiness—even the pursuit of foolishness. But if you are after a functional article of footwear, then open your eyes, start demanding it and don't be shy. The best advice is "buyer beware." As the famous newscaster Walter Cronkite might have concluded: "And that's the way it is—."

Achilles Tendonitis

Achilles tendonitis can be caused by an acute trauma, and occasionally an athlete will tear or rupture the Achilles tendon during training or competition, but this is an infrequent occurrence. Most Achilles tendon problems come from training over-loads and training errors. For example, an athlete who dramatically increases mileage or conducts quality work without a sufficient warm up, might become injured. Get the full story of what happened, and when. Inquire as to the athlete's history of injury, and then consider the individual's conformance, biomechanics, training practices and footwear.

Roads Aren't Made for Running

Always check for an anatomical leg length difference. However, it could be that a functional leg length difference exists due to the athlete often running across a grade. Sidewalks commonly decline about five degrees towards the curb. And to promote effective runoff and drainage, roads commonly decline from the crown or centerline by about five degrees toward the opposing curbs. Therefore, the only area an athlete can find a level grade on many modern roads is right down the middle. Obviously, running in this location is generally not advisable.

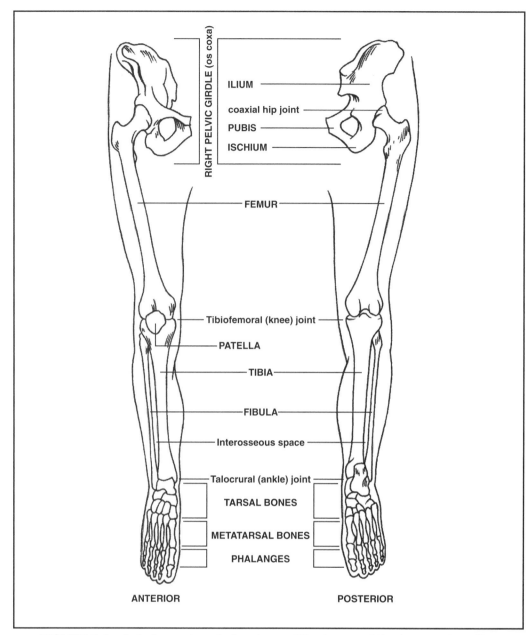

FIGURE 9.1—Anterior and posterior views of the bones of the lower extremities

Realize that over a relatively short distance, a grade of five degrees can result in a change in elevation of about 1/4 inch. When an athlete runs across a grade, the resulting functional leg length difference can displace and cause injury to the pelvis and lower back. Conversely, if an individual has an anatomical or true leg length difference, it is actually possible to compensate and neutralize the difference by selecting the proper position on the grade of a road or sidewalk upon which to run, but this is not the best solution. The introduction of a lift or orthotic by a trained medical professional can provide more appropriate relief.

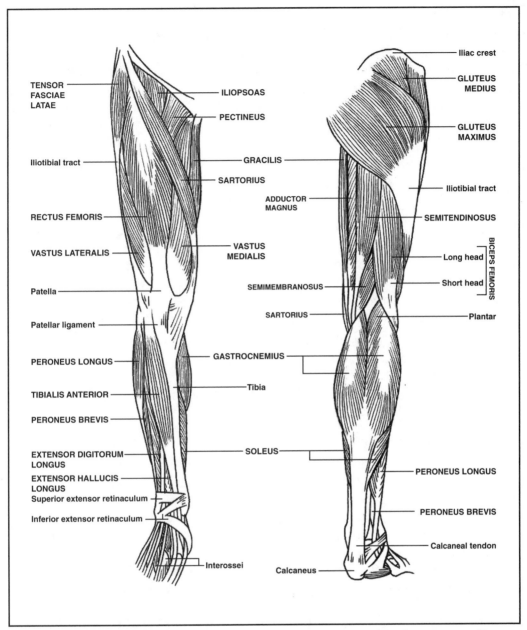

FIGURE 9.2—Anterior and posterior views of the muscles of the lower extremities

Warm-Up

Athletes need to properly warm up before performing high quality work. Breaking a sweat and attaining a pulse of 120 bpm are signs of a successful warm-up. However, even jogging two to three miles at an easy 1/4-effort, then running half a dozen stride-outs to break a sweat and attain a pulse of 120 bpm does not always provide an adequate warm-up for optimal performance. For better results, run three to four miles at 1/4-effort, and then include a faster segment close to your anaerobic threshold for about 2:30 to 3:00 minutes. Stride-outs can then follow this routine.

Tendons Like It Hot

In colder climates, or during the winter season, it is wise to protect the Achilles tendon. At times, the area between the collar of the shoe and the athlete's warm-ups can become exposed. The athlete's socks could sag or not be sufficiently heavy or windproof to protect the Achilles tendon. Further, the velocity of the lower limb and foot during running can exceed 50 mph. When an athlete is out in sub-zero weather, realize that the wind chill is being compounded at the hands and feet. A temperature gradient or cool area across the Achilles tendon can contribute to the onset of an injury.

Gimme Them Low Heeled Sneakers

Sudden or frequent changes in heel elevations can also lead to injury of the Achilles tendon. Occasionally, an athlete will run in training shoes with a relatively high heel, and then don a pair of racing flats or spikes without sufficient warm-up, stretching, or transition to the new footwear. The difference in the heel elevation between dress or casual shoes and athletic shoes can also cause problems. Attempt to minimize frequent changes in heel elevation, and insofar as possible, gradually progress the training loads when changing heel elevations.

Given the choice, gravitate towards footwear with lower heel elevation, since this normally lends itself to greater footwear stability and natural biomechanical function (Bates, James, and Osternig, 1979). Once an injury has occurred, it is often necessary to take pressure off the Achilles tendon by using a lift. The trick is to later phase out the use of the lift without re-injuring the tendon.

Time and Travel: As Things Speed Up Athletes Can Go Backwards

Injury to the Achilles tendon can also occur when, after hard exercise, an athlete must undergo a period of relative immobility. For example, perhaps the athlete runs a workout or engages in a competition, then travels in a vehicle for several hours. Given these circumstances, their connective tissue will often tighten up to a greater degree than normal. Traveling immediately after a hard workout or meet, even the following day, is not ideal. Whenever possible, travel on the second or third day after a hard training or racing effort. The worst situation occurs when an athlete performs hard exercise, then undergoes a period of relative immobility (where the initial warm-up is lost), and then later performs hard exercise again. This sometimes takes place when an athlete doubles or triples during a track and field meet, or participates in a multiple-stage relay event. These situations can be associated with a high risk of injury.

The Achilles Tendon and Shock

Excessive shock loading from repeated impact events can cause trauma to the Achilles tendon, and also disrupt the tendon's blood supply (MacLellan, 1984). The shock pulse or discontinuity from an impact event travels roughly at the speed of sound, approximately 1,600 meters per second in human soft tissue, and 3,200 meters per second in bone (Harris, 1988). The latter value is over three times faster than a high caliber rifle bullet! Further, sound has about five times more power in water than in air, and much of the human body consists of water.

One method the body uses to manage impact events is movement about a joint, associated with deflection and subsequent recovery in the manner of a spring, thus attenuating the impact event over time. An alternative method is to dampen the energy associated with an impact event and turn it into heat. Individual human muscles only dampen about 35% of the energy imparted to them (Greene and McMahon, 1979). The tendons provide a connection between bones and muscles in transferring loads, but they also become conduits for the shock pulse passing in and out of muscles. So-called "road-shock" can then be particularly stressful to tendons, which are less elastic and have a poorer blood supply than the muscles. Hard athletic shoes and hard roads are hard on the Achilles tendon.

Hard Shoes and Hard Surfaces

Athletic shoes with extremely low heel elevations, or forefoot to heel elevation differences less than 9-10 mm, can also place high loads on the Achilles tendon. This is due partly to the deflection of the fat pad on the heel. The fat pad normally deflects approximately 7-10 mm during impact. Within a pair of shoes this can contribute a negative heel elevation relative to the forefoot (Cavanagh, Valiant and Misevich, 1984). Many athletic shoes made during the 1960's and early 1970's had relatively hard soles, low heel elevations, and less than 9 mm difference in elevation between the forefoot and heel. Further, most runners in the United States train on hard asphalt. This was partly why Achilles tendonitis was such a common injury during that time (Cavanagh, *The Running Shoe Book*, 1980).

The most recent teachings of the athletic footwear industry comprise intellectual property. Accordingly, a number of United States patent documents will be cited and identified by their corresponding number. All of these documents can be found on the Internet at the U.S. Patent and Trademark website (www.uspto.gov). The fundamental idea behind the government granting a patent is the "exchange theory." In exchange for the net social welfare benefit generated when inventors disclose and teach their inventions to the general public, they are granted a certain commercial exclusivity for a period of seventeen to twenty years. Readers wishing to learn about footwear may refer to the patents about to be cited via the aforementioned website.

Today, Achilles tendon injuries are less frequent than in previous years, due in part to higher heel elevations, which take some of the loads off the tendon. There have also been improvements in cushioning and stability, particularly in the rearfoot area of athletic footwear. One example is U.S. Patent 4,506,462, granted to Peter Cavanagh, and assigned to Puma AG (See Figure 9.3).

Other teachings relating to differential cushioning in the rearfoot area include:

- U.S. 4,364,189, granted to Barry Bates, assigned to ASICS Corp.
- U.S. 4,731,939, granted to Rui Parracho et al., assigned to Converse, Inc.
- U.S. 4,817,304, granted to Mark Parker et al., assigned to Nike, Inc.
- U.S. 4,934,072, granted to Ray Frederickson et al., assigned to Brooks Sports, Inc.

- U.S. 5,046,267, granted to Bruce Kilgore et al., assigned to Nike, Inc.
- U.S. 5,197,206, U.S. 5,197,207, and U.S. 5,201,125, granted to Martyn Shorten, assigned to Puma AG.
- U.S. 6,029,374, granted to Herr, et al.
- U.S. 6,266,897, granted to R. Seydel, S. Luthi, R. Fumi, K. Beard, and O. Kaiser, assigned to Adidas-Salomon AG.

And also patents on which the author is an inventor, including:

- U.S. 5,425,184, U.S. 5,625,964, and U.S. 6,055.746, entitled "Athletic Shoe With Rearfoot Strike Zone," granted to Lyden et al., assigned to Nike, Inc. (See Figure 9.4)
- European Patent Application EP 0752216 A3, entitled "Footwear With Differential Cushioning Regions," by Lyden, assigned to Nike, Inc.
- U.S. 5,921,004, entitled "Footwear With Stabilizers," granted to Lyden, assigned to Nike, Inc.
- U.S. 6,449,878, granted to Lyden (see Figure 10.1)

Does The Shoe Bite?

If a portion of the Achilles tendon that may be in contact with the shoe becomes injured or painful, then look for a lump of material or for contact with the edge of a heel counter that could be irritating the tendon. The author once performed "shoe surgery" on an athlete's track spikes a few days before the U.S. Olympic Trials because he was suddenly having Achilles tendon problems. The athlete was apprehensive at the sight of his track spikes being modified with a razor blade, but the operation provided him with immediate relief.

In addition, check to see if the athlete is wearing shoes that are too small, and in particular, examine their track spikes. Runners will often gravitate toward a smaller shoe size to get a snug fit, especially when they have narrow feet or motion control problems. Again, dress shoes can sometimes be the real problem. Often the stiff collar of a dress shoe can impinge upon the tendon. This can easily happen if an individual has one foot larger than the other. In some instances, a bursa on the back of the calcaneus can become injured, rather than the Achilles tendon. In this case, the pressure on the general area needs to be reduced. If this condition persists, the bursa itself could become injured beyond repair and need to be surgically removed.

Flexibility and Strength

Check the individual's range of motion with respect to ankle and hip flexion. Stretching the calf muscles on an inclined platform is a sound training practice (Dellinger with Beres, 1978). What does the athlete do in the way of a stretching routine? Check the strength and condition of the athlete's calf muscles. Weak calf muscles can result in excessive loads being placed on the Achilles tendon.

United States Patent [19]

Cavanagh

[11] **Patent Number:** **4,506,462**

[45] **Date of Patent:** **Mar. 26, 1985**

[54] **RUNNING SHOE SOLE WITH PRONATION LIMITING HEEL**

[75] Inventor: **Peter R. Cavanagh**, Pine Grove Mills, Pa.

[73] Assignee: **Puma-Sportschuhfabriken Rudolf Dassler KG**, Herzogenaurach, Fed. Rep. of Germany

[21] Appl. No.: **387,667**

[22] Filed: **Jun. 11, 1982**

[51] Int. Cl.³ **A43B 7/16**
[52] U.S. Cl. .... **36/92**; 36/114; 36/30 R; 36/31; 36/129
[58] Field of Search .... 36/35 A, 34 R, 37, 129, 36/92, 32 R, 30 R, 31, 114

[56]   **References Cited**

U.S. PATENT DOCUMENTS

1,818,731	8/1931	Mattison	36/35 A
3,738,373	6/1973	Glancy	36/35 A
4,069,601	1/1978	Robbins et al.	36/32 R X
4,237,627	12/1980	Turner	36/129
4,316,332	2/1982	Giese et al.	36/37 X
4,364,188	12/1982	Turner et al.	36/129 X
4,364,189	12/1982	Bates	36/129 X

Primary Examiner—Werner H. Schroeder
Assistant Examiner—Tracy Graveline
Attorney, Agent, or Firm—Sixbey, Friedman & Leedom

[57]   **ABSTRACT**

A running shoe sole having a relatively thin outer sole layer of hard, wear-resistant material, a midsole layer resilient cushioning material and a heel sole layer, provided between the outer sole and midsole layers along approximately the rear half of the sole. In accordance with preferred embodiments, an outer, longitudinally extending portion of the heel sole layer spans approximately ⅔ of the width of the heel sole layer and is formed of a resilient cushioning material, while an inner portion spanning approximately the remaining ⅓ of the width of the sole layer is formed of a material that is of a hardness of approximately 10–20 shore durometer greater than that of the outer portion of the heel sole layer. This construction of the heel sole layer enables cushioning of the foot during lateral heel strikes occurring during running to be provided by the outer portion of the heel while the inner portion is able to act in a manner which limits pronation occurring thereafter.

8 Claims, 5 Drawing Figures

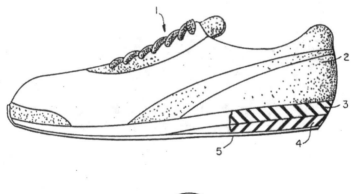

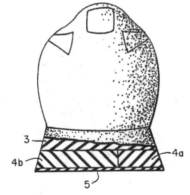

FIGURE 9.3—U.S. Patent 4,506,462

United States Patent [19]

Lyden et al.

[11] **Patent Number:** 5,425,184

[45] **Date of Patent:** Jun. 20, 1995

US005425184A

[54] **ATHLETIC SHOE WITH REARFOOT STRIKE ZONE**

[75] Inventors: **Robert M. Lyden; Gordon A. Valiant,** both of Beaverton; **Robert J. Lucas; Michael T. Donaghu,** both of Portland, all of Oreg.; **David M. Forland,** Battle Ground, Wash.; **Joel I. Passke,** Portland, Oreg.; **Thomas McGuirk,** Portland, Oreg.; **Lester Q. Lee,** Gaston, Oreg.

[73] Assignee: **Nike, Inc.,** Beaverton, Oreg.

[21] Appl. No.: **38,950**

[22] Filed: **Mar. 29, 1993**

[51] Int. Cl.^{6} A43B 13/20

[52] U.S. Cl. .... **36/29; 36/114;** 36/59 C

[58] Field of Search .... 36/102, 88, 103, 114, 36/25 R, 28, 29, 34 R, 35 R, 35 B, 59 C

[56] **References Cited**

U.S. PATENT DOCUMENTS

D. 27,361	7/1897	Waters .	
30,037	7/1868	Ausdall .	
D. 86,527	3/1932	Klein .	
D. 115,636	7/1939	Sperry .	
D. 136,226	3/1943	Wright .	
248,616	10/1881	Shepard	36/68
D. 278,851	5/1985	Austin	D2/320
280,791	7/1883	Brooks .	
D. 288,027	2/1987	Tonkel	D2/320
D. 288,028	2/1987	Chassaing	D2/320
D. 296,152	6/1988	Selbiger	D2/320
D. 298,483	11/1988	Liggettt et al.	D2/320
D. 301,658	6/1989	Hase	D2/320
D. 305,955	2/1990	Hase	D2/320
D. 307,351	4/1990	Kayano	D2/320
D. 311,810	11/1990	Hatfield	D2/320
D. 315,442	3/1991	Kilgore et al.	D2/320
D. 318,170	7/1991	Hatfield	D2/320
D. 319,532	9/1991	Mitsui	D2/320
D. 320,690	10/1991	Lucas	D2/320
D. 321,584	11/1991	Mitsui	D2/277
D. 321,973	12/1991	Hatfield	D2/320
D. 321,977	12/1991	Kilgore et al.	D2/320
D. 322,511	12/1991	Lucas	D2/320
D. 324,762	3/1992	Hatfield	D2/318
D. 324,941	3/1992	Hatfield	D2/320
D. 325,289	4/1992	Aveni	D2/314
D. 326,557	6/1992	Gardner	D2/319
D. 326,762	6/1992	Kiyosawa	D2/277
D. 329,528	9/1992	Hatfield	D2/314
D. 329,534	9/1992	Worthington	D2/320
D. 329,536	9/1992	Lucas	D2/320
D. 329,739	9/1992	Hatfield	D2/318
D. 329,936	10/1992	Lucas	D2/314
D. 329,939	10/1992	Bailey	D2/320
D. 330,800	11/1992	Lucas	D2/320
D. 334,279	3/1993	Teague	D2/314
D. 334,650	4/1993	Teague	D2/314
D. 335,015	4/1993	Lozano	D2/314

(List continued on next page.)

FOREIGN PATENT DOCUMENTS

0083449 7/1983 European Pat. Off. .

(List continued on next page.)

OTHER PUBLICATIONS

The Air Structure shoe, Spring 1991 Nike Footwear, pp. 8–9, 12–13.

(List continued on next page.)

Primary Examiner—Bryon P. Gehman
Assistant Examiner—Ted Kavanaugh
Attorney, Agent, or Firm—Banner, Birch, Mckie & Beckett

[57] **ABSTRACT**

An athletic shoe has a sole with a rearfoot strike zone segmented from the remaining heel area by a line of flexion which permits articulation of the strike zone during initial heel strike of a runner. The line of flexion is located to delimit a rearfoot strike zone reflecting the heel to toe running style of the majority of the running population. In addition to allowing articulation of the rearfoot strike zone about the line of flexion, the sole incorporates cushioning elements, including a resilient gas filled bladder, to provide differential cushioning characteristics in different parts of the heel, to attenuate force applications and shock associated with heel strike, without degrading footwear stability during subsequent phases of the running cycle. The line of flexion may be formed by various means including a deep groove, a line of relatively flexible midsole material, and a relatively flexible portion of a segmented fluid bladder.

47 Claims, 5 Drawing Sheets

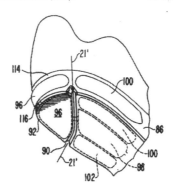

FIGURE 9.4—U.S. Patent 5,425,184

Wreck and Roll: Motion Control Out of Control

It may cause confusion to simply refer to any inward rotation of the foot—in particular, of the midfoot and forefoot—as pronation, because this word is generally used to describe rearfoot motion. Only recently has reliable three-dimensional equipment become available that may enable researchers to one day well understand rotation of the midfoot and forefoot. In this book, pronation will describe inward rotation associated with articulation of the sub-talar joint, and inward rotation will describe midfoot and forefoot motion.

During the 1960's and early 1970's Achilles tendon injuries were sometimes caused in part by low heel elevations and inadequate cushioning. Presently, the majority of Achilles tendon injuries are associated with motion control problems. Inward rotation of the foot (or pronation) and outward rotation (or supination) can place torque on the Achilles tendon (See Figure 9.5). Rearfoot pronation of the calcaneus (or heel) and inward rotation of the midfoot is associated with internal rotation of the tibia and lower leg. This internal rotation imparts a twist on the Achilles tendon. However, the use of proper shoes can reduce this motion.

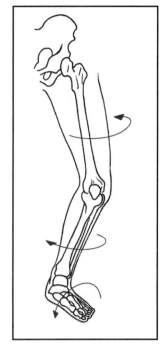

FIGURE 9.5
from Cavanagh, 1980

When running in many commercial athletic shoes, runners commonly exhibit 12-14° of rearfoot pronation (Edington, Frederick, and Cavanagh, 1990). Typically, when athletes run barefoot on grass, only about seven to eight degrees of rearfoot pronation occurs—that is, inward rotation of the calcaneus associated with articulation of the sub-talar joint. And they also tend to have less inward rotation of the midfoot and forefoot (See Figure 9.6).

In brief, the cushioning provided by higher heel elevations—and the longer effective lever arm created by the sole of athletic footwear—can double rearfoot pronation. Running barefoot on grass, an athlete can experience approximately the same magnitude of shock as running in well-cushioned shoes on asphalt (Unold, 1974). Moreover, an athlete running in sand can experience even less than on grass. So, in a perfect world we would all be "down under" in Portsea, Australia, running in the sand dunes where Herb Elliott trained. A practical alternative is to train on natural surfaces in athletic shoes having a relatively low heel elevation (See Figures 9.7 and 9.8).

Many of the athletic shoes made in the 1960's and early 1970's had soles too hard for running high mileage on asphalt streets, but otherwise adequate for running on natural surfaces. European runners at that time normally ran on natural surfaces, and that was the consumer on whom Adidas, AG, the major manufacturer of the time, was primarily focused. Because they did not pay attention to those individuals running on asphalt in the United States, companies such as Nike, Inc. came to the fore.

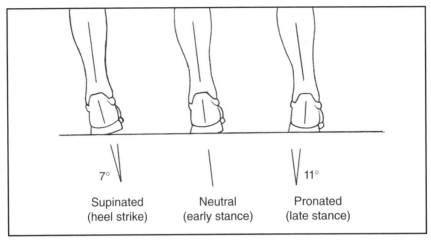

FIGURE 9.6

Numerous running shoes of this era included a foxing strip, or band of rubber bonded around the perimeter of the sole: the Converse All Star basketball shoe, the Adidas Olympia and Gazelle. This had the effect of stiffening the edges of the sole. It was undesirable for those areas of the sole receiving sudden impact loading when running on asphalt, but was beneficial in areas requiring motion control.

As discussed in detail in U.S. Patent 5,921,004, one of the fundamental weaknesses of the soles of many athletic shoes manufactured in the last twenty years is that most exhibit an edge effect—that is, when compressed they are approximately 30% less stiff about a substantial portion of the perimeter relative to the middle of the sole. Check for yourself if you trust your fingers. If an athlete experiences substantial inward or outward rotation, such footwear will do little to arrest this tendency. Instead, the article of footwear can actually facilitate it. For this reason, the author alternated running shoes having an edge effect (for running on asphalt) with shoes having a foxing strip (for running on natural surfaces). Thus, he attempted to have the best of both worlds. This practice eliminated the experience of knee pain and injury common during the 1960's and early 1970's.

The following two patents teach ways of reducing stiffness in a central portion of the rearfoot area of the sole to enhance stability and cushioning—U.S. Patent 4,043,058, granted to Geoffrey Hollister, et al., and U.S. Patent 4,364,189 granted to Tom Clarke et al., assigned to Nike, Inc. Conversely, the next two patents teach ways of stiffening up the edges of a sole relative to the central portion—U.S. Patent 4,302,892, granted to Jaroslav Adamik, and U.S. Patent 4,288,929, granted to Edward Norton, assigned to New Balance Athletic Shoes, Inc. Some of these teachings can counteract the edge effect apparent in many modern athletic shoes, but they do not find their way into athletic footwear on a regular basis. Moreover, positioning a relatively stiff foam material in the lateral rear corner of the sole can sometimes compromise both cushioning and rearfoot stability. Again, see the patents directed towards optimizing both cushioning and stability, cited on pages 275-276.

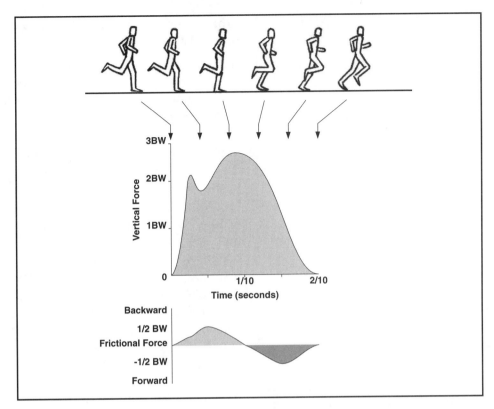

FIGURE 9.7—Ground reaction forces in body weight units during running (from Cavanagh, 1980)

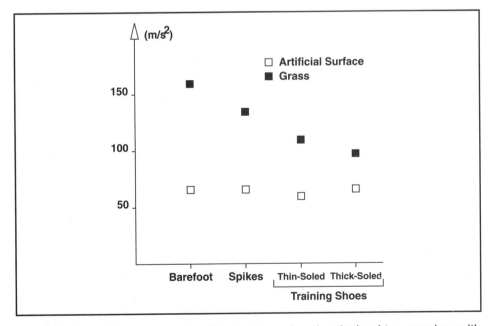

FIGURE 9.8—Mean values for the heel acceleration in heel-toe running with different footwear on grass and synthetic surface for 5 subjects, 10 trials each at a running velocity of about 4 m/s (from Unold, 1974)

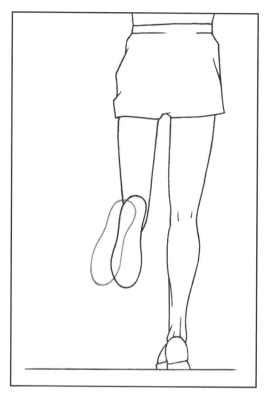

FIGURE 9.9—Rear view of runner showing pronation and resulting whip

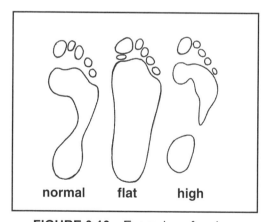

normal   flat   high

FIGURE 9.10—Examples of arches

What Happens on the Ground Determines What Happens in the Air

The presence of a whip—that is, a circular deviation of an athlete's foot and lower leg during the so-called "flight phase" when the foot is in the air—can indicate a motion control problem. In this regard, what happens on the ground determines what happens in the air. For example, if the runner's foot rotates inward and does not recover to a more neutral position by toe-off, then the ground reaction force of this action will normally cause the foot to displace laterally upon toe-off, causing a visible circular whip during the flight phase. This whip normally imparts a twist to the Achilles tendon, and also works against the lateral side of the knee (See Figure 9.9).

Check Conformance

Check the athlete's conformance for any potential structural dispositions to injury. What is the athlete's Q-angle from the hip? Is the individual bow-legged? Does the athlete have normal, flat, or high arches? See Figure 9.10 for examples of each.

Often, individuals with flat feet have a *forefoot varus* condition. When their foot is in a non-weight-bearing neutral position, their forefoot has the first toe in an elevated position relative to the fifth toe. In order to compensate for this and bring the first toe to the support surface during weight-bearing, the subtalar joint must articulate, causing pronation, that is, the individual's heel tilts inward. An athlete with flat feet can also load the midfoot area about the navicular and medial longitudinal arch to a greater degree than other individuals. Accordingly, the athlete can become injured by using a curve lasted shoe (which does not provide support in this area). Instead, the individual may benefit from arch supports and orthotic posting of the medial longitudinal arch by a trained medical professional. Those with normal arches tend to have a more neutral stance. However, those with high arches often have a

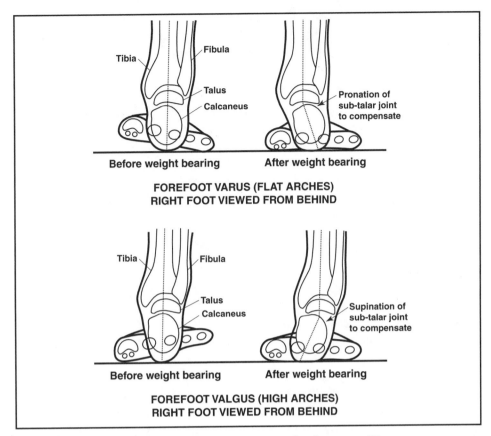

FIGURE 9.11—Forefoot varus and valgus conditions

forefoot valgus condition. When their foot is in a non-weight-bearing neutral position their forefoot has the fifth toe elevated relative to the first toe. And in order to compensate for this and bring the fifth toe to the support surface during weight-bearing, the sub-talar joint must articulate, causing supination, that is, the heel tilts outward. Those having high arches normally benefit from arch support under the medial longitudinal arch, the transverse and lateral longitudinal arch, and in particular, the midfoot area proximate the cuboid between the calcaneus and proximal head of the fifth metatarsal. An individual with either flat feet or high arches tends to experience greater rotation of the foot, and this can impart a twist to the Achilles tendon. To reduce the amount and rate of rotation that may be injuring the tendon, the individual might obtain more substantial arch support or a corrective orthotic—and perhaps a straighter lasted shoe (See Figure 9.11).

Seeing is Believing

The wear pattern on a runner's shoe can provide significant clues regarding the individual's biomechanics. To check their running form, videotape the individual running from the front, back, and sides. For the best results, videotape outdoors whenever possible. Despite what the lab researchers might claim, athletes do not run the same on treadmills. Athletes running on a level treadmill generally do not use their hamstrings to the same degree as when running outdoors. And, experienced rearfoot strikers tend to use a flatter technique at footstrike and alter their way of going by loading the shoe more anteriorly, thus more closely resembling a midfoot or forefoot striker.

Injured athletes who are rehabilitating on a treadmill will later have to re-adapt to race well outdoors. The same phenomenon is observed with horses trained on treadmills. Tom Ivers, an author and equine trainer, has trained thoroughbreds on treadmills for many years. When horses come off a treadmill-training program, they are unable to race well on a natural surface. However, after a few weeks of training, including some uphill gallops, the required neuromuscular re-training and fitness of the hindquarters are brought far enough along to accomplish favorable racing results. The muscles in the hindquarters of a horse generally correspond to the hamstrings and gluteus muscles in humans (Ivers, 1994).

Things to Do

The best advice for a minor tendon injury of any kind is to let it rest. Comparing muscles to tendons in the early phase of healing, muscles respond to more aggressive forms of therapy such as light strength work and moderate stretching, but tendons for the most part need to rest. Tendons have much poorer blood supply than muscles, and take longer to heal. Athletes should take Vitamin C, since it promotes healing of connective tissue. Apply an ice massage to the affected area for at least 20 minutes before bedtime, and wear socks to bed in order to keep the area warm. This will speed up the local metabolic rate. Before taking the first step in the morning, athletes should draw out the ABCs with their affected foot, and perhaps use a heel lift with that first step. Further, a warm towel should be placed on the affected area first thing in the morning. In addition, it will help to carefully conduct some easy strength training exercises early in the morning, such as riding a stationary bicycle. Athletes should maintain an appropriate flexibility routine, but when afflicted with a tendon injury, runners should beware of over-stretching, and in particular, when they are not fully warmed up. They are well advised to run on soft but stable surfaces, and to wear long socks and sweats. In general, athletes should not be running without their warm-ups unless it is at least 60° Fahrenheit. Do not play the hero by braving the cold. This demonstrates ignorance or just plain foolishness. Replace athletic footwear that could be causing the problem. When in doubt, throw them out. Again, beware of wearing dress shoes, changing heel elevations frequently, and remedy any instability problems. Practice anonymous and random acts of kindness. This has merit and is reward enough in itself. Moreover, it will also make you feel better, and when you feel better, you heal faster.

Knee Injuries and Chondromalacia

Patello-femoral tracking problems and chondromalacia became the epidemic of the late 1970's and early 1980's. One of the underlying causes was a common practice of manufacturers at the time to incorporate heel flare, with the intention of enhancing footwear stability. The midsoles on many shoes flared out and became

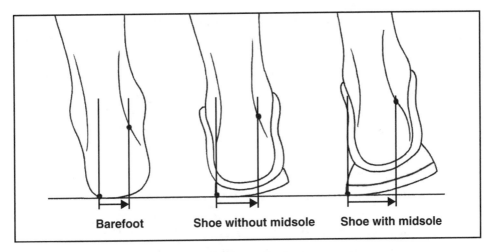

FIGURE 9.12—Rear view showing lever arm phenomenon

progressively wider, starting at the junction with the shoe upper and moving down towards the outsole. Instead of providing stability, this effectively increased the length of the lever arm extending from beneath the center of the heel towards the lateral side of the sole (See Figure 9.12). The increased length of this lever arm commonly resulted in greater pronation, and also a higher rate of pronation. Meanwhile, higher heel elevations were also introduced to improve cushioning, and this also tended to undermine stability. As a result, runners then suffered a relatively high incidence of tendon injuries near the knee (Nigg and Morlock, 1987).

Manufacturers have since reduced the amount of flaring used in the soles of athletic footwear. Further, attempts were made by Peter Cavanagh, then with Puma AG, and also Kenneth Misevich, with Etonic Athletics, Inc., to round the lateral edge of the sole in order to reduce this lever effect (as taught in U.S. Patent 4,449,306, and U.S. Patent 4,557,059, respectively). These attempts worked well in a laboratory setting on a treadmill, and when running on a flat surface. However, such footwear tended to facilitate inversion sprains when individuals ran on uneven surfaces, or improperly used the shoes for lateral movement sports. Today, most athletic footwear incorporate a slight bevel inclined at approximately 2-15° in the lateral rear corner of the sole.

Cavanagh also taught the use of softer foam material along the lateral side of the sole to decrease the lever effect and enhance cushioning (in U.S. Patent 4,506,462, assigned to Puma AG). This approach proved to be sound and has endured. Barry Bates, formerly with ASICS Corp., taught the use of firmer midsole foam on the medial side to reduce pronation (U.S. Patent 4,364,189). Later introduction of devices such as the Footbridge® also served to limit compression of the medial side of the sole, and thereby rearfoot pronation (U.S. Patent 5,046,267, Bruce Kilgore et. al, assigned to Nike, Inc.). The author is associated with patents (U.S. Patents 5,425,184, 5,625,964, and 6,055,746, assigned to Nike, Inc.) that teach the use of a groove delimiting a rearfoot strike zone, and a gas-filled bladder having relatively low stiffness in compression, to enhance both cushioning and stability. This can reduce the effective length of the lever arm and the magnitude of the force imparted thereby. Much like the independent suspension found in many automobiles, the rearfoot strike zone as a whole can deflect and articulate. In addition, just like a tire, the gas-filled bladder is then placed near the point of impact for effective vibration isolation. In brief, reducing the relative stiffness of the rear lateral corner of the sole can decrease rearfoot pronation, and also the rate of pronation, thus providing relief to an athlete having an injured knee.

What's Their Deal?

Again, check the runner's conformance for conditions that might make the individual more prone to injury (e.g., a large Q-angle, substantial rearfoot or forefoot varus or valgus, bowed legs, and either high or low arches). Determine the individual's range of motion and strength while searching for a muscle imbalance. Notice the visible wear pattern on the training shoes. Observe and videotape the individual's running technique from all sides. Look for greater than normal pronation, tibial and femoral rotation, and the presence of a whip. Given a patello-femoral tracking problem, relatively straight lasted shoes may be beneficial.

Muscle Imbalances

A tracking problem of the patella can be caused by instability below the knee, but also by muscle imbalances associated with faulty running technique. What is the cause? With recreational runners, the following scenario may apply. They do not frequently run faster than 6:30 per mile, and often run at about the same speed on relatively level terrain. They are not only heel strikers, but also heel runners. They have learned to let the present generation of well-cushioned shoes do a lot of the work for them when running on hard asphalt. They often do not exhibit substantial hip extension or ankle flexion. They may have overdeveloped lateral quadriceps, but underdeveloped medial quadriceps, and hamstrings. This muscle imbalance can result in the patella being pulled into an orientation where it mistracks and rubs with more force than it should in the wrong place. In time, this can roughen the cartilage underlying the patella and cause chondromalacia.

Knee Extensions and Walking Squats to the Rescue

Normally, the quick fix for a patello-femoral tracking problem is to strengthen the medial quadriceps. The best way to accomplish this is to perform knee extensions, and in particular, to work the last 30° while pointing the toes outwards. If done properly, this single exercise probably does more than any other to correct a wandering patella. Leg presses, step-ups and 1/4-squats can also be done, but get things under control first with knee extensions. Walking squats—that is, stepping forward with one foot to do a "lunge," then stepping forward again with the other foot and repeating the sequence—simultaneously strengthens the medial quadriceps and hamstrings, and also enhances hip extension and ankle flexion. Begin by taking 10 steps in this manner, and then provide a full recovery. At the beginning, do not take a long lunge or dip with the opposite knee so deeply that it touches the ground. Do not perform more than three sets of 10 steps. If athletes do too much, they could be sore beyond belief over the next two days. When they are able to take a fuller lunge step and touch the ground slightly with the opposite knee, then they are beginning to get into better shape. In a short time, fit athletes should be able to do this with a 15-pound barbell behind their head. And they can later progress by adding more weight. However, it is rare even for highly conditioned athletes to perform this exercise with more than 50 pounds on their back.

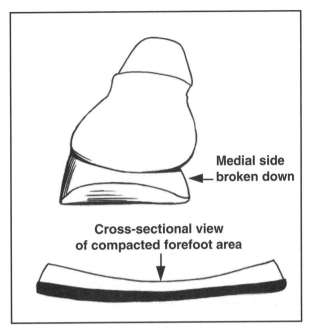

FIGURE 9.13

After leg extensions and walking squats, the most effective exercise to improve range of motion, and correct muscle imbalances is simply to go back to nature. Begin by walking and then running barefoot on a natural grass surface. Athletes who have had patellar tracking problems for years, and bounced from one form of therapy to the next, have recovered after a month of walking and running on golf courses.

Knee Joint Problems

Problems with the medial and lateral menisci, ligaments, or tendons, are generally the result of instability below the knee. What is happening below the knee needs to be identified and resolved. Normally, it is a case of too much inward rotation of the tibia and outward rotation of the femur. The toes are the primary forefoot mechanism for stabilizing inward rotation of the foot, whereas the connective tissues of the medial longitudinal arch and posterior tibialis are the primary midfoot mechanism. If neither of these successfully controls rotation, then unusually high loads will be passed on to the Achilles tendon and joint capsule of the knee.

Of course, the manifest injury at the knee needs to be treated. Obtain an accurate and concise history of the injury. Has the individual been running across a grade, or on steep uphills or downhills—and is this deviating their normal footpath? Is there a biomechanical problem? Does the runner pronate or supinate excessively? The presence of a whip will often work against the knee. Again, check the runner's conformance for conditions that make her or she more prone to injury (e.g., a large Q-angle, substantial rearfoot or forefoot varus or valgus, bowed-legs, and either high or low arches). Determine the individual's range of motion and strength while searching for a muscle imbalance. Notice the wear pattern on the runner's training shoes. Observe and videotape the individual's running technique from all sides.

Get Out of Dying Shoes Before They Take You with Them

The degradation of a shoe sole can also cause knee problems. Often, the midsole will break down on the medial side, and also become compacted under the ball of the foot. (See Figure 9.13). This is generally not apparent on the outside of the shoe. Rather, look inside the shoes for compressed areas of foam material under the ball of the foot. Is there a pronounced bowl shaped depression there? The fact that many athletic shoes are made with foam midsoles already having a bowl shape in the forefoot area when viewed in cross-section along the transverse axis, probably does not help matters. This configuration may promote a smooth transition, and also help to offset the "edge effect," that is, the reduced stiffness often found at the edges of conventional midsoles made of foam material, but it probably promotes faster degradation of the central portion of the forefoot area where peak loads are commonly experienced. Does the shoe sit flat on a tabletop, or is the forefoot area of the sole deformed into a rounded, bowl shape? Sometimes the lugs located more centrally in the outsole will wear down first, and this also contributes to the formation of a bowl shaped footbed. This particular degradation of athletic footwear is often connected with knee problems. Such a shoe, when set on a tabletop and prodded from any direction, will oscillate to and fro. This is not a stable situation. Eject! Eject! Get out of dying shoes before they take you with them. New shoes, and perhaps shoes having firmer midsoles are in order. Curve lasted shoes are generally contraindicated for those with knee problems (See Figure 9.13).

What is Cheap, Light and Won't Last as Long as it Used To?

Most athletic shoes manufactured today use an ethylene vinyl acetate (EVA) closed cell foam material. This material is lightweight and inexpensive. It is not as heavy as the open-celled polyurethane foam often used in the late 1970's and early 1980's. However, EVA foam normally takes a compression set and breaks down faster than polyurethane foam—and the latter generally breaks down faster than higher quality, heavier, and more expensive foam rubber materials. The consumer is then getting an economical, lightweight and disposable shoe. When running 100 miles a week and swapping between two different pairs of training shoes, an athlete could reasonably expect to get six weeks, or about 300 miles, out of a pair of shoes—and it is probably not advisable to attempt more.

Iliotibial (I-T) Band Syndrome

Downhill running often contributes to the onset of an I-T band injury. Further, running downhill on streets having a transverse grade makes for an even more dangerous situation. Racecourses that include this condition are potentially hazardous to runners, particularly if this stretch comes late in the race when they are fatigued.

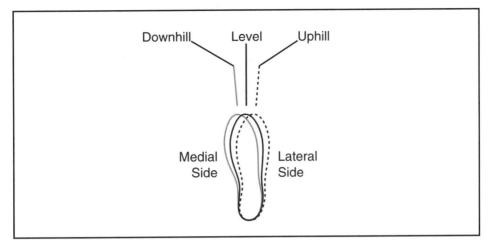

FIGURE 9.14—Deviated footpath running uphill and downhill

The Foot bone is Connected to the Leg Bone, the Leg Bone...

As Figure 9.14 shows, downhill running causes a medial deviation of footpath—that is, an individual's forefoot points inward (medially) more than normal. When running downhill there is more time for footfall after heelstrike, and this gives an opportunity for the foot to turn more medially. Often this inward deviation of footpath brings greater than normal rearfoot pronation, inward rotation of the tibia, and outward rotation of the femur. At the same time, greater than normal load bearing and braking can be taking place. As a result, the knee's lateral aspect can be over-loaded, and the IT band can suffer trauma as it is strained, abraded, and suffers micro-tears in the area near the lateral condyle of the femur. In contrast, uphill running causes the footpath to deviate just the opposite way—that is, the forefoot tends to point outward (laterally) to greater degree, and this tends to stress connective tissue on the inside (medial side) of the knee.

However, other things can also place unusual stress on the IT-band. Those who have a large Q-angle from wide hips, are bow-legged, supinate, or are midfoot and forefoot strikers, are more vulnerable. Again, note the runner's arch characteristics and any varus or valgus conditions. Is the individual running across a grade? Is there a visible whip? As always, check the wear pattern on the runner's athletic shoes, and in particular, look to see if the lateral side of the sole has broken down. Perhaps the stiffness of material on the lateral side of the shoe is not sufficient for the individual. Large or heavy runners should be especially attentive to this. The same stiffness of foam material or midsole device does not suit all.

Also look for excessive wear on the medial side of the forefoot (See Figure 9.15). This indicates instability, since individuals suffering I-T band syndrome will sometimes load their shoes transversely from the medial to the lateral side more than normal. Often, they have extremely tight quadriceps, particularly the lateral quadriceps muscle. These athletes will need to stretch this area well before and

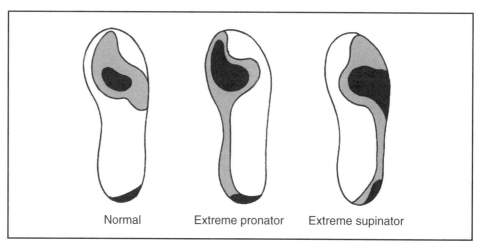

FIGURE 9.15—Adapted by permission, from T. Noakes, 1991, *Lore of Running*, 3rd ed., Champaign, IL: Human Kinetics, page 493.

immediately after training sessions. However, the quadriceps and I-T band are getting tight for a reason, namely, due to the way they are being used when the athletes run. So it will be helpful to videotape the athletes running from all angles, and share with them suggestions on how to improve their running technique. Often, correcting the situation requires specific exercises to improve their range of motion and strengthen the weaker muscle groups.

Plantar Fasciitis

Runners often refer to virtually any injury in the area of the arch as plantar fasciitis. Since there are multiple layers of connective tissue in this area of the foot that are difficult to isolate and discriminate, this broad definition will be accepted at face value. Obviously, there are a host of training errors, as well as a number of anatomical or biomechanical reasons why some individuals might be predisposed to getting plantar fasciitis. However, whereas Achilles tendonitis was perhaps the epidemic of the 1960's and early 1970's, and knee pain the epidemic of the late 1970's and early 1980's, plantar fasciitis was the epidemic of the late 1980's and 1990's—even to the present day. The former problems seem to have coincided with changes in shoe design. This more recent epidemic is probably no different. The question is why?

Heel Elevations Have Gotten Higher

One of the changes made in athletic footwear over the last twenty years has been an increase in heel elevation. The annual *Runner's World* shoe reviews used to rate the cushioning of the various shoes against one another, and everyone in the industry wanted to win the big cushioning showdown. The industry attacked the problem of cushioning and came to understand it reasonably well. Many manufacturers increased heel height to enhance the cushioning provided by conventional foam materials. Some also increased heel height to facilitate insertion of new devices such as fluid or gas filled bladders in order to improve the cushioning of athletic shoes. However, higher heel elevations can introduce greater potential for instability.

When the Gizmo Fails

In the search of new technology, and in order to feed the insatiable marketing and consumption monster, many footwear manufacturers have introduced various devices into the soles of athletic shoes. A few of these gizmos work, but most do not—that is, they do not provide any better cushioning or stability than footwear made from conventional foam material. Simple is sometimes better. From the standpoint functionality and performance as opposed to fashion, many of the best athletic footwear values are presently found in the sixty to eighty dollar price range.

Athletes should also consider what happens when the gizmo fails in their athletic shoe. If a component inside the midsole fails, They might not recognize it. This is especially true of devices encapsulated in foam. Athletes may never recognize that a problem exists with the shoe, and might continue to run on faulty footwear for some time before making the discovery. As a result, athletes may mistakenly assume that an injury they suffered was due to a training error or chance, when it was actually defective footwear.

Generally, when a gizmo fails it reduces the stiffness of the midsole in the affected area and the wearer's foot then penetrates further into the midsole. When running, this can cause a functional leg length difference, which is well known to cause injury. Moreover, if the runner's heel or forefoot penetrates further into the midsole, then the plantar fascia can become impinged (e.g., upon a plastic part inside the midsole, or upon the conventional foam material underlying the arch area). The failure of a gizmo can also sometimes create a dysfunctional ledge in the arch area of the midsole upon which the plantar fascia can impact.

Stiffness Problems

Athletic shoes with relatively thick soles can be relatively inflexible. Depending on the configuration and intended use of the footwear, an inflexible sole can sometimes work against the plantar fascia. Flex grooves, such as those taught by E.C. Frederick et al. (U.S. Patent 4,562,651) and by the author (U. S. Patent 5,384,973) have been used to reduce the stiffness of athletic shoe soles. However, footwear that are too flexible in the wrong places can also cause problems. Athletes can check a shoe by placing the toe and heel between their hands and compress it to see where it bends. If it bends under the arch area instead of the ball of the foot near the metatarsal-phalangeal joints, then they could be in for a problem. Athletic footwear that include a cut-away or weakened area underneath the arch can be susceptible to this problem because they will sometimes flex in this area instead of beneath the ball of the foot.

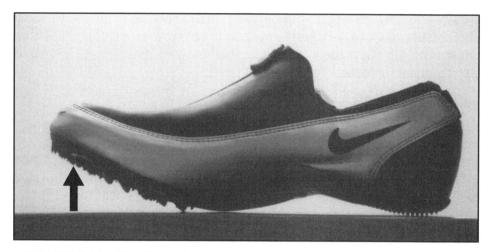

FIGURE 9.16—Nike Zoom Celar track spike including substantial toe spring.

Toe Spring

Toe spring refers to the degree to which the sole of a shoe appears to curl upward in the forefoot area (See Figure 9.16). It can be roughly measured between the bottom of the sole and a flat underlying surface. The origin of toe spring derives from inflexible Dutch wooden shoes that required this configuration to be functional. It can give a relatively inflexible sole the ability to provide a smooth transition during the gait cycle.

Due to increases in the thickness of midsoles during the 1970's and 1980's, many athletic shoes have become less flexible. Toe spring has been widely used as a partial remedy. Transverse flex grooves have also been introduced to facilitate dorsiflexion of the toes. However, when wearing athletic footwear, it can be difficult or impossible for a wearer to stand on the ground and move the toes to a neutral or flat position as when barefoot. This situation can be dysfunctional, depending on the intended use of the footwear. Conventional walking and running shoes intended for normal use at relatively slow speeds should generally include little toe spring, because this best provides for stability and cushioning. However, it can be advantageous to include greater toe spring in footwear intended for running at high speeds. For example, a racing flat intended for the marathon can include more toe spring than a training shoe for running long, slow, distance work. Also, track spikes for sprinters can include more toe spring than those intended for middle distance and distance runners. Substantial toe spring in a sprint spike is functional because sprinters normally make most surface contact with their forefoot while sprinting. Thus, a sprint spike with substantial toe spring can facilitate a more rapid transition and less ground contact time. Unfortunately, the correct use of toe spring is not always well understood or implemented. Cosmetically, toe spring provides many athletic shoes with a sporty, automotive look. As a result, too many shoes include substantial toe spring at the present time. This is probably not a healthy situation. Peter Cavanagh questioned the widespread introduction of toe spring in athletic footwear during the early 1980's (Cavanagh, *The Running Shoe Book*, 1980).

A patent granted to the author (U. S. Patent 5,384,973, assigned to Nike, Inc.) contains relevant discussion of toe spring, and discloses the use of numerous longitudinal and transverse lines of flexion to enhance the functionality of conventional athletic shoes. This teaching and the competitive response of other footwear manufacturers have led to dramatic changes in the midsole and outsole configuration of athletic shoes. Whereas the forefoot area of athletic shoes once generally resembled a slab of foam material completely covered by an outsole, they now commonly include numerous grooves and segments to improve both cushioning and stability.

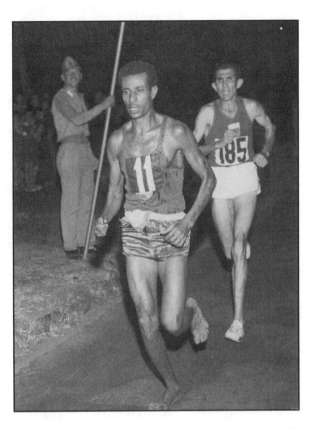

PHOTO 9.2—Abebe Bikila running barefoot in the marathon, 1960 Olympic Games. Photo from Hulton/ Getty Images.

Abebe's Legendary Feet

Another cause of plantar fasciitis can stem from a runner having poorly conditioned feet. Abebe Bikila won the 1960 Olympic Games marathon in Rome while running barefoot. Athletes can sometimes be enlightened about the need to condition their feet by attempting to run barefoot for two miles on asphalt. The problem will not be blisters on their tender feet. Instead, the intrinsic muscles of their feet will become exhausted. Few athletes do anything to train their feet, but rather imagine their feet to be in good condition simply because they run a great deal. This is not the case. Many runners exhibit a limited range of motion in their ankle and toes, and also have weak intrinsic foot muscles. When confined to the "splint" of a running shoe, the foot (which is the most basic piece of equipment needed for distance running) can in fact be the least conditioned.

Get Back to Nature

The simple answer is to get back to nature. Asphalt and athletic shoes are recent inventions. Whenever it is practical and possible, walk and run barefoot on a grass surface. However, gradually increase both the distance and intensity of the barefoot workouts (See the discussion in Chapter 2). Generally, it is difficult to find a natural surface where one can run safely. When on school grounds, it is always wise to first jog a lap while wearing shoes and inspect the area for any hazardous material. If athletes can at least warm-up and warm-down while running barefoot on the infield grass, it will pay big dividends by preventing injury and enhancing their running technique.

Listen for the Canaries

The initial injury that commonly sets plantar fasciitis into motion is a slight strain to muscle, tendon or fascia in the medial longitudinal arch. If rested, it will often clear up within three to four days. Athletes often completely ignore the earliest symptoms of the developing problem. They fail to pay heed to the initial muscle strain, and that is truly when the canaries stop singing. If athletes do not rest the injury, then the resulting loss of elasticity and the body's defensive reflexes will often induce greater stiffness in the arch area, and a more serious injury. Running will only make things worse. Nip plantar fasciitis in the bud. It is far better to resolve the little muscle strain by taking three to four days off than to ignore it and conduct a hard workout on the injury. If athletes make that mistake, they may face a more serious injury. The injury will normally travel towards the origin of the plantar fascia, and eventually reach it at the calcaneus. At this point, disruption of the bone surface (or periosteum) can occur, and result in the development of a bone spur. Appropriate therapy includes rest, ice massage, wearing socks to bed to keep the affected area warm, taking Vitamin C, performing ankle ABCs before taking the first step, and placing a warm towel on the affected area in the morning.

Arch Support is Essential

The aforementioned measures can help, but normally athletes will need a customized insole or lift to reduce both the mechanical loading and the plantar pressure being placed on the plantar fascia. To relieve pain and avoid further local trauma, a hole can be made in the insole or lift to accommodate the swollen or affected area. This can be especially beneficial if the injury has progressed to the origin of the plantar fascia on the bottom of the calcaneus, or heel. The author once advised Air Jordan® designer Tinker Hatfield to use this technique with Michael Jordan when he was afflicted during the NBA Championships, and it provided such immediate relief that Jordan requested his golf shoes be made in the same manner. Athletes can go months or even years with symptoms of plantar fasciitis unless they remedy inadequate arch support. In this regard, flimsy women's dress or casual shoes without arch support can sometimes be the problem for female athletes. It is sometimes advisable for women to discontinue wearing these types of shoes during the day.

Regardless of gender, the introduction of a customized insole or orthotic device can go a long way toward resolving plantar fasciitis. Unfortunately, most of the insoles provided in present athletic footwear are relatively flat, and lack arch support. In contrast, some of the insoles provided in previous decades were of superior quality, and frequently included a generic shaped latex rubber foam arch support. Insoles with cupped formations about the heel and sides of the foot were also sometimes commercially available (e.g., in the Lydiard EB Brütting AG brand shoes, and also those made by Etonic Athletics, Inc.). However, most manufactur-

United States Patent [19]

Lyden

[11] **Patent Number:** 5,632,057

[45] **Date of Patent:** May 27, 1997

[54] **METHOD OF MAKING LIGHT CURE COMPONENT FOR ARTICLES OF FOOTWEAR**

[76] Inventor: **Robert M. Lyden**, 16384 SW. Estuary Dr., Apt. #203, Beaverton, Oreg. 97006

[21] Appl. No.: **510,433**

[22] Filed: **Aug. 2, 1995**

Related U.S. Application Data

[63] Continuation of Ser. No. 275,642, Jul. 14, 1994, abandoned, which is a continuation of Ser. No. 74,771, Jun. 9, 1993, abandoned, which is a continuation-in-part of Ser. No. 976,407, Nov. 13, 1992, abandoned, which is a division of Ser. No. 805,596, Dec. 11, 1991, Pat. No. 5,203,793, which is a continuation-in-part of Ser. No. 714,971, Jun. 13, 1991, Pat. No. 5,101,580, which is a continuation of Ser. No. 410,074, Sep. 20, 1989, abandoned.

[51] Int. Cl.^{6} A43D 1/00; A43B 7/14

[52] U.S. Cl. .... 12/146 B; 12/146 M; 36/93

[58] Field of Search .... 12/146 B, 146 M; 36/93, 88, 89, 90, 92

[56] **References Cited**

U.S. PATENT DOCUMENTS

2,092,910	9/1937	Daniels	36/71
2,546,827	3/1951	Lavinthal	36/71
3,449,844	6/1969	Spence	36/44
3,786,580	1/1974	Dalebout	36/119
3,905,376	9/1975	Johnson et al.	36/154
4,139,337	2/1979	David et al.	425/2
4,183,156	1/1980	Rudy	36/44
4,211,019	7/1980	McCafferty	36/43
4,219,945	9/1980	Rudy	36/29
4,340,626	7/1982	Rudy	428/35
4,342,158	8/1982	McMahon	36/35 R
4,451,634	5/1984	Hatanaka et al.	528/24
4,674,206	6/1987	Lyden	36/88
4,780,486	10/1988	Lee et al.	522/14
4,817,304	4/1989	Parker et al.	36/114
4,831,064	5/1989	Varaprath et al.	522/99
4,874,640	10/1989	Donzis	36/92
4,876,806	10/1989	Robinson et al.	36/114
4,892,895	1/1990	Arai et al.	522/99
4,906,502	3/1990	Rudy	428/69
4,923,754	5/1990	Lee et al.	428/429
4,935,455	6/1990	Huy et al.	522/99
4,936,029	6/1990	Rudy	36/29
4,943,613	7/1990	Arai et al.	524/773
4,946,874	8/1990	Lee et al.	522/14
5,042,100	8/1991	Bar et al.	12/142 N
5,042,176	8/1991	Rudy	36/29
5,082,873	1/1992	Liles	522/86
5,083,361	1/1992	Rudy	29/454
5,084,489	1/1992	Liles	522/84
5,089,537	2/1992	Liles	522/84
5,101,580	4/1992	Lyden	36/93
5,124,212	6/1992	Lee et al.	428/429
5,128,880	7/1992	White	364/550
5,177,120	1/1993	Hare et al.	523/109
5,180,756	1/1993	Rehmer et al.	522/35
5,183,599	2/1993	Smuckler	264/22
5,183,831	2/1993	Bielat et al.	522/33
5,185,385	2/1993	Kanluen et al.	522/84
5,187,040	2/1993	Mueller-Hess et al.	430/157
5,203,793	4/1993	Lyden	36/88

OTHER PUBLICATIONS

Int'l Plastics Selector Adhesive Digest 1995 pp. 21–22, 271–291, and 677–678.

Primary Examiner—Ted Kavanaugh

[57] **ABSTRACT**

A method for making a conformable device including a light cure material for use in functional relation with an article of footwear in order to enhance conformance or fit, support, comfort, and cushioning. The present invention can serve to accommodate the unique anatomical features and characteristics of an individual wearer and finds application within numerous types of articles footwear (44).

20 Claims, 11 Drawing Sheets

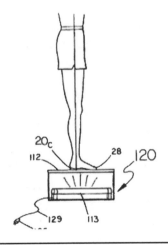

FIGURE 9.17—U.S. Patent 5,632,057

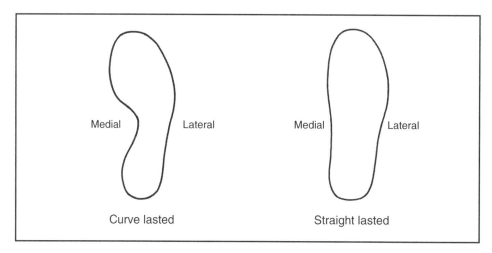

FIGURE 9.18—Curved versus straight lasted shoes

ers are currently not spending the money to provide consumers with a quality arch support and insole. If you want a better product, then demand it, and vote with your dollars. Dollars and public goodwill are what corporations understand.

An insole providing arch support can substantially improve the fit of a shoe and reduce inward and outward rotation of the foot (Cavanagh, *The Running Shoe Book*, 1980). Improving conformance under the plantar aspect of the foot can also effectively increase the surface area of the midsole being worked. A well-designed insole can then reduce local plantar pressures, and enhance cushioning, stability, comfort, and overall performance. The general public would benefit greatly from an insole providing enhanced conformance and support. Relatively few people actually require correction and prescription orthotics. When in doubt, seek out a qualified medical professional. Approximately 20% of the population have a high risk of injury when they engage in exercise without proper orthotic correction. Generally, a semi-rigid or flexible orthotic is preferable to a rigid and inflexible orthotic. The connective tissue of the plantar fascia requires adequate room to flex during exercise, like the more visible muscles and tendons of the hand and arm. The use of rigid orthotics, or those with too much correction, can sometimes impede the plantar fascia and cause a problem. A patent granted to the author addresses the need for a fast, effective and relatively inexpensive method of providing custom insoles (U.S. Patent 5,632,057). This patent teaches the use of a light table to photocure a conformable insole under the wearer's foot in approximately one minute (See Figure 9.17).

Straight versus Curved Lasts

The late Bill Bowerman and Arthur Lydiard once debated the merits of straight versus curve lasted shoes, with Bowerman favoring straight lasted, and Lydiard favoring a more curve lasted shoe (see Figure 9.18). They were both correct. When running at relatively slow speeds, about 80% of distance runners are rearfoot strikers, that is, they impact the lateral rear corner of the shoe sole. The center of plantar pressure then passes more or less up the middle of the sole

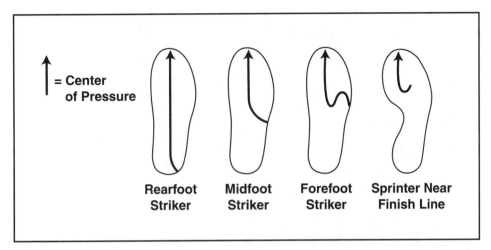

FIGURE 9.19—Center of Pressure

before exiting between the big toe and second toe (See Figure 9.19). A straight lasted shoe is normally more stable for those who run at relatively slow speeds, and also for those who have flat arches or motion control problems. Curve lasted shoes provide less medial support while running at slow speeds, and generally, they should be avoided by those individuals having flat arches or motion control problems.

However, when running at progressively higher speeds, athletes normally become midfoot and forefoot strikers. The center of pressure will then travel inward, and sometimes also rearward in the midfoot or forefoot area, before exiting between the big toe and second toe. Therefore, when athletes run at higher speeds in a curve lasted shoe, the loads tend to be shifted away from the medial side. With increasing speed, many also tend to abduct (or point the forefoot more laterally) and place more load on the big toe. Accordingly, a curve lasted shoe then may not undermine stability when athletes are moving at higher speeds, and rather, can actually facilitate movement. Curve lasted shoes tend to provide superior performance when runners are midfoot or forefoot strikers, and when they are running faster than 6:00/mile pace. Nevertheless, the vast majority of the public does not do a significant portion of their running under 6:00 /mile pace, and that is approximately the speed at which most individuals transition from being a rearfoot striker to more of a midfoot or forefoot striker. So, when in doubt, play it relatively straight. Some individuals simply prefer the fit provided by one or the other configuration. Most manufacturers today are making so-called semi-curve lasted shoes, which effectively split the difference.

Neuroma

Nerve tissue can sometimes become impinged or bruised in the foot, particularly between the metatarsals. A neuroma consists of swollen and possibly enlarged nerve tissue. It can be caused by acute trauma, such as being kicked while playing soccer, or even by running or jumping on hard surfaces. Overtightening

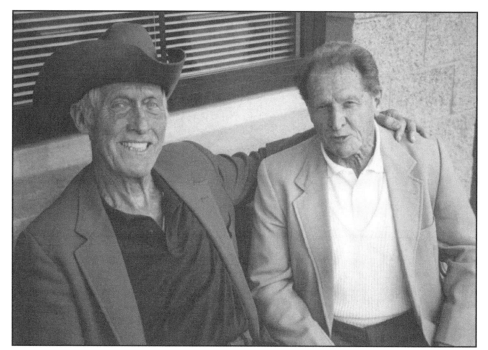

PHOTO 9.3—Bill Bowerman and Arthur Lydiard at Hayward Field, Eugene, Oregon, 1996. Photo courtesy of Nobuya Hashizume.

the laces of athletic shoes, especially track spikes, can narrow the foot and cause the metatarsals to impinge upon a nerve. Again, check if the forefoot of the athletic shoe has degraded and includes a bowl shaped impression under the ball of the foot. This can cause the metatarsals to migrate towards one another and induce a fallen transverse arch, thus entrapping and injuring a nerve.

Shin Splints

Often, the first time young distance runners participate in high school cross-country or track, they will get shin splints. It is a case of too much too soon. The transition from complete inactivity to running a few miles each day constitutes a leap from zero to several thousand impacts and repetitions—each involving approximately two and a half body weights. Beginners also tend to have faulty running technique, and are easy prey to motion control problems. Often, they are neither aerobically conditioned, nor muscularly strong. Further, their running form often degrades markedly because no motor memory has yet been instilled to maintain optimal biomechanics when they are fatigued. Young athletes returning from a run are sometimes physically and mentally exhausted.

The best prevention is to make certain that young runners begin with low mileage, wear good footwear, and run slowly on forgiving surfaces. Once shin splints arise, runners are often stuck with them for a while—that is, if they continue with an exercise program without taking a rest. Shin splints will often stay with athletes for an entire season, but will disappear after a month of rest. The use of ice and anti-inflammatory drugs can make athletes feel better, but time and rest is what they really need to get better. The problem is not normally encountered thereafter, provided they continue a nominal level of training. The equivalent of shin splints in a horse is called bucked shins, and this also happens when too much is attempted too soon.

True shin splints are an inflammation of connective tissue between the tibia and fibula. However, athletes will refer to virtually any pain along the medial edge of the tibia as shin splints. This is usually a form of tendonitis near the point of origin for the muscles of the lower leg, where the muscles transition into tendon tissue or where the tendons attach to bone. Hot spots on the bone are then common. These can develop into stress fractures, but the latter will generally not show up on X-rays until 10 to 14 days after the injury is noticed. Again, excessive pronation and tibial rotation can cause shin splints. Young athletes just beginning to train, or individuals who have recently increased their training dramatically are especially vulnerable. In any case, individuals having a motion control problem, and in particular, excessive pronation, could need correction.

Inversion Sprains and Peroneal Injury

Inversion sprains and peroneal injuries are not often associated with running. Perhaps, the exception being when a runner turns an ankle while running across a grade, or accidentally steps into a pothole during cross-country. However, during the track and field season, this injury most often happens when several athletes play pick-up basketball after practice. Commonly, the victim will make a vertical leap and come down upon another player's foot, thus spraining an ankle. However, if none of these circumstances seem to fit, then determine whether the lateral side of the sole is too soft for the individual, or has suffered degradation. Further, observe the runner's conformance, and be on the lookout for bowed legs or a rearfoot varus condition. Is the athlete a supinator, or running on a road with a grade? Any one of these conditions, and certain combinations, will increase the risk of an inversion sprain.

Bunions

Lateral deviation of the big toe at an early age is a problem directly associated with the use of conventional footwear (Staheli, 1991). Native peoples do not have a laterally deviated big toe. Instead, their big toe lines up directly with the first metatarsal (Hoffman, 1905, James, 1939, Sim-Fook and Hodgson, 1958). Even later in life, the foot has some capacity to change and adapt. Those who stop wearing restrictive shoes and start walking and jogging barefoot will generally improve their range of motion and strength—and their big toe will tend to align itself more medially. A laterally deviated big toe can decrease one's ability to stabilize the foot against inward rotation, and can thereby cause a whip, since it may not be able to maintain the foot in a balanced position during toe-off. In particular, if the foot is inwardly rotated at toe-off, the ground reaction forces generally cause lateral movement of the foot as it begins the flight phase, and this can result in a whip.

A confining shoe upper that causes the big toe to deviate laterally, can contribute to the formation of a bunion. Further, the combination of a confining shoe upper and excessive pronation (which abnormally stresses the joint capsule of the big toe) can greatly accelerate the formation of a bunion. Women more frequently have problems with bunions. Many women think they are supposed to have small feet, and better yet, small, pointy feet. So they wear small, pointy dress shoes, which is the modern day equivalent of foot binding. This gives them bunions and ugly, painful feet. However, the present generation seems to better understand that shoes ought to be made to actually fit the human foot and provide plenty of room for the toes.

Posterior Tibialis

Just as the toes are the primary stabilizer regarding inward rotation in the forefoot area, the posterior tibialis is the primary stabilizer with respect to inward rotation in the midfoot area. Again, to a lesser degree, the intrinsic muscles of the foot, particularly those in the medial longitudinal arch, can also stabilize the medial aspect of the midfoot. Moreover, the tendon of the posterior tibialis can become overworked and inflamed when an individual has a motion control problem. Beware of soreness near the insertion, at the bend near the protuberance below the ankle, and also near the origin on the medial side of the tibia. An injury to the posterior tibialis will often travel in a direction from the point of insertion to the origin. If the injury has reached the origin, then a hot spot can develop and eventually cause a stress fracture of the tibia. Athletes with flat feet are the most vulnerable—they often have forefoot varus. In any case, injury to the posterior tibialis is normally caused by over-pronation, an excessive rate of pronation, and inward rotation of the midfoot. If an athlete has flat feet, it is best to avoid curve lasted shoes. Orthotics, or insoles that provide adequate arch support, can stabilize the medial longitudinal arch, and prevent an injury to the posterior tibialis, or alternately, can facilitate recovery.

The Hip Joint

Injuries involving the hip are less frequent than problems with the foot, lower leg and knee. The latter structures can usually isolate any motion control problems before they reach the hip. However, if an athlete is suddenly afflicted with a hip injury, check to see whether the individual has been running downhill or on a slippery surface. Downhill running can induce greater than normal hip extension and cause a slight tearing of the connective tissue near the hip joint. If one is looking from the side at an athlete facing to the right, the affected area is usually just behind and above the joint at about 10 o'clock. Running on a slippery surface at high speeds can cause the same condition. A "slip-and-jerk" reaction takes place. Perhaps the athlete has been running on wet barkdust, mud or snow.

Maybe the individual has been running on a downhill at speeds faster than 5:20/ mile, or across a significant grade. Check the runner's shoes for a failed gizmo or breakdown. These are potentially hazardous circumstances and combinations.

Again, check the athlete's conformance for an excessive Q angle, bowed legs, or a leg length difference. Look for overdeveloped and tight quadriceps, as well as limited hip extension. The individual may have weak hamstrings, lower abdominals, gluteals, internal and external rotators of the hip, and vastus medialis muscles. Videotape and view the runner's biomechanics from several angles. Is there excessive medial or lateral rotation of the upper and lower legs? Is there excessive motion at the knee? Does the athlete exhibit a whip?

A hip injury is often deep and difficult to locate or isolate with ice or heat therapy. The best medicine is prevention. Avoid the high-risk conditions mentioned above. An individual with a minor injury should always conduct a pre-warm up and full range of motion exercises before running. The injury will normally respond to strengthening the internal and external rotators of the hip. However, do not conduct these exercises to the point of eliciting pain. Discontinue the exercise before the area becomes fatigued and pain is experienced. If an athlete pushes things to the point of causing pain, then the individual may be taking two steps forward and one step backwards. Given a hip injury, easy bicycling can be of help, particularly during the early stages of rehabilitation. Another beneficial exercise for strengthening and healing the hip area is skating at moderate speed with a conservative technique. Swimming is normally beneficial, but it can sometimes aggravate a hip injury, thus an individual should first test matters and then be careful to exercise in moderation.

Sciatic Nerve

The sciatic nerve is actually composed of several nerves, which emerge both from the lumbar vertebrae and the sacrum, at L4, L5, and S1-4. A sciatic nerve problem generally manifests itself as a pressure, pain, or numbness in the lower back, sacrum, or buttocks. Most frequently, sciatica is felt in the left or right buttocks a couple of inches above the ischial tuberosity, or so-called "sit bone." The pain will often radiate down the back of the leg. If sciatica begins during training, the athlete should cease the activity immediately in order to catch it early. If the individual stops and conducts suitable therapeutic exercises, he or she might be back in action the next day. However, a runner who fails to take appropriate measures could become seriously injured and put themselves out for a long time. Normally, in healthy young athletes with no history of a lower back or pelvic injury, sciatic nerve problems can generally be traced to excessive forward, that is, anterior pelvic tilt, a displaced sacroiliac joint, or a muscle spasm.

Gather the necessary information to determine what happened and when. Did the sensation or injury develop following a workout? Perhaps the individual had a long aircraft flight, was sitting slumped on a sofa for several hours watching television, or slept in a strange position? If athletes sleep on their back in too soft a bed, then the sinking of their buttocks into the mattress can induce anterior pelvic tilt. Sleeping on a firm futon or placing pillows behind their knees can reduce anterior pelvic tilt. Even if athletes sleep on their side, a too soft or broken down bed can still cause their lower back to be misaligned. Athletes who normally sleep on their side might want to place their arms around a pillow positioned parallel to their torso. Otherwise, some might rotate too much at their shoulders, and that could place a lot of stress on their lower back. If athletes habitually sleep on their side, then placing a pillow between their knees might also help. Again, athletes should sleep on a firm futon rather than too soft a bed. In this regard, the Australian coach Percy Cerutty suggested that athletes sleep on wooden bunks to improve their posture and vital capacity.

Check the individual's anatomical conformance, particularly in the back and pelvis. Compare the hip height of each iliac crest, and check for a leg length difference. Look also for a functional leg length difference due to a breakdown in one of the athlete's shoes. Is the athlete running on roads with a grade? Again, running across a five-percent grade can easily produce an effective leg length difference of 1/4-inch.

The most common problem is that the pelvis has tilted too far forward, that is, anteriorly, and is causing a nerve to become impinged in the lower back (See Figure 9.20). Generally, this is due to the athlete's quads being too strong and too tight relative to weak hamstrings and lower abdominals. Initially, an effective rehabilitation exercise could be to lie flat on your back on a hard, flat floor for about 30 minutes. At first, this may feel uncomfortable due to pressure being placed on the sacrum, and the small of your back might be in an over-extended position. However, as anterior pelvic tilt is reduced, your lower back will relax and flatten, and the pressure on the sacrum will re-distribute to the larger buttocks. During this exercise, you might hold your lower back in a flattened position and then relax, or alternately raise and hold each knee to your chest, and then relax. Once you have restored the pelvis to its neutral position, strength training of the appropriate muscle groups needs to be conducted in order that proper posture be maintained. However, if an individual has any reason to believe that he or she could have a congenital defect or injury to the lower back, a medical professional should be consulted before attempting these exercises.

Rehabilitative training includes strengthening the hamstrings, vastus medialis, lower abdominals, and improving hip extension. All of these can be accomplished by doing walking squats. Further, athletes often strengthen their upper abdominals, but tend to neglect their lower abdominals. Exercises that strengthen the lower abdominals include straight and bent knee sit-ups on an incline board, and L-sits. In addition, athletes can lie on their back and perform a bicycling action while sweeping their legs close to the floor in order to work their lower abdominals.

Runners tend to get sciatica when they suddenly and dramatically increase their mileage. Soreness in the lower back can sometimes be a false alarm for sciatica. Instead, it may be associated with the origins of the iliopsoas muscles, particularly the psoas major, which is a powerful flexor of the hip. An actual sciatic nerve problem can arise if the piriformis muscle goes into spasm, impinging the

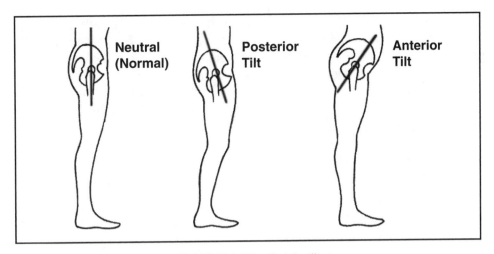

FIGURE 9.20—Pelvic tilt

sciatic nerve. Exercises that work the piriformis can often quickly relieve the spasm causing the impingement. Sciatica can also arise from a displaced sacroiliac joint. If the sacrum or ilia shift too much they can become slightly misaligned. A qualified physical therapist can often correct the problem via manipulation. Also, certain exercises can help to stabilize and restore the correct orientation.

An otherwise healthy individual with no history of back injury, may perform the dead lift exercise, using a barbell with light weights. The dead lift can often clear up the warning twinge or spasm from a developing sciatic problem that is being caused by a slightly displaced sacroiliac joint, or piriformis muscle that has gone into spasm. This exercise should only be considered if the injury is not advanced. Find someone who knows proper technique and learn how to perform the dead lift correctly. The barbell should be grasped with one palm turned in and the other out. The barbell should rest against the athlete's shins and be dragged upward, along the front of the shins, then across the knees and quads as if it were glued to them. The athlete's head should face forward and upward during the lift. It is important to use a weight belt when performing this exercise. The movement to the up position should finish with a pelvic thrust to prevent the pelvis from rotating forward. And the athlete's back should not be flexed relative to the pelvis—both should remain relatively straight and aligned. The movements then take place mostly between the legs and the pelvis, not the pelvis and the back. The entire exercise should be done slowly, taking approximately a count of six to the up position. On reaching the up position, the athlete should either hand off or drop the weights. This can be done using rubber weights and dropping them on an elevated platform, or by dropping the weights into sand. Under no circumstances should the athlete return to the start position, bend over, or lower the weights. It is important that concentric muscle contractions take place, not eccentric. If the athlete instead lowers the weights while returning to the start position, the net positive effect will generally be zero, or the problem could actually become worse.

The athlete should first attempt an easy effort of six to 10 repetitions with light weight, then wait several hours or even a day to judge the reaction. If the response is positive, then add a little more weight and conduct two or three sets of 10 reps. Wait a day, and then repeat the session. If the problem indeed involves a spasm of the piriformis muscle and/or displaced sacroiliac joint, the athlete will often feel that something positive has been accomplished within a few minutes, and certainly within one hour of the exercise. If an athlete later feels a twinge coming on and heads it off with a couple of sets, it will often be gone within a few hours. However, an individual who chooses to ignore the warning twinge and runs anyway will risk more serious injury.

For healthy young athletes, the author has found this exercise to be the single most effective technique for heading off a sciatic problem. It works the hamstrings, but also the gluteus minimus, medius, and the piriformis muscles. The exercise causes these muscles to shorten, thus stabilizing and causing the pelvis to tilt backward into correct position. When these muscles contract, the practical effect is to shorten the distance between their origins and insertions, and this reduces anterior pelvic tilt. A physical therapist might refer to this exercise as a muscle energy or stabilization technique, whereas a coach or trainer would simply hold this to be a part of a balanced strength training program.

Compartment Syndrome

Distance runners rarely experience compartment syndrome. Those who do will not likely recognize what is happening or know what to do about it, and that can be dangerous. In this condition, a muscle (perhaps developing too rapidly) outgrows its confining muscle sheath and becomes constricted during exercise. As the muscle fills with blood, becoming hot and pumped during exercise, it enlarges and begins to cut off its own blood supply. The symptoms are rigor and pain resembling a muscle cramp. The affected muscle can become hard to the touch, as if it were being voluntarily flexed. If this occurs, the athlete should stop training immediately, and then ice and elevate the affected part. If the muscle does not relax within a few minutes, the athlete must get to a physician as quickly as possible. Get the athlete to an emergency room STAT by dialing 911. If left untreated, the loss of circulation can kill the affected muscle tissues. Sometimes surgery is needed to relieve the pressure by slicing the muscle sheath. This is not a problem, and in time it will normally repair itself. Young athletes going through a growth spurt who are beginning to exercise heavily can be susceptible to this syndrome. Another group that may experience this problem are those using illegal hormones and steroids, because these substances induce abnormally rapid gains and losses of muscle mass. Play with matches and you will probably get burnt.

Stress Fractures

It takes bone tissue at least five to six weeks to adapt to a new level of training stress. Dramatic changes in training quantity or quality can place an athlete at risk. Bone tissue is not a perfectly rigid material. Instead, it bends or flexes to some degree when loaded. The long bones of the legs are especially vulnerable to rotational (or torsional) loading. As the foot pronates and rotates inward, the tibia is loaded and also rotates inward. At the same time, the femur rotates outward. These torsional loads on the long bones can result in stress fractures.

Sometimes the precipitating event is damage to the bone surface (or periosteum) where a tendon originates. A lot of energy is conducted through the point of origin, and sometimes the site is not adequately robust. With continued loading, a hot spot or stress fracture can develop. Hot spots can be observed immediately using Magnetic Resonance Imaging (MRI), but this procedure is expensive and sometimes unavailable. A stress fracture can sometimes take seven to 14 days to appear on a conventional X-ray. Often, if a stress fracture is present, a tuning fork placed upon the affected long bone will elicit pain. An athlete with a stress fracture will need at least five to six weeks to recuperate. However, depending on the age of the athlete, and the location, type, and severity of the injury, it can take as long as 12 weeks for the bone to mend. The most common stress fractures suffered by runners are to the metatarsals, sesamoids, tibia, and fibula. Fractures to the femur, pelvis, or vertebrae do happen, but these are relatively rare. Women more frequently experience stress fractures. This is due in part to their lighter bone structure, but it can sometimes also stem from an eating disorder.

Eating Disorders

If a coach is training a young female athlete conservatively and she does not appear to have faulty technique or motion control problems, yet she suffers reoccurring injuries (such as shin-splints or stress fractures of the tibia, fibula, or metatarsals of the foot), then the coach may actually be seeing the symptoms of an eating disorder. Exercise creates a higher demand for calcium, phosphorus and other essential minerals. If an athlete is not eating adequately or keeping food down, these minerals will be drawn from bone tissue. After ruling out other possibilities, the coach should seriously consider the possibility of an eating disorder, and then refer the athlete to professional help. As a coach, do not attempt to also assume the role of a clinical psychologist or medical doctor regarding arousal addiction and eating disorders. Those two hats present a potential conflict of interest. This condition is potentially life-threatening, and a coach is not qualified to practice in this area unless trained as a medical doctor or clinical psychologist.

Muscle Strains

The best medicine is an ounce of prevention. An athlete can avoid muscle pulls by maintaining well-conditioned, flexible muscles, and adopting sound training practices. However, if a muscle strain does occur, the affected area should be iced and elevated immediately. Do not apply heat or massage until the next day, or perhaps even the second or third day—that is, until the bleeding and inflammation has stopped and the healing process begun. After the desired range of motion has been restored, the fastest way to rehabilitate an injured muscle is with easy and well-controlled strength training. If an injured athlete does little or no rehabilitative activity, then even after having rested for a week or two he or she may still be at square one. However, with a suitable rehabilitation program, an athlete will normally be back in training much sooner, and the injury will heal better. Given a serious muscle strain, seek out the assistance of a medical doctor and a qualified physical therapist.

In this chapter a number of common orthopedic injuries have been briefly addressed. However, recognize that the most frequent injury suffered by athletes is not to their physical structure, but rather to their metabolism as the result of over-training (See the discussions in Chapter 1 and Chapter 6). Entire books have been written on the subject of athletic injuries—and also about running shoes. This chapter has touched on some important points, but not every possible topic of interest could be addressed in detail. Again, when you have questions about your health or that of someone for whom you are responsible, always consult a qualified medical professional such as a doctor, podiatrist, or physical therapist. Also, recognize that many knowledgeable and sincere individuals—whether researchers, coaches, or medical professionals—will sometimes differ in their opinions and past experiences. We are all unique individuals. And no two sets of circumstances are ever identical. Listen to your body, and in the words of the Delphic Oracle: **Know Thyself.**

I went to Penn State and asked the people who were rating shoes about balance and spring. Well, they didn't know what I was talking about. How can they rate shoes if they don't know even the most elementary things? They're not experts.

—Arthur Lydiard

References

Adamik, Jaroslav, U.S. Patent 4,302,892, *Athletic Shoe and Sole Therefor*, 1981.

Bates, Barry, U.S. Patent 4,364,189, *Running Shoe with Differential Cushioning*, 1982.

Bates, Barry, and S. L. James, L.R. Osternig, "Foot Function During the Support Phase of Running," *American Journal of Sports Medicine*, Volume 7, 1979, page 328.

Catlin, M.E., and R.H. Dressendorfer, "Effect of Shoe Weight on the Energy Cost of Running," *Medicine and Science in Sports*, Volume 11, Number 1, 1970, page 80.

Cavanagh, Peter, *The Running Shoe Book*, Mountain View, California: Anderson World, 1980.

Cavanagh, Peter, U.S. Patent 4,449,306, *Running Shoe Sole Construction*, 1984.

Cavanagh, Peter, U.S. Patent 4,506,462, *Running Shoe with Pronation Limiting Heel*, 1985.

Cavanagh, Peter, and M.A. LaFortune, "Ground Reaction Forces in Distance Running," Journal of *Biomechanics*, Volume 13, 1980, pages 397-406.

Cavanagh, Peter, and M.L. Pollock, J. Landa, "A Biomechanical Comparison of Elite and Good Distance Runners," *Annals of the New York Academy of Sciences*, Volume 301, 1977, pages 328-345.

Cavanagh, Peter, and G.A. Valiant, K.W. Misevich, "Biological Aspects of Modeling Shoe/Foot Interaction During Running," *Sport Shoes and Playing Surfaces*, E. C. Frederick, Editor, Champaign Illinois: Human Kinetics, 1984.

Cheskin, Melvin, and K.J. Sherkin, B. Bates, *Athletic Footwear*, Fairchild Publications, 1989.

Chopra, Deepak, *The Seven Spiritual Laws of Success*, San Rafael, California: Amber-Allen Publishing, 1994, page 84.

Clarke, T.E., and E.C. Frederick, L.B. Cooper, "Biomechanical Measurement of Running Shoe Cushioning Properties," *Biomechanical Aspects of Sports Shoes and Playing Surfaces*, B.M. Nigg and B.A. Kerr, Editors, Calgary, Alberta: University of Calgary, 1983, pages 25-33.

Clarke, T.E., and E.C. Frederick, C.L. Hamill, "The Effect of Shoe Design Upon Rearfoot Control in Running," *Medicine and Science in Sports and Exercise*, Volume 15, Number 5, 1983, pages 376-381.

Clarke, T.E., and M.A. LaFortune, K.R. Williams, P. Cavanagh, "The Relationship between Center of Pressure and Rearfoot Movement in Running," *Medicine and Science in Sports and Exercise*, Volume 12, Number 2, 1980, page 192.

Clarke, T.E., et al., U.S. Patent 4,439,936, *Shock Attenuating Outer Sole*, 1984.

Clement, D., and J. Taunton, J.P. Wiley, G. Smart, K. McNicol, "The Effects of Corrective Orthotic Devices on Oxygen Uptake During Running," *Proceedings of the World Congress on Sports Medicine*, L. Prokop, Editor, Vienna: World Congress on Sports Medicine, 1984, pages 648-655.

Daniels, Jack, "A Physiologist's View of Running Economy," *Medicine and Science in Sports and Exercise*, Volume 17, Number 3, 1985, pages 1-23.

De Clercq, D., and P. Aerts, M. Kunnen, "The Mechanical Characteristics of the Human Heel Pad During Footstrike in Running: An In Vivo Cineradiographic Study," *Journal of Biomechanics*, Volume 27, Number 10, 1994, pages 1213-1222.

Dellinger, Bill, and George Beres, *Winning Running*, Chicago, Illinois: Contemporary Books, Inc., 1978, pages 228-229.

Edington, C., and E.C. Frederick, Peter Cavanagh, "Rearfoot Motion in Distance Running," *Biomechanics of Distance Running*, Peter Cavanagh, Editor, Champaign, Illinois: Human Kinetics Books, 1990, pages 135-164.

Frederick, E.C., "Measuring the Effects of Shoe and Surfaces on the Economy of Locomotion," *Biomechanical Aspects of Sports Shoes and Playing Surfaces*, B.M. Nigg and B.A. Kerr, Editors, Calgary, Alberta: University of Calgary, 1983, pages 93-106.

Frederick, E.C., "Physiological and Ergonomics Factors in Running Shoe Design," *Applied Ergonomics*, Volume 15, Number 4, 1984, pages 281-287.

Frederick, E.C., and T.E. Clarke, J.L. Larsen, L.B. Cooper, "The Effects of Shoe Cushioning on the Oxygen demands of Running," *Biomechanical Aspects of Sports Shoes and Playing Surfaces*, B.M. Nigg and B.A. Kerr, Editors, Calgary, Alberta: University of Calgary, 1983, pages 107-114.

Frederick, E.C., and J.T. Daniels, J.W. Hayes, "The Effect of Shoe Weight on the Aerobic Demands of Running," *Proceedings of the World Congress on Sports Medicine*, L. Prokop, Editor, Vienna: World Congress on Sports Medicine, 1984, pages 616-625.

Frederick, E.C., and E.T. Howley, S.K. Powers, "Lower Oxygen Demands of Running in Soft-Soled Shoes," *Research Quarterly for Exercise and Sports*, Volume 57, Number 2, 1986, pages 174-177.

Frederick, E.C., et al. U.S. Patent 4,562,651, *Sole with V-Oriented Flex Grooves*, 1986.

Frederickson, Ray, et al., U.S. Patent 4,934,072, *Fluid Dynamic Shoe*, 1990.

Gamow, Rustem Igor, and Hugh Herr, U.S. Patent 5,367,790, *Shoe and Foot Prosthesis with a Coupled Spring System*, 1994.

Greene, Peter, and Thomas McMahon, "Reflex Stiffness of Man's Anti-Gravity Muscles During Kneebends While Carrying Extra Weights," *Journal of Biomechanics*, Volume 12, 1979, pages 881-891.

Hamill, C.L., and T.E. Clarke, E.C. Frederick, L.J. Goodyear, E.T. Howley, "Effects of Grade Running on Kinematics and Impact Force," *Medicine and Science in Sports and Exercise*, Volume 16, 1984, page 165.

Harris, Cyril B., Editor, *Shock & Vibration Handbook*, 3rd edition, New York: McGraw-Hill Book Company, 1988, page 44-10.

Herr, Hugh, et al., U.S. Patent 5,701,686, *Shoe and Foot Prosthesis with Bending Beam Spring Structures*, 1997.

Herr, Hugh, et al., U.S. Patent 6,029,374, *Shoe and Foot Prosthesis with Bending Beam Spring Structures*, 2000.

Hoffman, P., M.D., "Conclusions Drawn From a Comparative Study of the Feet of Barefooted and Shoe-Wearing Peoples," *The American Journal of Orthopedic Surgery*, Volume 3, Number 2, October, 1905, pages 105-136.

Hollister, Geoffrey, et al., U.S. Patent 4,043,058, *Athletic Training Shoe Having Foam Core and Apertured Sole Layers*, 1977.

Hoppenfeld, Stanley, M.D., *Physical Examination of the Spine & Extremities*, San Mateo, California, Appleton & Lange, 1976.

Ivers, Tom, *The Fit Racehorse II*, GrandPrairie, Texas: Equine Research, Inc., 1994.

James, Clifford, "Footprints and Feet of Natives of the Solomon Islands," *The Lancet*, December 30, 1939, pages 1390-1393.

James, S. L., and B. T. Bates, L. R. Osterning, "Injuries to Runners," *American Journal of Sports Medicine*, Volume 6, 1978, pages 40-50.

Kerr, B.A., and L. Beauchamp, V. Fisher, R. Neil, "Footstrike Patterns in Distance Running," *Biomechanical Aspects of Sport Shoes and Playing Surfaces*, B. M. Nigg and B. A. Kerr, Editors, Calgary, Alberta: University of Calgary, 1983, pages 135-142.

Kilgore, Bruce, et. al, U.S. Patent 5,046,267, *Athletic Shoe with Pronation Control Device*, 1991.

Kim, Hee-Jin, *Dōgen Kigen: Mystical Realist*, Tuscon, Arizona: University of Arizona Press, 1987.

Lyden, Robert, European Patent Application EP 0752216 A3, *Footwear with Differential Cushioning Regions*, published 1997.

Lyden, Robert, U.S. Patent 5,384,973, *Sole with Articulating Forefoot*, 1995.

Lyden, Robert, U.S. Patent 5,632,057, *Method of Making Light Cure Component for Articles of Footwear*, 1997.

Lyden, Robert, U.S. Patent 5,921,004, *Footwear with Stabilizers*, 1999.

Lyden, Robert, U.S. Patent 6,449,878, *Article of Footwear Having a Spring Element and Selectively Removable Components*, 2002.

Lyden, Robert, et. al., U.S. Patent 5,425,184, *Athletic Shoe with Rearfoot Strike Zone*, 1995.

Lyden, Robert, et. al., U.S. Patent 5,625,964, *Athletic Shoe with Rearfoot Strike Zone*, 1997.

Lyden, Robert, et. al., U.S. Patent 6,055,746, *Athletic Shoe with Rearfoot Strike Zone*, 2001.

Misevich, Kenneth, U.S. Patent 4,557,059, *Athletic Running Shoe, 1985*.

MacLellan, Gordon, "Skeletal Heel Strike Transcients, Measurement, Implications and Modifications," *Sport Shoes and Playing Surfaces*, E. C. Frederick, Editor, Champaign, Illinois: Human Kinetics, 1984, pages 76-86.

McCraken, Grant, *Culture and Consumption: New Approaches to the Symbolic Character*, Indiana: Indiana University Press, 1988.

McMahon, T.A., and P.R. Green, "The Influence of Track Compliance on Running," *Journal of Biomechanics*, Volume 12, 1979, pages 893-904.

McMahon, T.A., *Muscles, Reflexes, and Locomotion*, Princeton, New Jersey: Princeton University, 1984.

McMahon, T.A., "Spring-Like Properties of Muscles and Reflexes in Running," *Multiple Muscle Systems: Biomechanics and Movement Organization*, J. M. Winters and S.L.-Y. Woo, editors, Springer-Verlag, 1990, pages 578-590.

McMahon, T.A., and George Cheng, "The Mechanics of Running: How Does Stiffness Couple with Speed," *Journal of Biomechanics*, Volume 23, Supplement 1, 1990, pages 65-78.

Nigg, B. M., "Biomechanical Aspects of Running," *Biomechanics of Running Shoes*, B. M. Nigg, Editor, Champaign, Illinois: Human Kinetics Publishers, 1984, pages 1-26.

Nigg, B.M., and M. Morlock, "The Influence of Lateral Heel Flare of Running Shoes on Pronation and Impact Forces," *Medicine and Science in Sports and Exercise*, Volume 19, 1987, pages 294-302.

Noakes, Tim, *Lore of Running*, 3rd Edition, Champaign, Illinois: Human Kinetics, 1991, page 493.

Norkin, Cynthia C., and Pamela K. Levangie, *Joint Structure and Function*, 2nd Edition, Philadelphia, Pennsylvania: Davis Company, 1992.

Norton, Edward, U.S. Patent 4,288,929, *Motion Control Device for Athletic Shoe*, 1981.

Parker, Mark, et al., U.S. Patent 4,817,304, *Footwear with Adjustable Viscoelastic Unit*, 1989.

Parracho, Rui, et al., U.S. Patent 4,731,939, *Athletic Shoe with External Counter and Cushion Assembly*, 1988.

Seydel, R., and S. Luthi, R. Fumi, K. Beard, O. Kaiser, U.S. Patent 6,266,897, *Ground-Contacting Systems Having 3-D Deformation Elements for Use in Footwear*, 2001.

Shorten, Martyn, "The Energetics of Running and Running Shoes," *Journal of Biomechanics*, Volume 26, Supplement 1, 1993, pages 41-51.

Shorten, Martyn, U.S. Patent 5,201,125, *Shoe, Especially a Sport or Rehabilitation Shoe*, 1993.

Shorten, Martyn, U.S. Patent 5,197,206, *Shoe, Especially a Sport or Rehabilitation Shoe*, 1993.

Shorten, Martyn, U.S. Patent 5,197,207, *Shoe, Especially a Sport or Rehabilitation Shoe*, 1993.

Shorten, Martyn, and G.A. Valiant, L.B. Cooper, "Frequency Analysis of the Effects of Shoe Cushioning on Dynamic Shock in Running," *Medicine and Science in Sports and Exercise*, Volume 18, 1986, pages S80-81.

Shorten, Martyn, and Darcy S. Winslow, "Spectral Analysis of Impact Shock During Running," *International Journal of Sport Biomechanics*, Volume 8, Number 4, November 1992, pages 288-304.

Shorten, Martyn, and S.A. Wootton, C. Williams, "Mechanical Energy Changes and the Oxygen Cost of Running," *Engineering in Medicine*, Volume 10, Number 4, MEP, Ltd., 1981, pages 213-217.

Sim-Fook, Lam, and A. Hodgson, "A Comparison of Foot Forms Among the Non-Shoe and Shoe-Wearing Chinese Population," *The Journal of Bone and Joint Surgery*, Volume 40-A, Number 1, January 1958, pages 1058-1062.

Stacoff, A., and X. Kaelin, "Pronation and Sportshoe Design," *Biomechanical Aspect of Sport Shoes and Playing Surfaces*, B. M. Nigg and B.A. Kerr, Editors, Calgary, Alberta: University of Calgary, 1983, pages 143-151.

Stacoff, A., and X. Kaelin, J. Denoth, E. Stuessi, "Running Injuries and Shoe Construction: Some Possible Relationships," *International Journal of Sport Biomechanics*, Volume 4, 1988, pages 342-357.

Staheli, Lynn, "Shoes for Children: A Review," *Pediatrics*, Volume 88, Number 2, August 1991.

Unold, E., "Erschuetterungsmessungen beim Gehen und Laufen auf verschiedenen Unterlagen mit verschiedenem Schuhwerk." *Jugend und Sport*, Volume 8, 1974, pages 280-292.

PART III

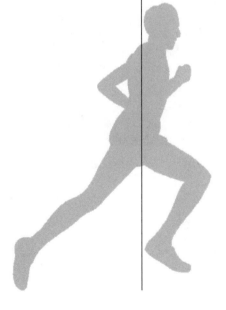

SPECIAL CONSIDERATIONS FOR DISTANCE RUNNERS

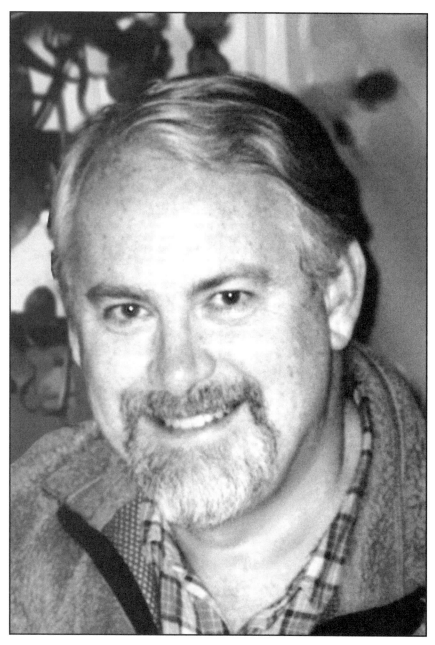

PHOTO 10.1—E. C. "Ned" Frederick at his home in New Hampshire, 2000.
Photo courtesy of Ned Frederick.

CHAPTER 10

SHOE WEIGHT AND MECHANICAL EFFICIENCY

The weight and mechanical efficiency of an article of footwear can significantly impact athletic performance, particularly at national and international levels of competition. How much do your track spikes and racing flats weigh? How much does additional shoe weight cost a distance runner in terms of performance? How much does the mechanical efficiency of a shoe or running surface affect athletic performance?

Shoe Weight

E.C. (Ned) Frederick is probably the most knowledgeable person in the United States on this subject. Ned found that 100 grams added to each shoe equated to an increased energy cost of 1.2% of an individual's oxygen uptake while running at racing speeds (Frederick, Daniels, Hayes, 1984). How does this translate into ounces? Given 28.35 grams in an ounce, 100 grams would roughly equal 3.5 ounces. Accordingly, 1.2% divided by 3.5 ounces equals .342% as the approximate energy cost per ounce of additional shoe weight.

After reviewing the methodology of various studies on this subject, the author estimates that the actual energy cost of carrying an additional ounce on a shoe would be a bit higher in the practical application. Rather, it would affect performance by about .5% of VO_2 maximum. The reason being that in a lab setting weight can simply be added to a shoe, but additional weight in a commercial product is often associated with disadvantageous changes in the structure and function of athletic footwear. Further, most of these studies were conducted on level treadmills, which can solicit changes in a person's running technique, reducing the amount of work in hip extension. This can be overcome by inclining a treadmill to require greater effort during hip extension, but this introduces another variable.

With the use of the tables found in *Oxygen Power* (Daniels and Gilbert, 1979) and a calculator, the energy cost of carrying an extra ounce of weight on an athletic shoe can be estimated. A change in shoe weight of one ounce (corresponding to a .5% change in oxygen uptake or VO_2 maximum) is worth at least approximately:

- 1 second in a 1,500 meters performance of 3:35
- 4 seconds in a 5,000 meters performance of 13:20
- 8 seconds in a 10,000 meters performance of 27:45
- Over 30 seconds in a marathon

These are large margins in national or international competitions.

The spikes that Bill Bowerman made for Steve Prefontaine weighed between three and four ounces. Commercial size 9 track spikes or racing flats commonly weigh between 6.5 to 7.5 ounces, but clearly, it is possible to have equally functional and durable footwear weighing between 4.0 and 5.5 ounces. It is sometimes possible to modify a commercial shoe and reduce shoe weight by two full ounces, thus the time savings shown above could potentially be doubled.

Mechanical Efficiency

In addition to its weight, an athletic shoe's mechanical efficiency should also be considered. Athletic shoes function as a spring, thereby storing and returning energy over time. But they also act as a dampener, undergoing hysteresis and transforming mechanical energy into heat. The characteristic ratio of the spring and dampening qualities of most athletic shoes is about 50/50, but can range from 40/60 to 60/40. Often, the price for using a stiffer spring is greater transmission of shock and vibration, and reduced cushioning effects. However, at times an athlete may wish to sacrifice cushioning in favor of maximizing mechanical efficiency. For example, sprinters are sometimes wise to remove soft insoles from their track spikes when competing on elastomeric track surfaces, because cushioning is associated with deflection, and deflection takes time. Moreover, all things being equal, reducing the elevation of a sprinter's foot relative to the track surface will result in less time and energy being lost to rotation and stabilizing movements.

Some racing flats with non-homogenous shoe sole compositions can provide good cushioning and high mechanical efficiency. For example, some shoes use a relatively soft foam material in the lateral rear corner, or "rearfoot strike zone," but include stiffer foam materials on the medial side and in the forefoot area. In fact, some athletic footwear can actually provide an energy savings by reducing the oxygen uptake used in protecting the runner from shock and vibration—a phenomenon known as the "cost of cushioning." Frederick was able to demonstrate an improvement in performance corresponding to a change in oxygen uptake of 1.3% in subjects running at racing speeds while using a NIKE AIR® racing flat (Frederick, Clarke, Larsen, and Cooper, 1983). For athletes capable of running 2:09 in the marathon, a 1.3% improvement of their oxygen uptake would result in a time saving of approximately 90 seconds—thus a performance of 2:07:30 would be possible. Obviously, increasing the mechanical efficiency of athletic shoes can result in substantial improvements in athletic performance.

The question of mechanical efficiency and the "cost of cushioning" can also influence efforts to reduce shoe weight. Stripping a track spike or racing flat down to about four ounces can work well for cross-country and road race events shorter than 8,000 meters. However, because of the increased stress placed upon the body when cushioning is reduced, extremely light shoes can be a risky proposition at distances between 10,000 meters and the marathon. The ideal racing flat for short distance events may be unsuitable for longer distance events because it can permit greater transmission of shock and solicit biomechanical adjustments that diminish performance and delay recovery from exercise.

Springs and Performance

The current USATF Rulebook, Apparel Rule 71 (essentially the same as IAAF Rulebook, Rule 143) reads as follows:

> a) A competitor may compete in bare feet or with footwear on one or both feet. The purpose of shoes for competition is to give protection and stability to the feet and a firm grip of the ground. Such shoes, however, must not be constructed so as to give the competitor any additional assistance, and no spring or device of any kind may be incorporated in the shoes. A shoe strap over the instep is permissible.

However, all of the materials and devices presently used in the soles of athletic footwear—including rubber, foam, thermoplastic, carbon fiber composites, and gas-filled bladders—comprise both a spring and a dampener. One question would concern the mechanical efficiency provided by a given component in an article of footwear, and the potential competitive advantage conferred by so-called spring devices. Several variables greatly complicate this question, such as the body mass and characteristic running technique of a given individual. Insofar as a shoe provides either too stiff or too soft a spring for the needs of a distance runner, it will not provide the wearer with advantageous performance. Further, the suitability of a shoe including a spring also depends on the rate of loading, thus the particular speed an individual is running. To achieve optimum mechanical efficiency, an athlete requires a softer spring when running slowly, but a stiffer spring when running at faster speeds.

Athletic shoes are not all the same, and the differences can significantly impact performance. A single generic commercialized product cannot provide all athletes with equal mechanical efficiency. No two footwear products, or individuals are alike. Most commercial athletic shoes have been developed and wear-tested for a generic size 9 male weighing between 140 and 165 pounds. Accordingly, athletes differing in body mass, running technique, and speed will normally experience differences in their mechanical efficiency and running economy when using the same make and model of footwear. Since the geometry and stiffness of conventional footwear cannot be customized, it is simply not possible for everyone to enjoy an equivalent level of performance. Athletes should experiment with a number of shoes to understand which characteristics provide them with the best results. A promotional athlete is sometimes in the position to order custom footwear. Recognize that the support surface upon which the athlete performs also constitutes a part of the mechanical system. However, the most important part of the mechanical equation is the human body, which normally contributes and manages over 97% of the energy during athletic performance.

When Adidas-Salomon AG approached the IAAF with a track spike incorporating a full-length carbon fiber spring element for possible use by sprinters during the 2000 Olympic games, the IAAF ruled it was permissible. The claimed enhancement of performance was between one and four percent, roughly corresponding to one second/400 meters (Nielsen, 2000). This was potentially the most significant development with respect to human performance in track and field since the introduction of the modern elastomeric track surface.

However, this was not an entirely new development. Nike, Inc. had previously used a carbon fiber composite element that was visible on the bottom of Mike Powell's long jump spikes during the 1992 Olympic Games. Also, other footwear manufacturers—including Etonic Athletic, Inc., Brooks Sports, Inc., and Mizuno, Inc.—have used like materials in footwear that have been previously commercialized. In particular, Hugh Herr and Igor Gamow are co-inventors on patents directed towards spring elements for use in footwear (U.S. Patents 5,367,790, 5,701,686, and 6,029,374). Moreover, the author has also filed several patent applications relating to selectively removable and replaceable spring elements for use in making customized articles of footwear that can provide an individual with enhanced cushioning, stability, and running economy (See Figure 10.1, U.S. 6,449,878). In brief, the traditional materials and methods of making athletic footwear are presently in the process of transformation and a new paradigm is beginning to emerge (Kerdok, Biewnere, McMahon, Weyand, Herr, 2001, and Herr, Huang, Langman, Gamow, 2002).

It is thus becoming more difficult to provide simple advice on the functional qualities that an athlete should look for in footwear. When searching for a conventional shoe construction, select a product with an appropriate design and cushioning characteristics for optimizing your running technique. Also, select a shoe that dissipates heat well, is relatively lightweight, and provides good traction and overall performance given the anticipated environmental conditions. Again, athletes need to confirm their footwear selection at least three months before a major championship competition. Moreover, for optimal biomechanical adaptations to accrue, distance runners should train at least twice a week in the make and model of footwear that they have selected.

Orthotic Devices

The use of an orthotic (or insert) device can increase efficiency and enhance performance, but only when the overall weight of the resulting shoe remains nearly constant (Clement, Taunton, Wiley, Smart, and McNicol, 1984). The transport of weight at the end of an individual's foot—which can be moving at nearly 50 mph—consumes limited energy. For some athletes, lightweight orthotics for use in their racing spikes or flats can be an essential piece of equipment, as this can save those runners having atypical conformance or motion control problems from injury, and so facilitate recovery from competition. However, regarding the possible beneficial effect of using orthotics upon athletic performance, runners should consider themselves lucky to break even.

Running Surfaces

Surface variations can also dramatically affect the efficiency of the larger mechanical system comprising the human body, athletic shoe, and underlying

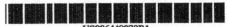
(12) **United States Patent** (10) **Patent No.:** US 6,449,878 B1
Lyden (45) **Date of Patent:** Sep. 17, 2002

(54)	**ARTICLE OF FOOTWEAR HAVING A SPRING ELEMENT AND SELECTIVELY REMOVABLE COMPONENTS**			

(76) Inventor: **Robert M. Lyden**, 18261 SW. Fallatin Loop, Aloha, OR (US) 97707

(*) Notice: Subject to any disclaimer, the term of this patent is extended or adjusted under 35 U.S.C. 154(b) by 0 days.

(21) Appl. No.: **09/523,341**

(22) Filed: **Mar. 10, 2000**

(51) Int. Cl.[7] A43B 13/28
(52) U.S. Cl. 36/27; 36/38
(58) Field of Search .... 36/27, 28, 30 R, 36/38, 7.8

(56) **References Cited**

U.S. PATENT DOCUMENTS

75,900	A	3/1868	Hale et al.	36/28
RE9,618	E	3/1881	Nichols	36/27
298,844	A	6/1884	Glanville	
318,366	A	5/1885	Fitch	
324,065	A	8/1885	Andrews	36/37
337,146	A	3/1886	Gluecksmann	36/7.8
357,062	A *	2/1887	Buch	
413,693	A	10/1889	Walker	
418,922	A	1/1890	Minahan	
427,136	A	5/1890	Walker	36/7.8 X
620,582	A	3/1899	Goff	

(List continued on next page.)

FOREIGN PATENT DOCUMENTS

AT	33492	6/1908		
CA	1115950	1/1982	....	36/6
CH	425537	5/1967		
DE	59317	3/1891		
DE	620963	10/1935		
DE	2419870	11/1974		
DE	250156	7/1976	.....	A43B/13/26
DE	2543268 a1	3/1977	.....	A43C/15/16

DE	2851535 A1	4/1980	....	A43B/13/26
DE	2851571 A1	5/1980	....	A43B/13/26

(List continued on next page.)

OTHER PUBLICATIONS

Runner's World, Fall 2000 Shoe Buyer's Guide, Sep., 2000.
Patent application No. 09/228,206, filed Jan. 11, 1999 by Robert M. Lyden entitled "Wheeled Skate with Step–in Binding and Brakes".
Patent application No. 09/570, 171, filed May 11, 2000, by Robert M. Lyden entitled "Light Cure Conformable Device for Articles of Footwear and Method of Making the same".
8 Photos of NIKE Secret Prior Art Published Oct., 2000.
2 Pages, DuPont Website Information Re:ZYTEL© and Nike Track Shoes dated Feb. 2, 2001, published Oct., 2000.
K. J. Fisher, "Advanced Composites Step into Athletic Shoes," *Advanced Composites*, May/Jun. 1991, pp. 32–35.
Product Literature from L.A. Gear regarding the Catapult Shoe Design.
Discovery, Oct. 1989, pp. 77–83, Kunzig.

Primary Examiner—Ted Kavanaugh
(74) *Attorney, Agent, or Firm*—Westman, Champlin & Kelly, P.A.

(57) **ABSTRACT**

The article of footwear taught in the present invention includes a spring element which can provide improved cushioning, stability, running economy, and a long service life. Unlike the conventional foam materials presently being used by the footwear industry, the spring element is not substantially subject to compression set degradation and can provide a relatively long service life. The components of the article of footwear including the upper, insole, spring element, and outsole portions can be selected from a range of options, and can be easily removed and replaced, as desired. Further, the relative configuration and functional relationship as between the forefoot midfoot areas of the article of footwear can be readily modified and adjusted. Accordingly, the article of footwear can be customized by a wearer or specially configured for a select target population in order to optimize desired performance criteria.

30 Claims, 9 Drawing Sheets

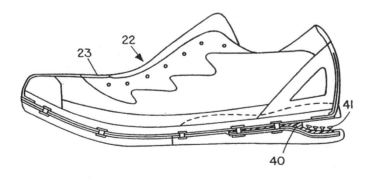

FIGURE 10.1—U.S. Patent 6,449,878

running surface. The most celebrated experiment in this regard being the tuned track at Harvard University (McMahon, Green, 1979). And not all portions of a given track surface are alike. Prior to a track and field competition, the Australian coach Percy Cerutty had the habit of bouncing a golf ball on different areas of the track to determine where the surface was alive and where it was dead.

The elastomeric tracks now available to athletes will generally aid distance performances by approximately .5 to one second/400 meters, whereas they commonly reduce performances in the sprinting events by .1 second/100 meters relative to hard asphalt-like tracks. Different road and cross-country course conditions can also dramatically influence running efficiency. On softer courses, it is sometimes wise to use footwear with firmer cushioning, and vice-versa. Further, athletes should prepare for the type of course conditions and surface footing expected in an upcoming major championship. They will then be able to adapt and optimize their running technique prior to the competition.

Many coaches and athletes never question the possible effects of the weight and efficiency of athletic footwear—or the impact that orthotics and running surfaces have on performance. This is a serious mistake. The practical effect of any one of these variables can be substantial.

If you can doubt at points where other people feel no impulse to doubt, then you are making progress.

— Chang Tsai

References

Catlin, M.E., and R.H. Dressendorfer, "Effect of Shoe Weight on the Energy Cost of Running," *Medicine and Science in Sports*, Volume 11, Number 1, 1970, page 80.

Cavanagh, Peter, and M.A. LaFortune, "Ground Reaction Forces in Distance Running," *Journal of Biomechanics*, Volume 13, 1980, pages 397-406.

Cavanagh, Peter, and M.L. Pollock, J. Landa, "A Biomechanical Comparison of Elite and Good Distance Runners," *Annals of the New York Academy of Sciences*, Volume 301, 1977, pages 328-345.

Clarke, T.E., and E.C. Frederick, L.B. Cooper, "Biomechanical Measurement of Running Shoe Cushioning Properties," *Biomechanical Aspects of Sports Shoes and Playing Surfaces*, B.M. Nigg and B.A. Kerr, Editors, Calgary, Alberta: University of Calgary, 1983, pages 25-33.

Clement, D., and J. Taunton, J. P. Wiley, G. Smart, K. McNicol, "The Effects of Corrective Orthotic Devices on Oxygen Uptake During Running," *Proceedings of the World Congress on Sports Medicine*, L. Prokop, Editor, Vienna: World Congress on Sports Medicine, 1984, pages 648-655.

Daniels, Jack, "A Physiologists View of Running Economy," *Medicine and Science in Sports and Exercise*, Volume 17, Number 3, 1985, pages 1-23.

Daniels, Jack, and Jimmy Gilbert, *Oxygen Power*, Tempe, Arizona: Published Privately, 1979.

Frederick, E. C., "Measuring the Effects of Shoe and Surfaces on the Economy of Locomotion," *Biomechanical Aspects of Sports Shoes and Playing Surfaces*, B.M. Nigg and B.A. Kerr, Editors, Calgary, Alberta: University of Calgary, 1983, pages 93-106.

Frederick, E.C., "Physiological and Ergonomics Factors in Running Shoe Design," *Applied Ergonomics*, Volume 15, Number 4, 1984, pages 281-287.

Frederick, E. C., and T. E. Clarke, J. L. Larsen, L. B. Cooper, "The Effects of Shoe Cushioning on the Oxygen demands of Running," *Biomechanical Aspects of Sports Shoes and Playing Surfaces*, B.M. Nigg and B.A. Kerr, Editors, Calgary, Alberta: University of Calgary, 1983, pages 107-114.

Frederick, E. C., and J. T. Daniels, J. W. Hayes, "The Effect of Shoe Weight on the Aerobic Demands of Running," *Proceedings of the World Congress on Sports Medicine*, L. Prokop, Editor, Vienna: World Congress on Sports Medicine, 1984, pages 616-625.

Frederick, E.C., and E.T. Howley, S. K. Powers, "Lower Oxygen Demands of Running in Soft-Soled Shoes," *Research Quarterly of Exercise and Sports*, Volume 57, Number 2, 1986, pages 174-177.

Gamow, Rustem Igor, and Hugh Herr, U.S. Patent 5,367,790, *Shoe and Foot Prosthesis with a Coupled Spring System*, 1994.

Greene, Peter, and Thomas McMahon, "Reflex Stiffness of Man's Anti-Gravity Muscles During Kneebends While Carrying Extra Weights," *Journal of Biomechanics*, Volume 12, 1979, pages 881-891.

Herr, Hugh, et al., U.S. Patent 5,701,686, *Shoe and Foot Prosthesis with Bending Beam Spring Structures*, 1997.

Herr, Hugh, et al., U.S. Patent 6,029,374, *Shoe and Foot Prosthesis with Bending Beam Spring Structures*, 2000.

Herr, Hugh, and G. Huang, N. Langman, R. Gamow, "A Mechanically Efficient Shoe Midsole Improves Running Economy, Stability, and Cushioning," *Journal of Applied Physiology*, 2002 (in press).

Kerdok, A. and A. Biewnere, T. McMahon, P. Weyand, H. Herr, "Energetics and Mechanics of Human Running on Surfaces of Different Stiffness," *Journal of Applied Physiology*, Volume 92, 2001, pages 469-478.

Kerr, B.A., and L. Beauchamp, V. Fisher, R. Neil, "Footstrike Patterns in Distance Running," *Biomechanical Aspects of Sport Shoes and Playing Surfaces*, B. M. Nigg and B. A. Kerr, Editors, Calgary, Alberta: University of Calgary, 1983, pages 135-142.

Lyden, Robert, U.S. Patent 6,449,878, *Article of Footwear Having a Spring Element and Selectively Removable Components*, 2002.

Lyden, Robert, U.S. Patent 6,601,042, *Customized Article of Footwear and Method of Conducting Retail and Internet Business*, 2003.

MacLellan, Gordon, "Skeletal Heel Strike Transcients, Measurement, Implications and Modifications," *Sport Shoes and Playing Surfaces*, E.C. Frederick, Editor, Champaign, Illinois: Human Kinetics, 1984, pages 76-86.

McMahon, T.A., *Muscles, Reflexes, and Locomotion*, Princeton, New Jersey: Princeton University Press, 1984.

McMahon, T.A., "Spring-Like Properties of Muscles and Reflexes in Running," *Multiple Muscle Systems: Biomechanics and Movement Organization*, J. M. Winters and S.L-Y. Woo, Editors, Springer-Verlag, 1990, pages 578-590.

McMahon, T.A., and George Cheng, "The Mechanics of Running: How Does Stiffness Couple with Speed," *Journal of Biomechanics*, Volume 23, Supplement 1, 1990, pages 65-78.

McMahon, T. A., and P.R. Green, "The Influence of Track Compliance on Running," *Journal of Biomechanics*, Volume 12, 1979, pages 893-904.

Nielsen, Peter, "Tuned Shoes May Help Runners Break Olympic Records," *Reuters, http://reuters.com*, August 9, 2000.

Nigg, B. M., "Biomechanical Aspects of Running," in *Biomechanics of Running Shoes*, B. M. Nigg, Editor, Champaign, Illinois: Human Kinetics Publishers, 1984, pages 1-26.

Shorten, Martyn, "The Energetics of Running and Running Shoes," *Journal of Biomechanics*, Volume 26, Supplement 1, 1993, pages 41-51.

Shorten, Martyn, and S.A. Wootton, C. Williams, "Mechanical Energy Changes and the Oxygen Cost of Running," *Engineering in Medicine*, Volume 10, Number 4, MEP, Ltd., 1981, pages 213-217.

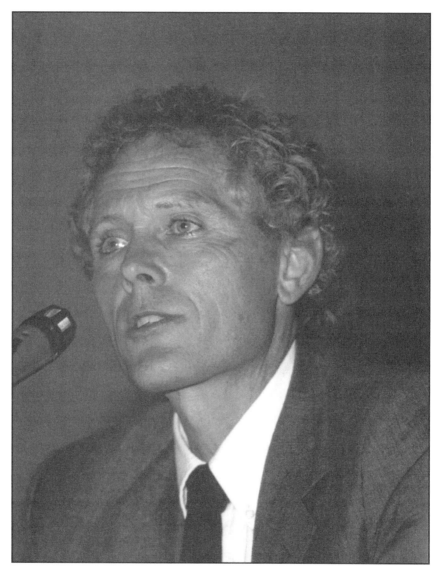

PHOTO 11.1—Jack Daniels, exercise physiologist, coach, and author, delivering a presentation in 1986. Photo from Victah Sailer / Photorun.

CHAPTER 11

IRON DEFICIENCY ANEMIA

This discussion of iron deficiency begins with several warnings. Iron is poisonous when taken in high doses. Iron supplements are one of the most frequent causes of household poisoning in children. Often, the pills are red and look like candy, and so iron supplements must be stored where children cannot get access. Further, athletes can sometimes lack sufficient iron, but one of the most common genetic disorders is hemochromatosis (affecting .3 to .5% of the population), which causes the affected individual to absorb too much iron (*Cecil Textbook of Medicine*, 1996). Accordingly, it is wise to consult with a physician before initiating any form of iron supplementation. Moreover, in extreme cases of iron deficiency anemia, an individual can require an injection under the care of a physician. Some of the products that have been developed must first be tested at 10% of normal dosage in an emergency room, because individuals can be allergic to the bovine serum containing the iron, and the reaction can cause anaphylactic shock.

Again, whenever iron deficiency anemia is suspected, first consult with a physician. In cases of iron deficiency anemia, the hemoglobin has priority with respect to the available iron. The level of iron stores will need to be determined by testing the serum ferritin because the hemoglobin content will be misleading. The values obtained in a serum ferritin test can vary a greatly from one individual to another. Moreover, an individual can have elevated serum ferritin values due to an inflammatory and infectious disease, or as the result of over-training. When in peak fitness, elite athletes might be wise to perform a serum ferritin test (as well as blood profile, blood lactate threshold and VO_2 max tests), as they would then have a basis of comparison if they would ever suffer a health problem.

In the abstract, the values obtained in a serum ferritin test could be anywhere in the range between 10 to 200 nanograms/milliliter (ml). However, the normal values differ considerably in populations of elite male and female distance runners. Since no definitive study on the subject of serum ferritin test values and distance runners has been published, the information in this chapter may then be of assistance to medical professionals. The author is indebted to Jack Daniels and other coaches for sharing their experiences concerning iron deficiency anemia. Moreover, several relevant references are cited at the end of this chapter.

Male distance runners normally maintain serum ferritin values over 60 nanograms/ml., but many individuals seem to be fine providing that they stay within the range of 30 to 60. When male athletes fall below 30 nanograms/ml., iron deficiency anemia can severely affect their aerobic ability. If athletes are on the low end of the 30 to 60 nanograms/ml. range, or abnormally lower than their usual profile, they will commonly experience good days alternating with bad days in training. Because of the wide range of individual variation, the serum ferritin test is often given several times in order to monitor an athlete's values. The average value recorded by approximately 30 elite male distance runners tested over several years by Jack Daniels (former exercise physiologist for club Athletics West) was about 60 nanograms/ml. But in order to illustrate the wide range of individual variability, one male 800 meters runner never tested much above 30 nanograms/ml., whereas a 5,000 meters specialist (who perhaps had hemochromatosis) was tested at 200 nanograms/ml.

Female distance runners experience a much higher incidence of iron deficiency anemia. Elite female distance runners are often close to borderline—thus they are generally well advised to take some form of iron supplement. The normal range of serum ferritin for women runners is lower than that of men. If a woman's serum ferritin test reads below 15 nanograms/ml., she will normally be seriously affected by iron deficiency anemia. Somewhere between 15 and 20 nanograms/ml. can be considered borderline and low. Values between 20 and 30 nanograms/ml. can be interpreted as normal. The average value of 30 elite female distance runners studied by Daniels was 26.8 nanograms/ml. (Daniels, Scardina, Hayes, and Foley, 1986). However, he felt that perhaps this group tested lower than normal and something closer to 30 nanograms/ml. might represent a healthier target value. On the other hand, it might be difficult for some female distance runners to attain a value of 30 nanograms/ml., even when taking iron supplements. Given the undesirable side effects of overdoing iron supplements, athletes should not think a higher value necessarily means that they will be healthier or capable of running faster. As long as female athletes test in the mid 20's and feel fine, then their serum ferritin levels are normally a non-issue (Daniels, 1987-1997).

Iron supplements are available in the form of ferrous gluconate or ferrous sulfate. A normal iron supplement dosage is about 150 milligrams/day, but under a doctor's prescription sometimes several times that amount can be taken. An overdose can lead to stomach cramps, constipation, or diarrhea. It is best to take iron supplements right after meals. Further, iron supplements are best absorbed when taken in conjunction with Vitamin C. Free iron in the body also plays a role in the actions caused by free radicals, thus athletes might be advised to take Vitamin E with iron supplements in order to counter possible undesired side effects (Berglund, 1992). They should avoid any form of caffeine within two hours of taking iron supplements, and this would include many soft drinks.

Athletes in torrid climates tend to encounter iron deficiency anemia more frequently since heavy perspiration tends to flush more iron and electrolytes out of their system. Further, athletes running in hard shoes or on hard surfaces can mechanically destroy more red blood cells than athletes training in well-cushioned shoes, or on natural surfaces (Falsetti, Burke, Feld, Frederick and Ratering, 1983, also Dressendorfer, Wade and Frederick, 1992). Shoes or insoles providing conformance including a cupped shape about the heel can also cause less mechanical trauma—including less damage to red blood cells (Jorgensen and

Ekstrand, 1988). Athletes should keep away from petroleum products, whether airborne or in topical applications because these can sometimes induce another form of anemia.

If an athlete's serum ferritin appears normal, anemia can still be present in one of several forms. To determine the nature and extent of the possible disorder, a physician may study a more comprehensive blood profile. One of the significant values is the hematocrit—that is, the percentage of particles in the blood by volume. The hematocrit is largely composed of RBC's (Red Blood Cells). The normal hematocrit range for women is $42 \pm 5\%$, and for males $47 \pm 7\%$. The RBC count is another important variable because red blood cells transport the hemoglobin that carries most of the body's oxygen to the cells. The normal count for males is approximately 5,400,000, and for females approximately 4,700,000 cells per cubic millimeter (Jacob and Francone, 1974). Changes in the red blood cells' MCV (Mean Corpuscle Volume) can indicate one of several forms of anemia. A physician can also examine the RET count—that is, the reticulocyte or infant red blood cell count. A change in the rate of RBC production can indicate a disorder, or the death of red blood cells due to an infection. A RET value of .5% indicates a slowing down of production, .5-1.5% the normal range, and 1.5% a speeding up of red blood cell production (Jacob and Francone, 1974). Physicians will also often test for hemoglobin, since it carries over 98% of the oxygen transported by the blood. The normal range for women is 12 to 14.5 grams/100 ml., and for males 14 to 16.5 grams/100 ml. (Martin, 1994). Other hemoglobin values include MCH—that is, Mean Corpuscle Hemoglobin by volume and weight.

Iron deficiency anemia is a relatively rare malady experienced by distance runners. Some athletes might then ask: How do you get it? The story of a high school athlete who became so afflicted can perhaps serve as a lesson for others so that they might avoid making the same mistakes. In the fall, the athlete had been successful in state and national cross-country championships. The individual then competed directly in a winter sport without taking a break. Despite being advised against this, neither the athlete nor the athlete's parents heeded the warning. Success and the need for entertainment can be a dangerous intoxicant. In truth, it had been a long, hard season, and the individual needed the break afforded by a period of post-season recovery. At the same time, the athlete was going through a growth spurt, but did not pay close attention to dietary needs. Moreover, the athlete also pursued an active social life. In short, this individual wanted to have it all.

Half way into the spring track and field season the athlete became tired and performance levels dropped. The runner was advised to see a doctor and have a serum ferritin test. The test came back with an abnormally low value. As a result, the athlete was diagnosed as having iron deficiency anemia, and was then provided with iron supplements. Within two weeks the runner was able to improve by ten seconds in the 1,600 meters, and a short while later managed to win the State Championship. However, the athlete's fitness did not approach the level attained six months earlier. The lesson that life often teaches is that you cannot have it all.

In sum, athletes who ignore their bodies and nature can succumb to iron deficiency anemia. Things do not just happen without a cause. Sometimes, when athletes experience health problems, what their body is really telling them is that they have made a mistake and need to take a break. When faced with adversity, if athletes take the opportunity to reevaluate their physical and mental approach, it might prove to be the significant breakthrough that they really need.

This chapter provides some basic information on iron deficiency anemia. Hopefully, athletes will be able to avoid or identify a potential problem early, and be able to ask some of the right questions. A naturopathic doctor or dietitian might say: "A handful of raisins a day, keeps iron deficiency away." However, any number of factors can contribute to an anemic condition, and athletes need expert medical attention whenever that possibility arises. Do not despair. Given proper medical care, most cases of iron deficiency anemia can be easily corrected within a relatively short time.

> *It is on disaster that good fortune perches; It is beneath good fortune that disaster crouches.*
>
> —Lao Tzu

References

Berglund, Bo, "High Altitude Training," *Sports Medicine*, Volume 14, Number 5, 1992, pages 289-303.

Cecil Textbook of Medicine, 20th edition, Philadelphia, Pennsylvania: W.B. Saunders, Co., 1996, pages 1132-1135.

Clement, D.B., and R.C. Asmundson, C.W. Medhurst, "Hemoglobin Values: Comparative Survey of the 1976 Canadian Olympic Team," *Journal of the Canadian Medical Association*, Volume 117, 1977, pages 614-616.

Daniels, Jack, *Conversations on Iron Deficiency Anemia*, 1987-1997.

Daniels, Jack, and Nancy Scardina, John Hayes, Peter Foley, "Elite and Subelite Female Middle- and Long-Distance Runners," *Sport and Elite Performers*, Daniel M. Landers, Editor, Champaign, Illinois: Human Kinetics Publishers, Inc., 1986, pages 57-72.

Dressendorfer, and R.H., C.E. Wade, E.C. Frederick, "Effect of Shoe Cushioning on the Development of Reticulocytosis in Distance Runners," *American Journal of Sports Medicine*, Volume 20, Number 2, 1992, pages 212-216.

Dufaux, B., and A. Hoederrath, I. Streitberg, W. Hollman, G. Assman, "Serum Ferritin, Transferrin, Haptoglobin, and Iron in Middle and Long Distance Runners, Elite Rowers, and Professional Racing Cyclists," *International Journal of Sports Medicine*, Volume 2, 1981, pages 43-46.

Falsetti, H.L., and E.R. Burke, R. Feld, E.C. Frederick, C. Ratering, "Hematological Variations after Endurance Running with Hard and Soft-Soled Running Shoes," *Physician and Sportsmedicine*, Volume 11, Number 8, 1983, pages 118-127.

Jacob, Stanley W., and Clarice A. Francone, *Structure and Function in Man*, 3rd Edition, Philadelphia: W.B. Saunders Company, 1974.

Jorgensen, U., and J. Ekstrand, "Significance of Heel Pad Confinement for the Shock Absorption at Heel Strike," *International Journal of Sports Medicine*, Volume 9, 1988, pages 468-473.

Martin, David E., "The Challenge of Using Altitude to Improve Performance," *NSA by the IAAF*, Volume 9, Number 2, 1994, pages 51-57.

Newhouse, I.J., and D.B. Clement, "Iron Status in Athletes: An Update," *Sports Medicine*, Volume 5, 1988, pages 337-352.

Tzu, Lao, *Tao Te Ching*, Translated by D.L. Lau, Middlesex, England: Penguin Books Ltd., 1963, page 119.

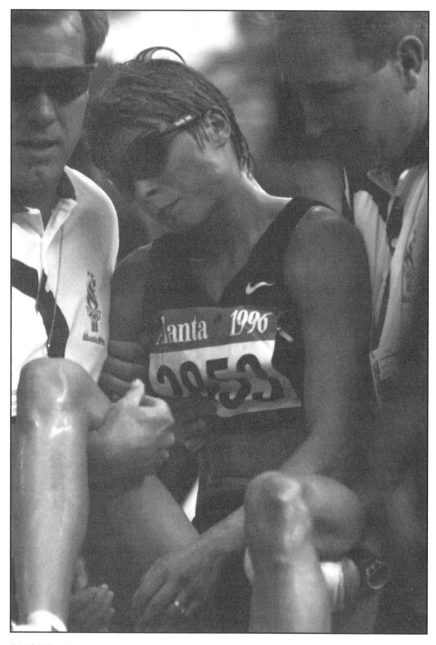

PHOTO 12.1—Anne Marie Lauck of the United States is carried from the track after the women's marathon in Atlanta, 1996 Olympic Games. Photo by Doug Mills, from AP/ Wide World Photos.

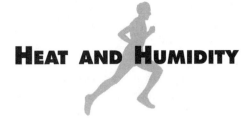

CHAPTER 12

HEAT AND HUMIDITY

Coaches and athletes need to appreciate several things about training and racing in conditions of high heat and humidity. The most important is that it can be dangerous. Training and racing in these conditions can cause heat cramps, heat exhaustion, and heat stroke. Generally, this level of distress does not arise when competing in events up through 1,500 meters, that is, unless it is a case of progressive exhaustion and dehydration over several days, as when conducting prelims, semis and a final. However, an athlete can fail to complete 3,000 meters in hot, humid weather conditions, and the risks are compounded in the longer distance events.

Heat Illness and Medical Emergencies

If an athlete shows signs of weaving about in a race, or otherwise becoming mentally disorientated, a coach is wise to act quickly. Do not wait to see the next lap, instead, pull the athlete off the course immediately. Failure to do so could result in a life-threatening situation. Alternately, the athlete's metabolism could be adversely affected, and the performances planned for the remainder of that athletic season could be compromised. Moreover, the athlete's future tolerance to hot and humid conditions could also become permanently impaired (Shapiro, et al., 1979).

Cool the individual down immediately, and if the available means are limited, first provide for the athlete's thirst, then cool the head, hands, feet and torso, in that order. If you are at a track and field facility and the steeplechase water hazard is filled, then go straightway for a dunk. Perhaps there is a hose available, or a shower facility nearby. Splashing or pouring water from a bottle can help, but this will not bring down elevated core temperatures as rapidly as will immersing the entire body in cool water. Sometimes an athlete can be directed to a cool shaded spot on the ground, and can then be soaked and briefly packed in ice. Obviously, fanning an athlete, or using an air conditioner can help to lower core temperatures, since much heat can be dissipated through respiration. In this regard, an automobile with air conditioning can provide on the spot assistance.

Heat illnesses include heat cramps (that is, muscle spasms induced by dehydration or loss of electrolytes), but also heat exhaustion and heat stroke. Heat cramps do not necessarily precede the onset of the latter two conditions, but with competitive athletes symptoms of heat exhaustion normally appear prior to the onset of heat stroke. Heat exhaustion is often caused by severe dehydration, and the individual will commonly manifest signs of shock. Common symptoms of heat exhaustion and shock therefore include: dizziness, fatigue, headache, faintness, paleness, nausea, vomiting, goosebumps and even chills. Placing something cold on the back of the neck can reduce feelings of nausea and sometimes prevent vomiting. If you can get an athlete to lie down, and then prop up the legs—this can increase the effective blood volume to the vital organs and will often relieve symptoms of shock within 15 minutes. After a long distance race, athletes are generally dehydrated (needing of water), hypoglycemic (needing a simple form of sugar) and in need of both electrolytes and simple proteins.

Our normal core temperature is approximately 98.6° Fahrenheit, which corresponds to 37° Celsius. The core temperature of athletes competing in hot and/or humid conditions can climb to over 104° F (or 40° C), and they would then likely suffer symptoms of heat exhaustion or heat stroke. When the athletes' blood volume is sufficiently reduced due to severe dehydration, they may actually stop sweating, and this can result in a dramatic increase of their core temperature. In cases of heat exhaustion and heat stroke, core temperatures can rise to between 106° and 110° F (or 41.1° and 43.3° C), thus creating a potentially life threatening situation. Symptoms of heat stroke include mental disorientation, confusion, unconsciousness, seizure, and comma. When in doubt, do not delay. Heat stroke is a life-threatening situation that merits an immediate emergency 911 call and treatment by a trained medical professional.

Heat loss can be accomplished by radiation, conduction, convection, and evaporation. By estimate, evaporation can accomplish about 80% of an athlete's heat loss (Costill, 1986). During a marathon, the body produces approximately 2400kJ of heat, and under ideal conditions, a loss of approximately three liters of sweat through evaporation would provide adequate cooling (Newsholme, Leech, and Duester, 1994). However, a change of merely one percent (caused by loss of fluids relative to an individual's body mass) can disturb the body's thermoregulation, largely controlled by the hypothalamus. So the loss of three liters of fluid (or several pounds) by a 150-pound athlete through dehydration during a marathon is more than enough to cause potential problems (Newsholme, Leech, and Duester, 1994).

Perhaps the most difficult and dangerous situation is when athletes compete in conditions of high heat and humidity. For example, when the USATF National Championships are held in locations like Indianapolis or New Orleans, you can expect some casualties in the 5,000 and 10,000 meters. In hot and humid conditions, the athletes' sweat hardly evaporates and only provides a small cooling effect: They can be soaking wet with perspiration and nevertheless suffer heat stroke. Regardless of the environmental conditions, do not suppose that athletes will stop perspiring when afflicted with heat stroke. If an individual becomes disorientated or loses balance, coordination, or consciousness, then presume the situation is life threatening and obtain professional medical attention immediately.

The American College of Sports Medicine issued a position statement concerning distance races in 1975, and suggested that races with a distance of 16k/10 miles or greater should not be conducted when the wet bulb globe temperature exceeds 82.4° F or 28° C (Fox and Mathews, 1981). David Costill has similarly suggested that distance races of 10,000 meters and longer should not be conducted when the wet bulb globe temperature exceeds 82° F (Costill, 1986). This guideline should apply to any event above 1,500 meters, and be adopted as a rule at the high school, collegiate, and national level.

The Acclimatization Process

How can athletes properly prepare for conditions of high heat and humidity? No doubt, it helps if their genealogy can be traced to a location reasonably close to the equator, or to a location having a torrid climate. It is also advantageous if they have had long-term exposure, or prior experience with these climatic conditions in the past. Of course, if the athletes presently train in a similar climate, things are simplified. However, the difficultly comes when a major competition will be held in a location predicted to be hot and humid, and the athletes are not acclimatized to such conditions. Athletes need at least nine to 10 days to acclimatize to hot and/ or humid conditions. However, if athletes put off acclimatization until the last nine to 10 days before the major competition, then the timing of this process will coincide with the nine-to-10-day worthwhile break and ascent to the desired time of peak performance. And with the exception of an under-distance time trial conducted three to five days prior to the competition, the athletes will not be performing hard work during the ascent. This scenario does not provide athletes with much practical experience, or the ability to judge their personal limitations when competing in these conditions.

Moreover, this acclimatization scenario introduces an undesirable stressor— that is, the burden of acclimatization—during the ascent to peak performance and thereby increases the training load at a time when just the opposite outcome is desired. Even with light or moderate training loads between 1/4 to 1/2-effort, recognize that nine to 10 days of acclimatization to heat and humidity will add at least an additional 1/4-effort to the overall equation. So athletes could unwittingly train at between 1/2 and 3/4-effort. This would completely defeat the purpose of the ascent preceding the major competition.

A more prudent course of action would be to include exposure to hot and humid conditions for a period of at least nine to 10 days during part of the sharpening period. The athletes could then carefully perform several of the 3/4-effort sharpening workouts. However, they should get away from hot and humid conditions for at least five to seven days and take care to recharge themselves (e.g., eat and drink properly, swim in cool water and avoid hot baths or saunas). In this way, they will become acclimatized and fully recover from the process. Thereafter, they should travel to the site of the competition and return to hot and humid conditions approximately seven to 10 days before the contest. They will then complete the acclimatization process, but now without undermining their

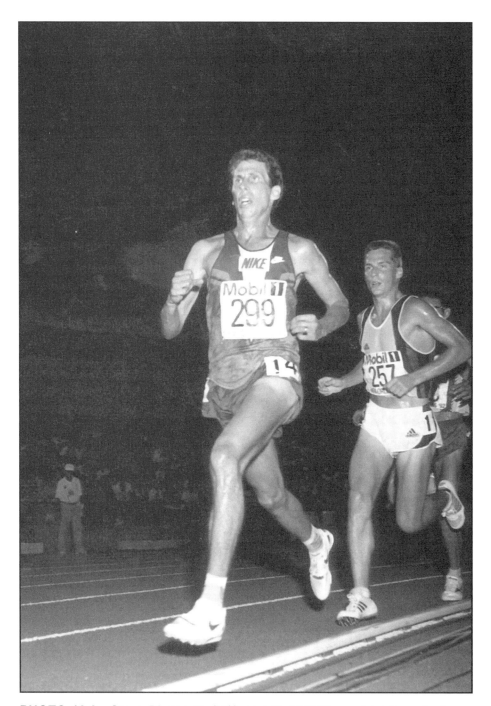

PHOTO 12.2—Steve Plasencia (left) and Todd Williams (right) contest one another, and the heat and humidity in New Orleans during the 10,000 meters at the 1992 Olympic Trials. Photo from Victah Sailer / Photorun.

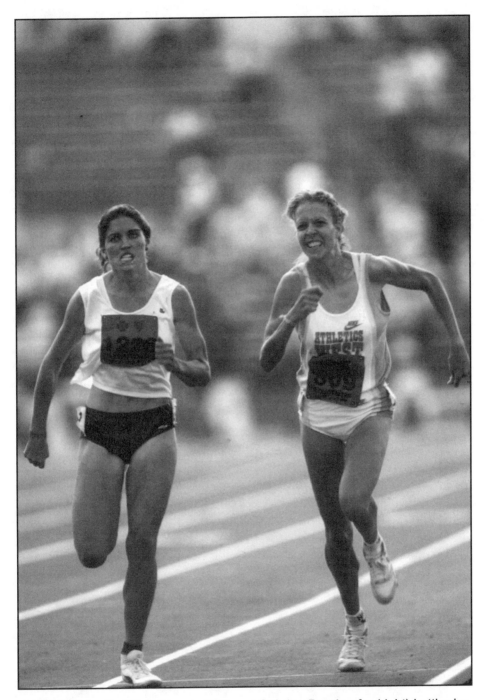

PHOTO 12.3—PattiSue Plumer (left) and Sabrina Dornhoefer (right) battle during the 3,000 meters in Indianapolis at the 1988 U.S. Olympic Trials. Dornhoefer collapsed at the finish line. Photo from Victah Sailer / Photorun.

competitive prospects. The worthwhile break preceding the peak plateau will then be easy, and they will be able to attain peak fitness. Aside from the method just described, unless athletes live in a hot and humid climate or have several months of exposure to these conditions, generally they should not assume a more dramatic acclimatization program, or otherwise flog themselves with heat and humidity training. In the latter case, they would be more likely to hurt, rather than help themselves.

If athletes are going to run the marathon event in a major competition, the only prudent course is to opt for an extended period of exposure to such climatic conditions. Acclimatization can be accomplished in less time, but not sound judgment regarding how various temperature, humidity, sun, cloud, and wind conditions affect their performance. In the marathon, if an athlete's guess is off in one direction or the other by four seconds per mile, it can mean the difference between winning the race or blowing up at 18 miles. And inexperienced athletes will not normally recognize that they are in trouble until it is too late.

There are some general considerations that coaches and athletes should attend to during the preceding period of acclimatization. Since acclimatization is a stressor, athletes should:

- Get more rest
- Drink more fluids
- Eat more carbohydrates in the course of more numerous smaller meals
- Take Vitamin C and a multivitamin with trace minerals supplements—since these can be depleted at a higher rate with more profuse sweating
- Watch for a decrease in body weight
- Monitor urine for color
- Check for an increase in the morning pulse rate
- Take salt incrementally with meals

When, after hard exercise, athletes drink more and more water without the feeling of their thirst being satisfied, this is due to a lack of salt. They should drink cool water at a moderate rate after exercising, and then avoid any diuretics, such as coffee, tea, alcohol, or canned carbonated soft drinks (which can contain the same). Make sure to keep well hydrated in the days prior to a major competition.

During the last few weeks of acclimatization, do not introduce greater stress by wearing sweats during training, or sit in a sauna. These methods, and training during the hottest part of the day, can be used early in the preparation, or as an alternative to direct acclimatization, but do not overdo it. As always in training, introduce the stress of acclimatization gradually over time. An hour or two of exposure each day is all that athletes need. They do not have to train or sleep in an incubator.

Time and Travel

Air travel places additional stress on athletes. For one thing, the cabin pressure on most commercial aircraft corresponds to 5,000 feet of altitude. If athletes are on a plane for the better part of one or two days, their metabolism can shift in the direction of acclimatizing to altitude. The cabin's air also tends to dehydrate passengers and crew. To get better quality air supply, it is advantageous to sit as far forward as possible. Following a plane trip, athletes should treat themselves as if they had been exposed to a hospital ward full of sick patients. Afterwards, as soon as possible, they should run for twenty minutes and take a shower. This will help stimulate their immune system and cleanse the lungs, sinuses, and skin.

Whenever possible, athletes should condition themselves to perform at the appointed hour of the competition. They need to be up and awake at least four hours before a competition. After rising, athletes should jog 15 to 20 minutes, then shower and eat breakfast. Many athletes eat a lighter than normal breakfast three to four hours before a competition. Try eating a normal breakfast sometime prior to a less important event and observe whether you have been cutting yourself short. Often, athletes find themselves a bit too hungry and actually too low on fuel when they eat a lighter than normal breakfast. Accordingly, sometimes it is best not to change your normal breakfast routine.

Travel across time zones presents a lot of other variables, but athletes can speed their recovery from jet lag by sticking to the new timetable on the first day. Light therapy can also be a great help. Athletes would do well to get up bright and early and to turn on every light available, but the quality of hotel lighting might not be sufficient. If possible, get outside for thirty minutes first thing in the morning and face the sun to take best advantage of the sunlight. Alternately, athletes might visit a sun tanning salon and take less than 15 minutes exposure to light therapy. However, make certain that the cooling fan normally provided is blowing, and wear a long sleeved shirt and pants to avoid receiving a sun tan or possible burn.

Heat, Humidity and Athletic Performance

When athletes are exposed to conditions of high heat and humidity their bodies will at first be a bit out of sorts. To provide for adequate cooling, blood must be diverted from working muscles to their skin. This decreases the oxygen available to the athlete's working muscles for performance, and thus effectively lowers their aerobic ability and anaerobic threshold. With acclimatization to heat and humidity: vasodilatation and cooling become much more efficient, the sweat response is faster and more robust, and blood plasma volume will increase. Athletes will then be able to perform well, but with diminished work capacity. Adverse climatic conditions always provide an opportunity, for those who know how to handle themselves correctly, to move up a bit relative to more talented athletes who do not.

Coaches and athletes also need to appreciate how much conditions of high temperature and humidity affect athletic performance at various competitive distances. To make an accurate estimate, you should always research the history of past athletic performances in similar conditions at the competition site. However, the following guidelines are provided for national caliber athletes competing at sea level in conditions equal to or greater than 70° F in combination with 70% humidity:

- There is no penalty to pay in events under 400 meters, and perhaps there is actually some advantage.
- In a single open 800 meters, the net effect is about zero, but with numerous preliminary heats, the practical effect will likely be a deficit of about two seconds.
- In the 1,500 meters, such conditions are worth a deficit of about four seconds.
- In the 3,000 meters, the deficit is about eight to 10 seconds.
- In the 5,000 meters, the deficit is about 20 seconds.
- In the 10,000 meters, the deficit is in the range of 60 to 80 seconds.
- In the marathon, the deficit is in the range of four to six minutes.

These guidelines are conservative and presume that athletes have acclimatized and prepared properly. Note that the deficits increase geometrically in relation to distance. Circumstances alter races, thus athletes should always reassess environmental conditions immediately prior to, and during the course of a competition.

Conduct on the Day of Competition

In conditions of high heat and humidity, athletes need to conduct themselves prudently on the day of competition. Consider taking the following positive steps: stay out of the heat and away from the sporting arena as long as possible; bring shade such as a light colored tent or umbrella; bring more ice water than needed and plan to sip a pint every fifteen minutes; bring several bags of ice in a cooler; locate a nearby shower facility; and, bring light colored clothing. Once exposed to the stressful environmental conditions, it is hardly possible to keep up with the need for rehydration. At the same time, beware of overdrinking out of nervousness, since you would then be constantly running to the bathroom and triggering an alarm reaction that would further tax your endocrine system.

As opposed to a conventional warm-up, athletes can actually benefit from a cool-down, completed about 30 minutes before the major contest. Despite their best efforts to minimize exposure on the day of competition, athletes will likely face the undesirable climatic conditions for several hours—that is, given the logistics associated with travel to the site, check-in, and so on. That being the case, whenever possible, they are well advised to take a cool, but not cold, shower as close as possible to race time, while still allowing adequate time to conduct a brief warm up. This will go a long way to rehydrate and freshen-up athletes for the coming event. Generally, in hot and humid climate conditions, a proper warm-up requires less than 30 minutes.

Normally, athletes should avoid electrolyte fluid replacement drinks during competition unless they have prior experience and control over the contents of the drink. Further, most commercially available electrolyte drinks need to be greatly diluted to be suitable for runners. Otherwise, the drink may later end up on their racing shoes and the pavement. The use of electrolyte fluid replacement drinks can be advantageous during the process of acclimatization and in the days prior to a major event, but on race day the prudent advice is—go with water. However, if the athletes will be competing in an ultra-distance event in torrid conditions, then they clearly need to perfect the contents of their electrolyte drink in the months prior to the competition.

In conditions of heat and humidity, do not be fooled by cloud cover, because it does not substantially reduce the need for hydration. And beware of prevailing winds in the presence of high temperatures since they can cause more rapid dehydration. Also, the energy lost when struggling against a headwind is not fully compensated for by a tailwind. Moreover, recognize that a headwind has an increased cooling effect, whereas a tailwind decreases the cooling effect.

Proper Equipment

The racing singlet should be white, and include relatively fine open mesh panels on the lower front, sides and back. The material should neither retain sweat so as to become heavy and sag, nor be incapable of saturation. Instead, a happy medium needs to be struck. Sometimes a light natural cotton fiber works well. Beware of many synthetic materials, and always first test a singlet under the conditions you expect to encounter. Many of the new so-called high technology synthetic fibers, which are supposed to breathe and do other sophisticated things, do not perform well in practical application. Let the buyer beware. Do not believe what you are told. Take the singlet with the wonder material and soak it in the sink, then check its weight when wet. Put it on and go for a run to see how long it takes to dry, and how it actually behaves on your body. Use the singlet in hot and humid conditions to be certain what it will do. Believe what you see, and what you know to be true after experimentation.

Athletic shorts should also be light colored, but not white, out of considerations of modesty, since they will likely become soaked and somewhat transparent. Make certain that the waistband is not too tight because this can restrict full respiration. Another restriction in the modern design of male athletic shorts is their inner liner, which functions much like an athletic support, not permitting the male private parts to be suspended in a natural manner. While good from the standpoint of modesty, this restriction can reduce heat dissipation. Further, abnormally high or low temperatures in this region can send the wrong message to the hypothalamus and trigger inappropriate physiological responses affecting temperature regulation. So, while not advising exhibitionism, male athletes might want to reconsider the extremely short, tight athletic shorts with restrictive inner liners that are most prevalent at the present time. Only in the last twenty-five years have athletic shorts with this kind of configuration become popular. The author's attempt to address these problems can be found in several granted utility patents (U.S. 6,243,879, U.S. 6,243,880, and U.S. 6,353,940).

Proper socks are a critical piece of equipment, especially when competing in the marathon. Thin socks with favorable qualities *vis-à-vis* heat dissipation and abrasion are best. The choice depends somewhat on the nature of the insole, but also the inside of the shoe upper. Figure out the shoe and sock combination well in advance and then have two spares of each available.

Many road racing shoes made at the present time have relatively thick, unbreathable uppers. To improve breathability, you can cut out portions of the sides, and punch holes in the central area of the forefoot of the shoe upper. Strip out the foam backing in the tongue, and replace the laces with water resistant ones. However, take care not to weaken the support structure of the shoe, or to do anything that will cause blisters. The spring stiffness and dampening performed by the soles of various footwear (and their thermal conductivity) are not all the same. Further, realize that dampening generates heat. Some light-weight shoes actually have foam midsoles that are too soft for many athletes. Such shoes may be light and provide good protection from shock loading, but can provide too soft a spring for effecting optimal performance. And high temperatures will tend to render the cushioning materials even softer. Efficiency is important in all distance events, but it is absolutely critical in the marathon.

Once again, how much do the athlete's racing shoes weigh? In this regard, you may wish to review Chapter 10, which discusses the effect of shoe weight and mechanical efficiency on athletic performance. Consider how conditions of high heat and humidity could influence the performance of athletic footwear. Whenever in doubt, *always* conduct a prior evaluation. Consider the worst-case scenario. If it rains, does the outsole afford good traction? In this regard, much is determined by the design and wettability characteristics of the outsole. Does the shoe or sock soak up moisture and then become much heavier? Does the shoe become too hot with prolonged running? Assume nothing and conduct appropriate experiments to find out what you need to know. Again, at least three months before a major competition, the athlete needs to select and start training in the correct shoe.

The human head can provide a major source of heat loss. A hat worn to shade dark hair from the sun must be of a kind that will not appreciably reduce heat loss. And unless athletes will be staring into the sun, they should avoid using sunglasses. Fashionable sunglasses have become popular with some elite athletes, since they are being compensated for wearing the products. While this may make some athletes *look* cool, it does not help them to *stay* cool. After athletes have completed a hard run, the area about their eyes will often appear to glow red. Accordingly, it is unwise to shield this area and reduce its ability to radiate and dissipate heat. The hands and feet can also provide substantial heat loss, thus cooling these areas as much as possible during a race can also positively influence an athlete's performance.

Race Conduct

Athletes should be conservative in the early pacing under conditions of high heat and humidity. They should treat the situation much as though they were running at altitude, or had suffered from a slight illness in the week prior to the competition. Since climate conditions then effectively diminish their aerobic ability and anaerobic threshold, athletes should not only be conservative in their energy use

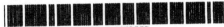

(12) **United States Design Patent** (10) **Patent No.:**   **US D467,055 S**

Lyden   (45) **Date of Patent:**   ** **Dec. 17, 2002**

(54) **ATHLETIC SHORTS**

(76) Inventor: **Robert M. Lyden**, 18261 SW. Fallatin Loop, Aloha, OR (US) 97007

(**) Term: **14 Years**

(21) Appl. No.: **29/144,574**

(22) Filed: **Jul. 6, 2001**

Related U.S. Application Data

(63) Continuation-in-part of application No. 29/116,513, filed on Dec. 29, 1999.

(51) **LOC (7) Cl.** **02-02**
(52) **U.S. Cl.** **D2/738**
(58) **Field of Search** D2/711–713, 731–732, D2/738, 742, 745; 2/400–408, 228, 236–238, 78.1, 78.2, 78.3, 76, 109, 110

(56) **References Cited**

U.S. PATENT DOCUMENTS

620,435 A	2/1899	Fisher
763,683 A	6/1904	Magoris 450/100
1,212,805 A	1/1917	Newman .... 2/401 X
1,277,839 A	9/1918	Birkenfeld 2/408
1,288,673 A	12/1918	Potterf .... 2/400 X
1,662,981 A	3/1928	Pazowski
1,737,882 A	12/1929	Hatch 2/237
1,861,383 A	5/1932	Ficcio
1,998,140 A	4/1935	Loew 2/403
D98,867 S	3/1936	Lee D2/716
2,034,312 A	3/1936	Rubin 2/228
2,128,876 A	8/1938	Boysen 2/237
2,216,897 A	10/1940	Zoob .... D2/712 X
2,232,246 A	2/1941	Klein 128/159
2,401,457 A	6/1946	Bryant 2/406
2,408,723 A	10/1946	Arpin et al. 2/224
2,411,922 A	12/1946	Keohane 2/82
2,419,867 A	4/1947	Woodman 2/224
2,623,210 A	12/1952	Chatfield 2/41

(List continued on next page.)

FOREIGN PATENT DOCUMENTS

CH	664878	4/1988	....	2/400
WO	89/07896	9/1989	....	2/403

OTHER PUBLICATIONS

US 5,915,536, 6/1999, Alberts et al. (withdrawn)
Allsop/Sims Vibration no date.
Calvin Klein Sport Brief Package, nd.
Seaquest Catalogue, nd.
Boxer Style Shorts, #8, p. 539, Sears Spring/Summer 1978 Catalog.
Internet printouts showing trunks worn by Muhammad Ali prio to Dec. 11, 1981 and Dec. 11, 1981, Nos. 7275–5 and 5709–9, publication date Dec. 11, 1981.

Primary Examiner—Louis S. Zarfas
Assistant Examiner—Robert A Delehanty
(74) *Attorney, Agent, or Firm*—Westman, Champlin & Kelly, P.A.

(57)   **CLAIM**

The design for athletic shorts, as shown and described.

DESCRIPTION

FIG. **1** is a front view of athletic shorts embodying my new design;
FIG. **2** is a right side view thereof, the left side being a mirror image of the right side view;
FIG. **3** is a rear view thereof;
FIG. **4** is a top view thereof; and,
FIG. **5** is a bottom view thereof.
The broken lines showing of interior environmental structure of the shorts in FIGS. **4** and **5** of the drawing views form no part of the claimed design.
The crosshatch shading shown in the drawings is understood to indicate fabric.
The area of the waistband including vertical lines indicates the inclusion of elastic material, and the area of the waistband devoid of vertical lines indicates the inclusion of non-elastic material.

1 Claim, 3 Drawing Sheets

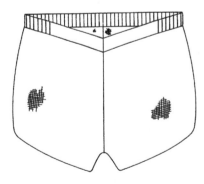

FIGURE 12.1—U.S. Design Patent 467,055

early on, but also as the race progresses. For example, an athlete would not be well advised to attempt numerous attacks in the form of surges or breakaways, but rather to make one decisive move when the opponents are vulnerable.

Recovery from Competition

Immediately after a race, athletes should drink cool, but not cold water. After hard exercise, it is normally not good to shock the overheated body with ice water. Accordingly, unless they suffer from heat exhaustion or heat stroke and face a medical emergency, athletes should not gulp down ice water or jump into cold water immediately after a workout or race. After taking some water, they should consume a citrus juice that includes a simple sugar such as pineapple-grapefruit juice, or a commercially available electrolyte and energy replacement drink. Athletes should then conduct a brief cool down lasting five to ten minutes, and finish by stretching while still warm. At that point, a cool shower or dip in a pool will do no harm.

If a meal is over an hour away, athletes should consume some additional carbohydrates with a high glycemic index such as glucose, fructose, honey, or bread, but then follow up with carbohydrates having a moderate glycemic index. A natural yogurt culture with fruit can sometimes help replace bacteria killed by high core temperatures, and also provide needed carbohydrates and protein. Generally, athletes find they can better digest smaller, more frequent meals in hot and humid conditions.

Upon arrival at a hotel, athletes should maintain the room at a moderate temperature, and perhaps cool it down over the period of an hour. Later in the evening, it may be possible to take an easy swim. Before going to bed, it is advisable to sit in a bathtub with several bags of ice packed above and below each leg. Despite any initial discomfort, packing the quads, hamstrings, and calves for 20 minutes in this manner will dramatically accelerate recovery. This procedure should be observed in the evening following competition whenever qualifying rounds are being undertaken.

When all is said and done, preparation for heat, humidity, and travel is just another training task. Athletes should not attach too much to the task, since that can disturb proper focus. Do not make it out to be more than what it is. Simply do what has to be done to prepare, and then forget about it. If worrisome thoughts should arise such as, "I wonder if I drank enough"—well, simply check to see that you have, and if so, do not further attach to the thought. Rather, simply let it go. Stay in the NOW.

> *When I look back on all these worries, I remember the story of the old man who said... that he had a lot of issues in his life, most of which never happened.*
>
> —Winston Churchill

References

Åstrand, Per Olaf, and Kaare Rodahl, *Textbook of Work Physiology*, Third Edition, New: York: McGraw-Hill Book Company, 1986.

Costill, David L., *Inside Running: Basics of Sports Physiology*, Carmel, Indiana: Cooper Publishing Group, LLC, 1986.

Costill, David L., *A Scientific Approach to Distance Running*, Los Altos, California: Tafnews Press, 1981.

Costill, David L., and W.F. Kammer, A. Fisher, "Fluid Injestion During Distance Running," *Arch Environmental Health*, 1970, 21, pages 520-525.

Daniels, Jack, *Daniel's Running Formula*, Champaign, Illinois: Human Kinetics, 1998.

Daniels, Jack, and Jimmy Gilbert, *Oxygen Power*, Tempe, Arizona: Published Privately, 1979.

Fox, Edward, and Donald Mathews, *The Physiological Basis of Physical Education and Athletics*, Third Edition, New York: Saunders College Publishing, 1981.

Gisolfi, C.V., Editor, "Symposium of the Thermal Effects of Exercise in the Heat," *Medicine and Science in Sports*, Volume 1, Number 1, 1979, pages 30-71.

Gisolfi, C.V., and J. Cohen, "Relationships Among Training, Heat Acclimatization and Heat Tolerance in Men and Women: The Controversy Revisited," *Medicine and Science in Sports*, 1979, 11, pages 56-59.

Hanson, P.G., "Heat Injury in Runners," *Physician Sportsmedicine*, Volume 7, Number 6, 1979, pages 91-96.

Humes, James C., *The Wit & Wisdom of Winston Churchill*, Forward by Richard M. Nixon, New York: HarperCollins Publishers, 1995.

Janssen, Peter G.J.M., *Training Lactate Pulse-Rate*, Oulu, Finland: Polar Electro Oy, 1987.

Lyden, Robert, U.S. Patent 6,243,879, *Anatomical and Shock Absorbing Athletic Pants*, 2001.

Lyden, Robert, U.S. Patent 6,243,880, *Athletic Shorts*, 2001.

Lyden, Robert, U.S. Patent 6,353,940, *Underwear*, 2002.

Lyden, Robert, U.S. Patent D467,055, *Athletic Shorts*, 2002.

Minard, D. "Prevention of Heat Casualties in Marine Corps Recruits," *Military Medicine*, Volume 126, 1961, pages 261-265.

Newsholme, Eric, and Tony Leech, Glenda Duester, *Keep On Running*, Chichester, England: John Wiley & Sons, Ltd., 1994.

Pandolf, K.B., and R.L. Burse, R. F. Goldman. "Role of Physical Fitness in Heat Acclimatization, Decay and Reinduction," *Ergonomics*, Volume 20, 1977, pages 399-408.

Piwonka, R.W., and S. Robinson, V.L. Gay, R.S. Manalis. "Preacclimatization of Men to Heat by Training," *Journal of Applied Physiology*, Volume 20, 1965, pages 379-384.

Saltin, B., and J. Stenberg, "Circulatory Responses to Prolonged Severe Exercise," *Journal of Applied Physiology*, Volume 19, 1964, pages 833-838.

Shapiro, Y., and A. Magazanik, R. Vdassin, G.M. Ben-Baruch, E. Shvartz, Y. Shoenfeld, "Heat Intolerance in Former Heatstroke Patients," *Annals of Internal Medicine*, Volume 90, Number 6, 1979, pages 913-96.

Walnum, Paul K., A.T.C., "Heat Illness and the Runner," *Track and Field Quarterly Review*, Volume 89, Number 2, 1989, pages 37-39.

Wyndham, C.H., and N.B. Strydom. "The Danger of Inadequate Water Intake During Marathon Running," *South African Medical Journal*, Volume 43, 1969, pages 893-896.

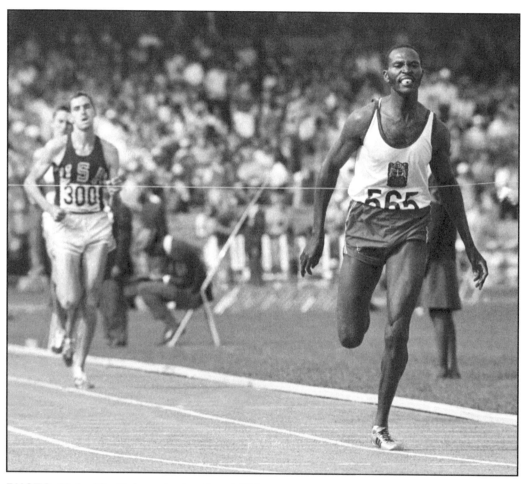

PHOTO 13.1—Kip Keino winning the 1,500 meters, 1968 Olympic Games. Photo by E.D. Lacey, from George Herringshaw & sporting-heroes.net.

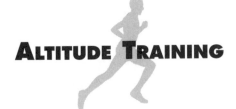

CHAPTER 13

ALTITUDE TRAINING

Altitude training first became a pressing topic of interest in track and field in connection with the 1968 Olympic games. Mexico City is at an altitude of 7,400 feet, and has a barometric pressure of only 580 mm of mercury, compared to 760 mm of mercury at sea level (Sparks and Bjorklund, 1984). This decrease of in ambient air pressure (approximately 23.5%) also meant a corresponding drop in air density. The lower air density reduced aerodynamic drag and provided a 1.7% improvement of performances in the sprint events (Ward-Smith, 1984). Certainly, the decrease in air density also aided performances in the jumping events: Bob Beamon's World Record in the long jump stood for over 20 years. Italy's Pietro Mennea's World Record at 200 meters was also set in Mexico City, and lasted from 1979 to 1996. However, the lower air pressure and density adversely affected performances in predominantly aerobic events. Performances in the 1,500 meters decreased by about three percent, or seven seconds. In the 5,000 meters, they suffered by about eight percent, or one minute. And in the 10,000 meters, they suffered by eight percent, or 2:30 (Sparks and Bjorklund, 1984). Athletes who were born, raised, and trained at altitude, such as Kip Keino of Kenya, had a substantial advantage, as did athletes who had acclimatized for performance at altitude.

Race Distance	Performance at Sea Level	Performance With 3% Altitude Adjustment
Men's 1,500m	3:40.5	3:46.6
Women's 1,500m	4:18.5	4:26.2
Men's 3,000m SC	8:42.0	8:57.6
Women's 3,000m SC	10:38.0	10:57.1
Men's 5,000m	13:47.0	14:11.8
Women's 5,000m	16:05.0	16:33.9
Men's 10,000m	28:50.0	29:41.9
Women's 10,000m	33:20.0	34:20.0

TABLE 13.1—2000 USATF Outdoor Qualifying Standards

Athletic Performance and Altitude

Coaches and athletes need to know how much altitude will affect performance in any given event. Table 13.1 provides the 2000 USATF outdoor qualifying standards, including a 3% allowance for events of 1,500 meters or longer, when contested in a facility at 4,000 feet or more. In addition, see Table 13.2 and Figure 13.1, which were created by Jack Daniels (Daniels, 1975, and 1979). Daniels is one of the most knowledgeable individuals in the United States on this subject, and an excellent coach. If you have a question about some aspect of altitude training not addressed in this chapter, the author suggests that you contact him through Cortland State University in the State of New York.

Race Tactics and Altitude

When runners compete at altitude, as in conditions of high heat and humidity, their aerobic ability and anaerobic threshold will be effectively decreased. A correct initial determination of race pace is therefore essential. Runners are wise to begin conservatively and to maintain an even pace they can sustain. Often, athletes who have done their homework will hang well behind in the first quarter of the race and not get into the thick of things until the third quarter. But at that point, they will pass numerous casualties who have misjudged their fitness and the conditions. Runners should not engage in numerous surge and breakaway attempts. They should take advantage of drafting the lead runners or pack, and then make a decisive move when the opportune moment arrives—or quickly cover the move of a competitor, and then finish with a well timed kick.

Athletic Performance and Moderate Altitude

Coaches and athletes often make the mistake of presuming that the altitude effect is not present when they travel to competitions at moderate altitude, such as three thousand feet above sea level. This is a grave mistake. It is there and athletes had better respect it.

Acclimatizing in Order to Compete Successfully at Altitude

Coaches and athletes need to know a few basic things about acclimatizing in order to race successfully at altitude. Several prescriptions are provided below to address the most probable scenarios coaches and athletes might encounter:

Scenario 1: Same or Next Day Competition at Altitude

If you face the prospect of having to travel to altitude and race without a period of acclimatization, then travel to the site as close to the time of competition as possible. If an overnight stay is necessary prior to a morning competition, then leave late on the day before. Eat lightly that evening and the next morning. Use as little energy as possible in order to maintain a slow metabolic rate. Do not conduct a long warm-up or go out fast in the race, but rather be conservative in the early going (Dales, 1997). This can apply to many other collegiate and professional sports. The athlete should fly into altitude either the night before or the day of the contest and compete directly—that is, if it is not possible to allow for at least five, and preferably nine to 10 days of acclimatization.

Race Duration Sea Level	Altitude 1,000 m (3280 ')	Altitude 1,500 m (4921 ')	Altitude 2,000 m (6561')	Altitude 2,250 m (7382')	Altitude 2,500 m (8202')
3 min	0:00.2	0:01.0	0:01.4	0:02.5	0:04.0
4 min	0:00.5	0:01.8	0:02.4	0:04.1	0:05.8
5 min	0:00.7	0:02.4	0:03.6	0:07.2	0:09.0
6 min	0:01.0	0:03.3	0:05.0	0:09.0	0:12.2
8 min	0:01.8	0:05.5	0:09.6	0:15.4	0:20.1
10 min	0:02.7	0:07.9	0:14.4	0:21.8	0:28.1
12 min	0:04.0	0:10.8	0:19.4	0:28.2	0:36.1
14 min	0:05.5	0:13.8	0:24.6	0:34.6	0:44.1
16 min	0:07.0	0:16.8	0:29.8	0:41.0	0:52.1
18 min	0:08.5	0:19.8	0:35.1	0:47.5	1:00.2
20 min	0:10.0	0:22.8	0:40.8	0:54.0	1:08.4
25 min	0:15.0	0:32.0	0:56.3	1:13.5	1:30.0
30 min	0:20.2	0:41.5	1:12.9	1:32.0	1:52.0
35 min	0:25.8	0:51.7	1:29.2	1:51.5	2:15.0
40 min	0:32.2	1:03.6	1:46.1	2:12.0	2:40.0
50 min	0:45.0	1:27.0	2:22.5	2:52.5	3:28.0
60 min	1:00.0	1:52.0	3:00.0	3:36.0	4:17.0
1.5 hr	1:45.0	3:10.0	5:00.0	5:47.0	6:50.0
2.0 hr	2:30.0	4:30.0	7:00.0	8:00.0	9:30.0
2.5 hr	3:30.0	6:00.0	9:10.0	10:30.0	12:15.0
3.0 hr	4:30.0	7:30.0	11:20.0	13:00.0	15:00.0

The table has been calculated for acclimatized athletes and the values provided should be added to the relevant sea level performances. Note: Unacclimatized athletes might lose up to twice the projected correction for altitude depending on the pace, terrain, and conduct of the competition.

TABLE 13.2—Adapted from Daniels, 1975

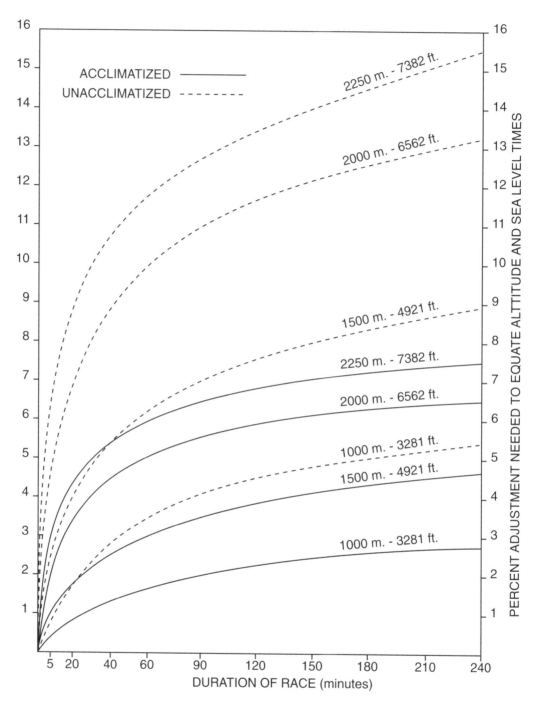

FIGURE 13.1—Adapted from Daniels, 1979

Scenario 2: When at Least 9-10 Days Are Available to Acclimatize

If a more extended period of acclimatization is possible, athletes should allow at least nine to 10 days to adjust. The acclimatization process does not advance to a substantial degree in the first 24 hours so as to dramatically compromise their working capacity. If athletes want a taste of what they will feel like when racing at altitude, then the first day is the time to do it. From purely a physiological standpoint, the athletes would not be well advised to conduct a workout or time trial at more than 1/2-effort in the first or second day, since a hard effort in the early days of exposure to altitude can cause an exercise-induced decrease in erythropoeitin and other adverse reactions that can hinder the acclimatization process (Berglund, 1992). However, if the athletes exert a hard effort anyway, much more can be gained in the domain of cognitive learning and mental callusing—and these will have a greater positive affect upon later performance at altitude. In particular, inexperienced athletes need to use the first or second day to find out how difficult racing at altitude will be (Daniels, 1984-1997). The altitude will impair their working capacity, but their metabolism will not yet be out of kilter from the changes soon to take place during the acclimatization process. Remember that normal cabin pressure in air travel effectively exposes athletes to the equivalent of about 5,000 feet of altitude. So athletes should start counting hours of exposure the minute the aircraft leaves the ground.

In an extended period of altitude acclimatization, the athlete's performance capability will most dramatically suffer between the first 24 through 72 hours of exposure. Thereafter, they will progressively improve as acclimatization continues through the ninth to 10th day. The morning pulse can be a good indicator of their progress. Figure 13.2 shows a typical heart rate response over the days of acclimatization.

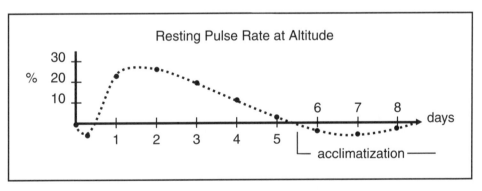

FIGURE 13.2—from Berghold, 1982

Scenario 3: When at Least Two Periods of Exposure to Altitude are Possible

Just as when acclimatizing to heat and humidity, athletes need to consider the increased workload imposed by altitude. Prior to a major competition at altitude, it is prudent to begin the acclimatization process prior to the nine-to-10-day worthwhile break leading to the seasonal peak performance. During this time, athletes normally decrease their training loads to less than 60% of their working capacity, and acclimatization would add at least 25% to the equation. Just as with heat and humidity, the additional training load imposed by acclimatization at this time would compromise the worthwhile break and suppress the ascent to peak performance. Instead, athletes should first acclimatize to altitude over a period of least nine to 10 days, then get away from altitude for not more than two to three weeks (so as not to lose substantial acclimatization), then return to altitude nine to 10 days prior to the competition. This way, the second period of exposure will not impose so substantial a workload on the athletes or suppress their potential performance.

Scenario 4: When an Extended Stay at Altitude is Possible

Athletes might seek to more fully acclimatize and compete at altitude, or to enhance their performance potential at sea level by exposure to altitude. In this case, a more lengthy stay at altitude is necessary. When athletes move from sea level to an altitude of 2,500 meters, then about 12 weeks of exposure to altitude is enough to fully acclimatize. Hemoglobin levels in athletes are commonly 50% higher than in sedentary individuals, but hemoglobin differences for individuals living at 2,500 meters are normally about 12% higher than those living at sea level, and athletes only gain about 1% for each week of exposure to altitude (Berglund, 1992).

J. A. Faulkner suggested an innovative training method (Faulkner, 1966), and Jack Daniels and Neil Oldridge subsequently proved it: athletes can enhance training by alternating two to three weeks of exposure to altitude with a week of training at sea level over an extended period of time (Daniels and Oldridge, 1970). Athletes can then conduct quality anaerobic work and performances at sea level and maintain a balanced training program. In fact, this can be an ideal way for distance runners to train. Flagstaff, Arizona, and Lake Tahoe, California, both provide athletes with the ability to train at altitude and yet escape from it periodically in less than two hours of driving time (Daniels, 1984 -1997). Further, the practice suggested by Daniels and Oldridge of alternating exposures to altitude and sea level would also tend to avoid training habituation and resulting stagnation. However, keep in mind that the harder the athletes train at altitude, the sooner they will need a worthwhile break.

Starting in the 1960's, many athletes began to use altitude training not only to compete to good effect at altitude, but also to aid their performances at sea level. To understand the principles behind this method, we need to look briefly into the physiology of acclimatization to altitude.

The 23.5% decrease in air density at 7,400 feet of altitude in Mexico City basically means that a liter of air has 23.5% fewer molecules of all the gases normally contained in ambient air. The same ratio of oxygen is still present, but there is 23.5% less of it, as well as the other gases, because of the reduced atmospheric pressure. The concentration of oxygen relative to the other atmospheric gases does not significantly decline until the elevation exceeds 10,000 feet.

In supercharging an automobile, the gas mixture injected into the combustion chamber is commonly pressurized between one to five psi—thus more molecules of fuel are packed into the confines of the combustion chamber prior to ignition. This illustrates what happens when athletes puff their cheeks and purse their lips while exhaling—they are placing backpressure on their lungs and performing the work of a supercharger.

At altitude, because there is less oxygen in each breath of air, athletes initially make up the difference by breathing more frequently. In fact, they will tend to hyperventilate, and this can lead to dizziness and nausea. Hyperventilation or a higher respiratory rate will expel higher than normal amounts of carbon dioxide, and this influences the acid-base balance of the body. The blood then becomes more alkaline, that is, it has a higher pH. Over time, this can reduce their ability to perform and use anaerobic power.

Altitude training can negatively impact preparation for the sprint events up through 800 meters, since these events primarily use anaerobic metabolism. Training at altitude can also compromise an athlete's ability to conduct quality-sharpening work in the longer distance events. This potential liability can be dealt with given the following training practices: maintain the desired goal pace when conducting shorter interval workouts at altitude, but simply take longer than normal recoveries. When running longer repetitions, shorten their length relative to sea level, and also provide extended recovery periods.

Altitude training also dehydrates athletes, but somewhat imperceptibly, since the air is much drier at higher elevations. Athletes will need to make doubly sure they are sufficiently hydrated, because they may not have the usual cue of profuse sweating to indicate the amount of dehydration. The most dramatic effect of altitude training is that it stimulates the production of more red blood cells, hemoglobin, and myoglobin, thus increasing the oxygen-carrying capacity of the blood and working muscles. Given a lengthy exposure to altitude, the number of mitochondria and capillaries present in muscle tissue will also increase.

Clearly, altitude training is not a bed of roses. The time, energy, expense and logistics of travel and dislocation must be considered. And there is something to be said about Percy Cerutty's criticism of altitude training. He found that there can be as much or more to gain by learning to breathe more deeply and fully as there is by going to altitude (Cerutty, 1970's). The pulmonary function of elite distance runners is greater than that of the average population (Martin, May, Pilbeam, 1986).

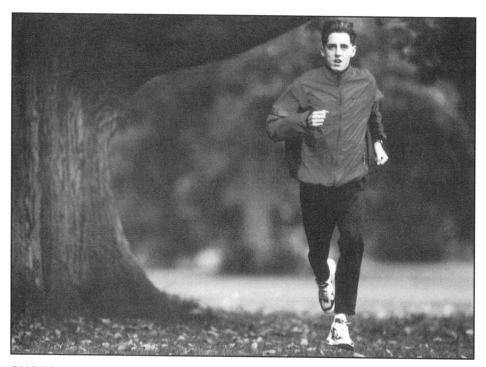

PHOTO 13.2—Karl Keska running in his native England. Photo courtesy of Karl Keska.

Nevertheless, in studying the careers of successful distance runners, altitude training clearly stands out as an important factor. It is a tool that can help athletes progress to the next level. And once they have attained a new level, their acquired performance potential does not evaporate if they decide to move away from altitude. True, they will lose the extra edge provided by additional hemoglobin and red blood cells, but not their fundamental performance capability. Steve Plasencia, a nationally ranked distance runner in the United States for over a decade, moved from Minnesota after college to live and train in Eugene, Oregon (419 feet). However, he would often conduct altitude training in Flagstaff, Arizona (7,000 feet) or Boulder, Colorado (5,400 feet) prior to a major national or international competition. Karl Keska, a graduate of the University of Oregon, also used a well-timed exposure to altitude in Boulder, Colorado prior to delivering his personal best performance for 10,000 meters at the 2000 Olympic games.

Racing at Sea Level After Descending from Altitude

Distance runners should come down from altitude and compete in the main event within the first three days of exposure to sea level. Athletes can race well on days one to three, but day four can be questionable, and by day five their performance will invariably suffer (Koch, 1999). Daniels relates that Jim Ryun descended from altitude and set the world record in the mile the next day (Daniels, 1984 -1997). Elite athletes in the long distance events sometimes feel that several days of exposure to sea level helps to re-adjust their respiratory rate. It may be an advantage to first conduct the under-distance time trial that is used to set up the athletes for a competition three to four days prior to the main event, and then descend to sea level and compete in the main event within a three-day period. Alternately, national and world-class athletes can descend and time trial at sea level approximately 72 hours prior to the main event.

Descending from Altitude When Acclimatizing to Heat, Humidity, or Time Change

Timing can be critical when athletes need to descend from altitude at an early date to prepare for a major competition at sea level. This is sometimes necessary when athletes train at altitude in relatively cool and dry conditions, but must acclimatize for competition in hot or humid conditions. Sometimes this is also necessary when they must travel extensively and adapt to a change in time zones. Research and practical experience suggest that upon descending from altitude, athletes will enjoy a favorable period of performance during the first three or four days. Then their performance capability regresses markedly until about the ninth or 10th day. Thereafter, their fitness will improve and can reach a second optimal period for performance between the 18th and 22nd day. Their fitness level will then gradually decline (Suslov, 1994, and Popov, 1994). This is the common perception of athletes who train at altitude and frequently race at sea level. Many variables could account for these findings. To understand which physiological changes are responsible, more controlled research studies need to be done.

The common perception is that the first window of opportunity, between days one and three, is superior to the second, between the 18th and 22nd day. But the latter option is best when athletes must also acclimatize to heat and humidity. Athletes might then consider the following: It can be advantageous to descend from altitude during the early part of the worthwhile break in the middle of the sharpening period. This places the move from altitude to sea level during a week of low training loads and enables them to compete at sea level in the scheduled weekend competition. They could then remain at sea level for the second seven-to-10-day work meso-cycle of the sharpening period and conduct the last two or three 3/4-effort sharpening sessions, which normally comprise repetition work-outs. They could recover from the last repetition workout over four to six days, then conduct an under-distance time trial or race three to four days before the major competition.

Altitude and the Advent of Artificial Performance Aids

It did not take long for those interested in exercise physiology to figure out that they could collect an athlete's red blood cells, plasma, or whole blood, and then preserve it for re-infusion at a later date. Shortly before a major competition, a portion of the blood would then be re-infused, and the athlete's performance could be considerably enhanced (Williams, 1981). This was called "blood boosting" or "blood doping," and it was done with Eastern Block distance runners as early as the 1960's. Blood doping permitted athletes to obtain some of the benefits of altitude training without the logistical problems of traveling and training at altitude several times during the months before a major competition. At the same time, the athletes were also able to conduct quality sharpening and anaerobic work at sea level. However, some athletes are believed to have died from complications associated with the procedure.

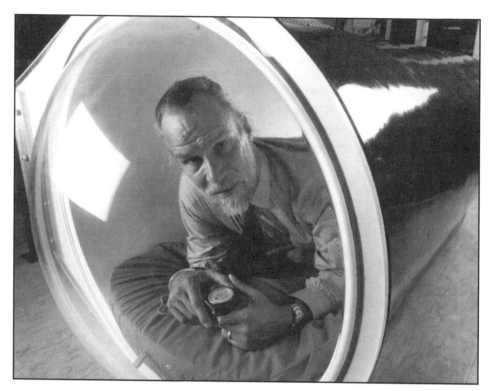

PHOTO 13.3—Igor Gamow, Associate Professor of Chemical Engineering at Colorado University, holding an altimeter inside a prototype altitude bed. Photo by Ken Abbott, Colorado University, and courtesy of Igor Gamow.

This method of doping became obsolete with the widespread availability of DNA-recombinant erthropoietin (RhEPO) as a prescription drug. The hormone erthropoietin is normally secreted by the kidneys in response to reduced oxygen in the body tissues, and it triggers the production of red blood cells. Unfortunately, there is no shortage of doctors willing to prescribe this substance for athletes. The use of RhEPO has also caused the death of numerous athletes. The blood can become too thick and viscous, thereby causing congestive heart failure. Athletes using RhEPO have taken still other drugs to thin their blood and reduce its ability to coagulate. However, a side effect of these drugs is that they can promote hemorrhaging.

The governing bodies in cycling and cross-country skiing have responded to the recent deaths by implementing pre-race tests of the athletes' hematocrit and hemoglobin. The normal hematocrit for males is approximately 47, plus or minus seven percent, thus a value slightly over 50 would not be judged abnormal (Jacob and Francone, 1974). In 1997, the *Union of Cycliste Internationale* (UCI) established a hematocrit limit of 50 for male athletes. If cyclists test over 50, then they are simply not allowed to compete since it is not considered safe. Some criticize this limit as being too low and likely to result in false positives (Martin, Ashenden, Parisotto, Pyne, Hahn, 1997). In 1996, the International Ski Federation (FIS) established a hemoglobin limit of 16.5 and 18.5 for female and male athletes, respectively. However, this limit is criticized as being too high. The International Olympic Committee has now approved RhEPO tests—they combine a urine-based method developed by a French laboratory and a blood sampling control devised in Australia. The introduction of blood sampling and tests for RhEPO constitutes a major step forward in the effort to curb the use of performance enhancing drugs (Koppel, 2000).

Nevertheless, there are other methods of simulating altitude, or otherwise stimulating red blood cell production. Igor Gamow, presently at the University of Colorado in Boulder, invented a device capable of saving mountain climbers from altitude sickness. Essentially, an ailing climber crawls into a bag and seals it shut, then the bag is inflated and pressurized. This has the effect of bringing the climber down from altitude to sea level while still on the side of a mountain. Gamow was also familiar with the use of hypobaric chambers in which the pressure can be reduced to below that at sea level, and he had contemplated the possible training effects from using them. Intrigued by the possibility, the author encouraged him to create a chamber that could be used by endurance athletes living at sea level to study the effects of sleeping high, and training low (be careful what you wish for). The altitude bed has been successfully used by endurance athletes, and is advertised on the web (altitudetraining.com). At night, an athlete can sleep in atmospheric conditions up to 14,000 feet, and by day perform quality anaerobic work as desired.

Shawn Wallace, a British pursuit cyclist who had first used Gamow's altitude bed, then developed the altitude tent. The altitude tent is designed to fit on top of a bed and comes in various sizes. There is room enough for two, and it is transportable. More information on the tent can be found at the website (altitudetent.com). It should be noted that the altitude bed and the altitude tent use different principles to simulate low oxygen conditions. The altitude bed creates a low-pressure environment similar to that found at altitude, whereas the altitude tent provides a lower percentage of oxygen at normal atmospheric pressure. At this time, which device and method gives the most benefit is unknown.

So-called "Altitude Houses" have also been springing up everywhere, which enable athletes to live a would-be normal life while simulating altitude conditions. To diminish the supply of oxygen, altitude houses sometimes use a greater than normal percentage of nitrogen in their artificial atmosphere, or alternately, the internal pressure of the house is simply reduced. A mobile unit, which puts the "Alps in a Winnebago," has also been developed in Norway (Seiler, 1997). There is now mounting evidence that "sleeping high and training low" can greatly enhance athletic performance, and not only in the distance events (Anderson, 1992).

However, the author does not advocate using any of these artificial devices or methods. Instead, national and world-class distance runners are best advised to train at altitude. As previously discussed in Chapter 3, running on long uphill grades provides a significant training benefit, and the best place to find such challenging terrain is at altitude. A synergistic training effect occurs when running on hilly terrain at altitude that cannot be duplicated by other means.

Moreover, the use of artificial devices flirts with the invisible line that separates the light side from the dark side. Clearly, the use of blood doping, RhEPO, steroid drugs, or other anabolic hormones crosses the line. The late Australian coach Percy Cerutty (1875-1975) would sometimes remind his athletes that running circles around a track was essentially a trivial pursuit, and utterly meaningless unless the activity contributed to cultivating their character (Masters, 1999). Occasionally, coaches and athletes need to step back and consider the big picture—and reflect on whether they enjoy peace of mind. Not everything in life can be measured by the stopwatch.

> *If you follow the present-day world, you will turn your back on the Way; if you would not turn your back on the Way, do not follow the world.*
>
> —Takuan Sōhō

References

Anderson, Owen, "Sleep-Don't Train-At Altitude," *Running Research News*, Volume 8, Number 3, May-June, 1992.

Bassett, D.R., and C.R. Kyle, L. Passfield, J.P. Broker, E.R. Burke, "Comparing Cycling World Hour Records, 1967-1996: Modeling with Empirical Data," *Medicine and Science in Sports and Exercise*, Volume 31, Number 11, November, 1999, pages 1665-1676.

Berghold, Franz, "Sport Medical Aspects of Hiking and Mountain Climbing in the Alps," *Schweizerische Zeitschrift fur Sportmedizin*, Volume 30, Number 1, March, 1982, pages 5-12.

Berglund, Bo, "High Altitude Training," *Sports Medicine*, Volume 14, Number 5, 1992, pages 289-303.

Cecil Textbook of Medicine, 20th edition, Philadelphia, Pennsylvania: W.B. Saunders, Co., 1996.

Cerutty, Percy, *Audio Tape Recording*, 1970's.

Clement, D.B., and R.C. Asmundson, C.W. Medhurst, "Hemoglobin Values: Comparative Survey of the 1976 Canadian Olympic Team," *Journal of the Canadian Medical Association*, Volume 117, 1977, pages 614-616.

Dales, George, *Conversations on Acclimatization to Altitude*, Kalamazoo, Michigan, 1997.

Daniels, Jack, "Altitude and Athletic Training and Performance," *American Journal of Sports Medicine*, Volume 7, 1979, pages 371-373.

Daniels, Jack, *Conversations on Altitude Training*, 1984-1997.

Daniels, Jack, "Equating Sea Level and Altitude Distance Running Times," *Track & Field Quarterly Review*, Volume 75, Number 4, 1975, pages 38-39.

Daniels, Jack, "Training Where The Air is Rare," *Runner's World*, June, 1980.

Daniels, Jack, and Neil Oldridge, "The Effects of Alternate Exposure to Altitude and Sea Level On World-Class Middle-Distance Runners," Medicine and Science in Sports, Volume 2, Number 3, 1970, pages 107-112.

Dill, D.B., and K. Braithwaite, W.C. Adams, E.M. Bernauer, "Blood Volume or Middle-Distance Runners: Effect of 2300m Altitude and Comparison with Non-Athletes," *Medicine and Science in Sports and Exercise*, Volume 6, 1974, pages 1-7.

Dufaux, B., and A. Hoederrath, I. Streitberg, W. Hollman, G. Assman, "Serum Ferritin, Transferrin, Haptoglobin, and Iron in Middle and Long Distance Runners, Elite Rowers, and Professional Racing Cyclists," *International Journal of Sports Medicine*, Volume 2, 1981, pages 43-46.

Editors of Market House Books Ltd., *The Bantam Medical Dictionary*, Revised Edition, New York: Bantam Books, 1990.

Faulkner, J.A., "Training for Maximum Performance at Altitude," *The International Symposium on the Effects of Altitude on Physical Performance*, Albuquerque, New Mexico, March 3-6, 1966, pages 88-90.

Faulkner, J.A., and Jack Daniels, B. Balke, "The Effects of Training at Moderate Altitude on Physical Performance Capacity," *Journal of Applied Physiology*, Volume 23, 1967, pages 85-89.

Frederick, E.C., and Jack Daniels, J. Hayes. "The Effect of Shoe Weight on the Aerobic Demands of Running," *Current Topics in Sports Medicine: Proceedings of the World Congress of Sports Medicine*, N. Bachl, L. Prokop and R. Suckert, Editors, Vienna: Urban & Schwartzenberg, 1983, pages 604-615.

Jacob, Stanley W., and Clarice A. Francone, *Structure and Function in Man*, 3rd Edition, Philadelphia, Pennsylvania: W.B. Saunders Company, 1974.

Janssen, Peter G.J.M., *Training Lactate Pulse Rate*, Oulu, Finland: Polar Electro Oy, 1987.

Koppel, Naomi, "IOC Approves EPO Tests For Sydney," *Associated Press*, August 1, 2000.

Koch, Damien, *Conversation on Altitude Training and Racing at Sea Level*, Fort Collins, Colorado, 1999.

Levine, B.D., and J. Stray-Gundersen, G. Duhaime, P.G. Schnell, D.B. Friedman, "Living High - Training Low: The Effect of Altitude Acclimatization / Normoxic Training in Trained Runners," *Medicine and Science in Sports and Exercise*, Volume 23, Supplement S25, 1991.

Martin, David E., and Donald F. May, Susan P. Pilbeam, "Ventilation Limitations to Performance Among Elite Male Distance Runners," *Sport and Elite Performers*, Daniel M. Landers, Editor, Champaign, Illinois: Human Kinetics, 1986, pages 121-131.

Martin, David T., and M. Ashenden, R. Parisotto, D. Pyne, A. Hahn, "Blood Testing for Professional Cyclists: What's a Fair Hematocrit Level?" *Sportsmedicine News*, March-April, 1997, http://www.sportsci.org/news/news9703/AISblood.html.

Masters, Roy, "The Secrets Herb Believes Can Make You Run A Little Faster," *The Sydney Morning Herald*, June 25, 1999.

Newhouse, I.J., and D.B. Clement, "Iron Status in Athletes: An Update," *Sports Medicine*, Volume 5, 1988, pages 337-352.

Popov, Ilia, "The Pros and Cons of Altitude Training," Published by the *IAAF*, Volume 9, Number 2, 1994, pages 15-21.

Seiler, Stephen, "Tighter Control on EPO Use by Skiers," *Sportsmedicine News*, Jan-Feb. 1997, http://www.sportsci.org/news/news9701/EPOfeat.html.

Sparks, Ken, and Garry Bjorklund, *Long-Distance Runner's Guide To Training And Racing*, New Jersey: Prentice-Hall, Inc., 1984.

Suslov, Felix, "Basic Principles of Training at High Altitude," published by the *IAAF*, Volume 9, Number 2, 1994, pages 45-50.

Svedenhag, J., and B. Saltin, C. Johanson, L. Kaijser, "Aerobic and Anaerobic Exercise Capacities of Elite Middle-Distance Runners after Two Weeks of Training at Moderate Altitudes," *Scandinavian Journal of Medicine and Science in Sports*, Volume 1, 1991, pages 205-214.

Takuan Sōhō, *The Unfettered Mind*, Translated by William Scott Wilson, New York: Kodasha International USA, Ltd. / Harper & Row, 1986.

Ward-Smith, A.J., "Air Resistance and Its Influence on the Biomechanics and Energies of Sprinting at Sea Level and at Altitude," *Biomechanics*, Volume 17, 1984, pages 339-347.

Williams, Melvin H., et al., "The Effect of Induced Erythrocythemia Upon 5-Mile Treadmill Run Time," *Medicine and Science in Sports and Exercise*, Volume 13, Number 3, 1981, pages 169-175.

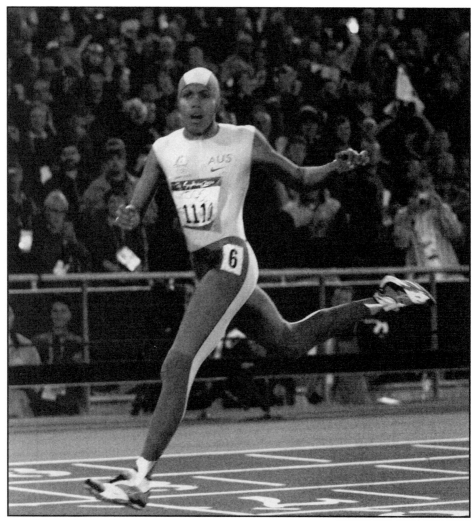

PHOTO 14.1—Cathy Freeman wins the 400 meters wearing aerodynamic apparel, 2000 Olympic Games. Photo by Thomas Kienzle, from AP/ Wide World Photos.

CHAPTER 14

AERODYNAMIC DRAG AND DRAFTING

Athletes and coaches need to respect the magnitude and practical effects of aerodynamic drag on running performance. The findings of technical experts on this subject generally agree with the consensus reached amongst knowledgeable coaches. In the absence of wind, drafting a lead athlete at less than or equal to one meter of separation is worth about one second/400 meters at sea level (Kyle, 1989). The additional energy cost of leading a race is then about one second/400 meters in the middle distance and distance events. If an athlete is going to attempt to lead and win the 1,500 meters right from the gun, then he or she had better be at least four seconds fitter than the rest of the field. And the athlete would have to be about eight seconds better in the 3,000 meters, 12 seconds in the 5,000 meters, 24 seconds in the 10,000 meters, and over 1:30 in the marathon. These are large margins at any level of competition.

Frequently a runner makes a break in a race, leaving behind a pack of two or more athletes. With respect to aerodynamic drag, the athlete leading the trailing pack is on par with the runner who has made the break. However, the athletes drafting the leader of the trailing pack are gaining one free second every 400 meters in terms of their relative energy cost. Unless the runner who has made the break can accumulate and sustain an advantage at the rate of one second/400 meters over the remainder of the race, her or she will be vulnerable in the closing stages of the race to athletes of equal ability who might attack from the trailing group.

If a runner takes the lead in the 5,000 meters at two miles, leaving behind a trailing pack of athletes, then he or she needs to accumulate a lead of four seconds and/or be that much more fit than the rest of the field in order to hold off a late attack. An athlete taking the lead in the 10,000 meters at four miles needs to accumulate and/or be about eight seconds more fit than the others in the field. And a runner taking the lead in the marathon at 18 miles needs to accumulate and/or be about 32 seconds more fit than the field. This realization can have a sobering effect on athletes who have never studied the phenomenon.

Several lessons can be drawn from this information. Sometimes patience is indeed a virtue. The lead is always a temptation. An athlete should not take the lead unless he or she is ready for the responsibility and possible penalty it may bring. A front-runner is sometimes well advised to take advantage of an honest early pace and use the surge tactics or preliminary breakaway attempts of other athletes to weaken and thin the field before making a decisive break. Many runners waste precious time and energy in a race by making inconsequential moves. Athletes will often assume the lead even when they do not intend to do anything with it, nor perhaps know what to do with it. Such theatrics may win the approval of some spectators, but they are foolhardy. However, recognize that nothing is fixed in strategy. Psychological dislocation is more important than physical dislocation, although one is generally associated with the other (Liddell-Hart, 1967). The decisive moment in a race can come in the first meter or the last.

Here is an estimate regarding the odds of an athlete winning the 1,500 meters, given a field of equally talented contestants, by attacking with:

400 meters to go—about 10%
300 meters to go—about 25%
200 meters to go—about 50%
150 meters to go—about 65%
100 meters to go—about 75%
 50 meters to go—about 85%

Some of the above is due to aerodynamic drag, which becomes more pronounced as athletes move at higher speeds. For example, let's say an athlete competing in the mile drafts for the first three laps, thereby saving about three seconds worth of energy over the first 1,200 meters, and then attacks with 400 meters to go. A second athlete, who has also drafted for the first three laps, then continues to draft the new leader for the next 300 meters. This second athlete accumulates a further energy savings of .75 seconds over the next 300 meters that can be used in the final kick with only 100 meters to go.

Does this mean an athlete should let others do all the work, sit back, and wait to kick? In truth, there can be two correct answers to this question, depending on the circumstances. If a runner is relatively inexperienced and substantially less fit than others in the field, then the answer is yes. However, if an athlete is as experienced and fit as others in the field, then the answer is no. For example, an athlete who wishes to excel will often need to contribute to the pacing in order to get a qualifying time or personal record. And unless a runner is alone in having a strong kick, simply sitting and waiting will not work. A complete athlete can win from the lead, win from the surge or breakaway, or win from the kick. Not every runner will have the natural talent or versatility to be able to do all of those things. But when an athlete can do all of these things, then he or she has developed a repertoire that makes for some exciting racing.

Obviously, there is plenty of room for sound judgment and intuition when racing. Certainly, when an athlete takes the lead in the third lap of a 1,500 meters race and wins (as Herb Elliott did in the 1960 Olympic games), or strikes early in a marathon (as Joan Benoit Samuelson did in the 1984 Olympics), it generally means they have superior physical fitness, but also the intelligence and courage to match.

The additional energy cost of running into a headwind is approximately proportional to the square of the wind speed. So unless you have a good reason, avoid doing all the work leading into the wind. Instead, it is better to trade off the lead. If you face competitors unwilling to do some of the work, then sometimes it

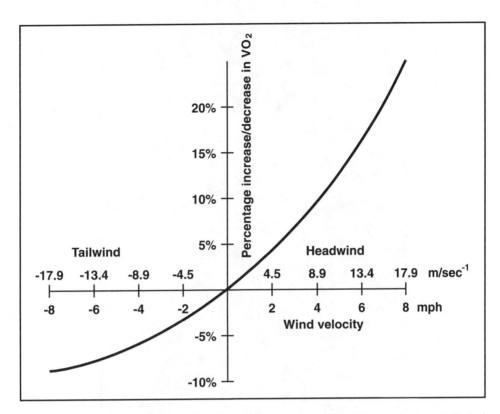

FIGURE 14.1—Change in VO_2 demand as a result of headwind or tailwind (% greater or lesser relative to calm air). Reprinted by permission, from J. Daniels, 1998, *Daniel's Running Formula*, Champaign, IL: Human Kinetics, page 184.

may be possible to move out to lane three, stop dead, and stand there with your hands on your hips. The psychological dislocation alone will probably be worth it. Wait till they go by and then sit on them. Runners are so conditioned to think they should never stop, and that lane one is the shortest course, that they sometimes fail to seize the obvious answer to this vexing problem. If the other athletes do not want to do their share of the work and lead, then sometimes you can maintain command of the race by making them lead.

An athlete can do a number of things to decrease aerodynamic drag. It is best not to run shoulder to shoulder with another athlete, as both athletes then increase their drag. It is better to run just off the shoulder of a lead runner, with the drafting athlete's left arm and leg synchronized with the right arm and leg of the lead runner so as not to make contact or impede. And if the tactical situation permits, it is best to follow directly behind one or more athletes as close as possible.

The torso generates less aerodynamic drag in the nude condition than when wearing a singlet, but obviously this is not always possible or conducive to modesty. Shorter or closely kept hair can also reduce aerodynamic drag. Accordingly, so-called "Benjamin Franklin" hairstyles can cost an athlete a healthy amount of time. However, it is possible for long hair secured behind the head to

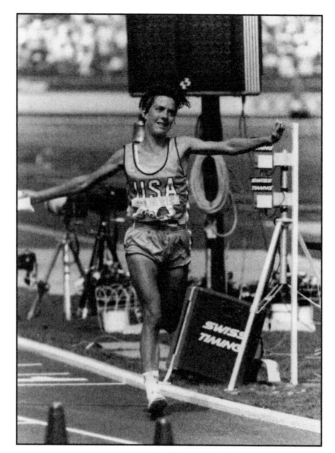

PHOTO 14.2—Joan Benoit Samuelson waves to the crowd after winning the marathon, 1984 Olympic Games. Photo from AP/Wide World Photos.

create a more tear-dropped shape that can actually slightly decrease drag. The common practice of women to draw their hair taught about the sides of the head into a trailing ponytail is sound. Accordingly, women should not go out and cut their hair unless it pleases them to do so. However, an elite male sprinter having substantial body hair would be well advised to consider the body shaving practiced by some swimmers.

Principles of Aerodynamic Drag

There are two types of aerodynamic drag: surface friction drag, and pressure-induced drag. The portion of total drag derived from surface friction is small compared to pressure-induced drag, but still a significant factor. Pressure-induced drag is created by a cylinder shaped object—that is, the human torso and limbs—blowing a hole through the fluid we know as air. Figure 14.2 illustrates some of the phenomena associated with pressure-induced drag. The boundary layer of air separates about the sides of the runner's torso, creating a turbulent wake. This results in the creation of a high-pressure area on the front of the torso, and a low-pressure area behind the runner.

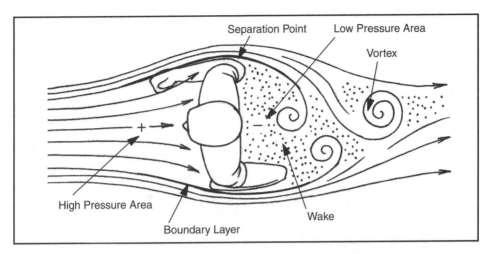

FIGURE 14.2—Top view of a runner, showing pressure-induced aerodynamic drag

Aerodynamic Drag: The sum of friction induced drag, which corresponds to the work done when a gaseous fluid (air) slows and produces heat when encountering a surface, and pressure induced drag, which corresponds to the work done in overcoming a build up of high pressure on the font of an object due to its blowing a hole in the gaseous fluid (air) and creating a wake of low pressure behind it. Pressure-induced drag is the most substantial contributor to the aerodynamic drag experienced when running. The formula for calculating pressure-induced drag is,

$$D = .5 \, (p) \, (Ap) \, (Cd) \, V^2$$

D = the force of drag in Newtons
p = air density (Kg/m^3)
Ap = the projected frontal area normal to the air stream (m^2)
Cd = the coefficient of drag, (the object's aerodynamic efficiency)
V = the velocity of the object in meters per second.

The variables in the equation for calculating pressure-induced aerodynamic drag merit further consideration. Accordingly, the practical effect of changes in the air density, projected frontal area, coefficient of drag, and running velocity will be briefly discussed.

Due to the presence of lower air density at altitude, there is less of a price to pay with respect to aerodynamic drag. A performance advantage of 1.7% was observed in the sprinting events at Mexico City (Ward-Smith, 1984). At the lower speeds of middle distance and distance events (that is, six to seven as opposed to 10 to 12 meters/second), the advantage would be approximately one quarter of that experienced in the sprint events, since velocity is squared in the formula for aerodynamic drag. Therefore, you can reasonably expect an advantage relative to sea level of only about .41%. This would be worth about .98 seconds in a 4:00 mile. So, instead of an energy savings of four seconds over the mile, drafting

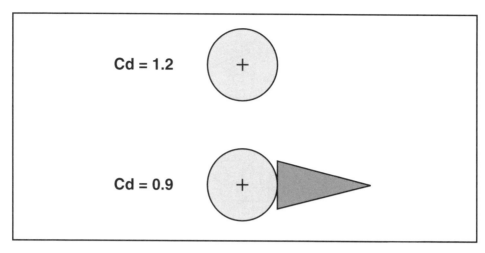

FIGURE 14.3—Adapted from Hoerner, 1965

athletes perhaps only gain about three seconds when competing at altitude. However, there is a greater penalty to pay for a misjudgment of pace and inefficient use of energy at altitude. In contrast, due to the higher air density associated with conditions of high humidity, athletes should then expect to pay a higher than normal price for leading.

The greater an individual's projected frontal area, the greater will be the resulting aerodynamic drag. In this regard, a shorter athlete with a slight build has an advantage over a larger athlete. The easiest way to reduce the projected frontal area is to draft another runner. And when confronted with headwinds, an athlete who leans forward will both reduce their projected frontal area, but also influence their coefficient of drag so as to become more aerodynamically efficient.

The coefficient of drag is a dimensionless number that expresses the aerodynamic efficiency of an object. In this regard, the human torso generally resembles a cylindrical shape, whereas the arms and legs have a more oval shape. As shown in Figure 14.3, modifying a cylindrical shape to a teardrop shape can significantly reduce its coefficient of drag and the resulting pressure-induced aerodynamic drag.

Other things being equal, the faster an athlete is running, the greater will be the resulting aerodynamic drag. Accordingly, aerodynamic drag can be a more significant factor with respect to the performance of sprinters than long distance runners, as sprinters can reach speeds exceeding 25 mph. And it is a much greater factor in the performance of speed skaters and cyclists who move at even higher speeds. In fact, about ninety percent of the work performed when bicycling on level terrain is expended to overcome aerodynamic drag.

The caveat to this discussion is that in certain circumstances the aerodynamic drag generated by an athlete can actually be reduced at higher speeds. What happens is complex, but can be simply explained as follows. When moving slowly, a cylindrical shaped object such as a runner's torso blows a relatively large hole in the fluid we know as air. The boundary layer then separates relatively

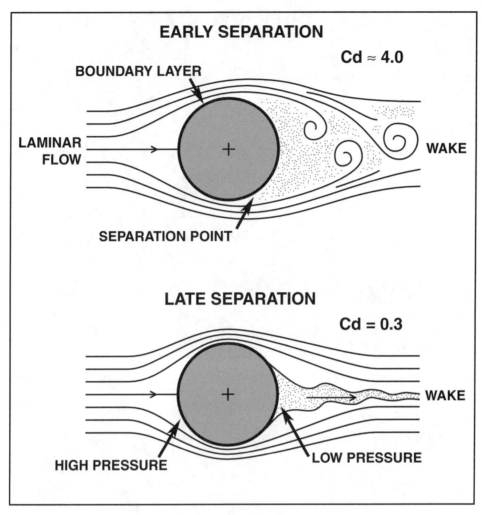

FIGURE 14.4—Adapted from Pugh, 1971

early, and this results in a large wake including random turbulence. However, as the runner's velocity increases, the boundary layer will separate later. And with the onset of fully developed turbulence, a dramatic narrowing of the athlete's wake can suddenly occur. There exists a dimensionless number called the critical Reynolds number that is associated with this threshold phenomenon. And the magnitude of the aerodynamic drag being generated can then dramatically decrease to only about 30% of its former value. Figure 14.4 illustrates the wake of two cylindrical shapes—one moving at a velocity below, and the other moving above the threshold associated with the critical Reynold's number.

Distance runners do not move at high enough speed to encounter this critical threshold, but sprinters can approach it under certain circumstances. In particular, the use of aerodynamic apparel can reduce an athlete's coefficient of drag so as to narrow the margin. However, speed skaters and especially bicyclists can move at speeds that enable them to reach the threshold with the aid of aerodynamic apparel.

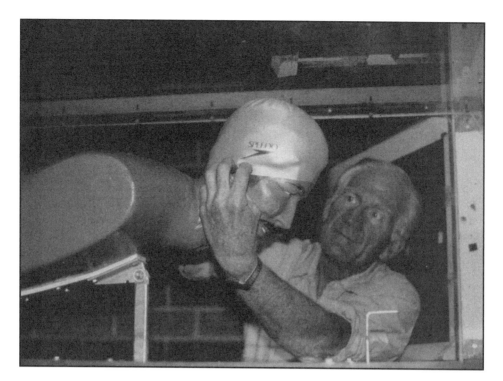

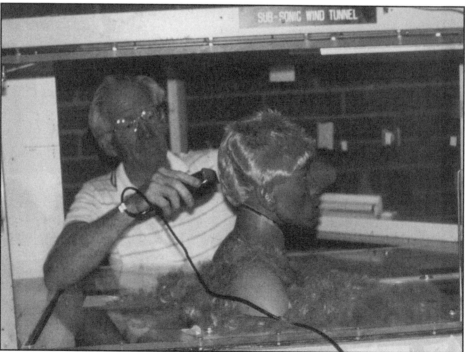

PHOTOS 14.3 and 14.4—Chester Kyle preparing models for wind tunnel testing, 1986. Photos courtesy of Chester Kyle.

Distance (m)	Avg. Speed (ms⁻¹)	Time Savings [s (I)]	Advantage* (m)		
			I	II	III
100	10.7	0.01	0.1	—	—
200	10.15	0.02	0.2	—	—
400	9.12	0.08	0.7	1.9	1.2
800	7.86	0.14	1.1	2.7	1.8
1,500	7.12	0.24	1.7	4.2	2.7
5,000	6.41	0.76	4.9	11.3	7.3
10,000	6.09	1.46	8.9	20.5	13.2
Marathon	5.50	5.70	31.3	70.2	45.4

TABLE 14.1—Advantage due to a 2% reduction in aerodynamic drag, using three different equations. From Kyle, 1986.

Aerodynamic Apparel

The present rules governing competition in track and field prohibit the use of apparel to unnaturally aid performance. However, practically speaking, even small variations in apparel design and construction can affect aerodynamic drag. In keeping with the spirit and letter of the rules, athletes then have latitude, by way of selecting appropriate apparel, to make prudent decisions that can impact their performance. Generally, a singlet made from a material with a tightly woven, smooth surface or a slick sheen rendered impenetrable to air works best to reduce friction drag. These materials can cause substantial heat build-up, and so although they can be used in the sprint events, they are not normally practical for distance runners. The one-piece stretchlastic body suits worn by sprinters, particularly suits with hoods covering the head, can and do reduce aerodynamic drag. The most knowledgable person in the United States on the subject of aerodynamic drag and athletic apparel is Chester Kyle of Weed, California. He has shown that even the difference between having short hair versus long hair can decrease aerodynamic drag by two percent (Kyle, "Athletic Clothing," 1986). Table 14.1 shows the effect of a two-percent-reduction in aerodynamic drag upon running performance calculated using three different equations.

Again, friction drag is a relatively small part of the total aerodynamic drag on a runner. The primary contributor is pressure-induced drag. An unusual thing can happen when a material having a fine surface roughness is positioned in just the right places. The introduction of surface roughness with a design that is capable of creating premature turbulence, or one that otherwise prevents the boundary layer from early separation about the sides of a runner's singlet and shorts, can narrow the wake and decrease pressure induced drag. Thus, if athletes need to include a fine mesh in their singlets in order to manage expected hot and humid conditions, it can be placed along the sides and back without so adversely affecting aerodynamic drag. And a well-designed singlet can slightly decrease drag. In this regard, the mere presence of a properly placed sewing seam, or a material having the surface roughness of fine woven wool is enough to change the resulting aerodynamic drag by a significant amount (Kyle, "Athletic Clothing," 1986, Brownlie, 1992).

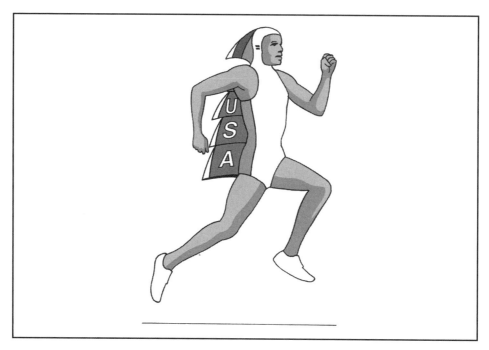

FIGURE 14.4

Aware of Kyle's work, the author designed a custom singlet for use by Steve Plasencia in the high heat and humidity encountered in Indianapolis during the 1988 U.S. Olympic Trials. A more radical design intended for sprinters included a dramatic V-shaped back to create a teardrop shape (See Figure 14.4). The apparel was tested on a bicycle by rolling with the acceleration due to gravity down a steep hill to attain a maximum speed of approximately 30 mph at the end of 100 meters. Most noticeable was the relative absence of turbulence, thus the pulling and flapping noise usually associated with conventional apparel was all but eliminated. The design shown in Figure 14.4 was found to be worth nearly a tenth of a second. The marketing strategy was to launch the "Godzilla Suit" at a major competition in Japan, and to create a sensation.

The author began working for Nike, Inc. as a regular employee in 1990, and later granted the company a non-exclusive license regarding certain aerodynamic apparel know-how and intellectual property. However, despite that fact Kyle, Len Brownlie and the author had shown the merit of such apparel, nothing really came of it until a decade later. By an unusual coincidence and turn of fate, Nike Vice-President Sandy Bodecker, who was aware of the research, married the Australian sprinter Cathy Freeman, and the rest is history.

Aerodynamic apparel has also had an impact on the outcome of speed-skating competitions, and the Tour de France. In this regard, the competition rules have not kept pace with the evolution of modern technology. In conclusion, aerodynamic drag and drafting can significantly affect athletic performance in the middle distance and distance events. It is important to appreciate and respect those forces which cannot be seen.

> *Pay attention even to trifles...*
> *Immature strategy is the cause of grief.*
> *That was a true saying.*
>
> —Miyamoto Musashi

References

Brownlie, Leonard R., "High Performance Sports Apparel," *NIKE Sport Research Review*, 1989, May-June, page 2.

Brownlie, Leonard R., *Ph.D. Thesis, Aerodynamic Characteristics of Sports Apparel*, Simon Fraser University, 1992.

Brownlie, Leonard R., et al., "The Influence of Apparel on Aerodynamic Drag in Running," *Annals of Physiological Anthropology*, Volume 6, Number 3, 1987, page 133.

Daniels, Jack, *Daniels' Running Formula*, Champaign, Illinois: Human Kinetics Publishers, 1998, page 184.

Davies, C.T.M., "Effects of Wind Assistance and Resistance on the Forward Motion of a Runner;" *Journal of Applied Physiology*, 1980, Volume 48, pages 702-709.

Gross, A., and C. Kyle, D. Malewicki, "The Aerodynamics of Human-Powered Land Vehicles," *Scientific American*, 1983, pages 142-152.

Hill, A.V., "The Air Resistance to a Runner," *Proceedings of the Royal Society of London*, Series B., pages 380-385.

Hoerner, S.F., *Fluid-Dynamic Drag*, Published by the author, 148 Busteed Drive, Midland Park, New Jersey, 1965.

Kyle, Chester R., "Athletic Clothing," *Scientific American*, Volume 254, 1986, page 106.

Kyle, Chester R., *Conversations on Aerodynamic Drag*, 1989, and 1997.

Kyle, Chester R., "Reduction of Wind Resistance and Power Output of Racing Cyclists and Runners Travelling in Groups," *Ergonomics*, 1979, Volume 22, Number 4, page 387.

Kyle, Chester R., and Vincent J. Caiozzo, "The Effect of Athletic Clothing Aerodynamics Upon Running Speed," *Medicine and Science in Sports and Exercise*, 1986, Volume 18, Number 5, page 511.

Kyle, Chester R., and R. Walpert, "The Aerodynamic Drag of the Human Figure in Athletics," *Unpublished Report to the U.S. Olympic Committee*, Colorado Springs, Colorado.

Liddell-Hart, B.H., *Strategy*, New York: Frederick A. Praeger Publishers, 1967.

Lyden, Robert, *Aerodynamic Apparel: Background for U.S. Patent Application and/or Trademark Protection*, publicly disclosed, 1989.

MacFarland, E., "How Olympic Records Depend on Location," *American Journal of Applied Physiology*, Volume 54, 1986, pages 513-519.

Musashi, Miyamoto, *A Book of Five Rings*, Translated by Victor Harris, Woodstock, New York: The Overlook Press, 1982, page 40.

Pugh, L.G.C.E., "Air Resistance in Sport," *Advances in Exercise Physiology*, E. Jokl, Editor, Basel, Switzerland: Karger, 1976.

Pugh, L.G.C.E., "The Influence Of Wind Resistance In Running And Walking And The Mechanical Efficiency of Work Against Horizontal Or Vertical Forces," *Journal of Physiology*, Volume 213, 1971, page 255.

Pugh, L.G.C.E., "Oxygen Intake in Track and Treadmill Running with Observations on the Effect of Air Resistance," *Journal of Physiology*, Volume 207, 1970, pages 823-835.

Shanebrook, J.R., and R.D. Jaszczak, "Aerodynamic Drag Analysis of Runners," *Medicine and Science in Sports*, Volume 8, Number 1, 1976, pages, 43-45.

Ward-Smith, A.J., "Air Resistance And Its Influence On The Biomechanics And Energies Of Sprinting At Sea Level And At Altitude," *Biomechanics*, Volume 17, 1984, pages 339-347.

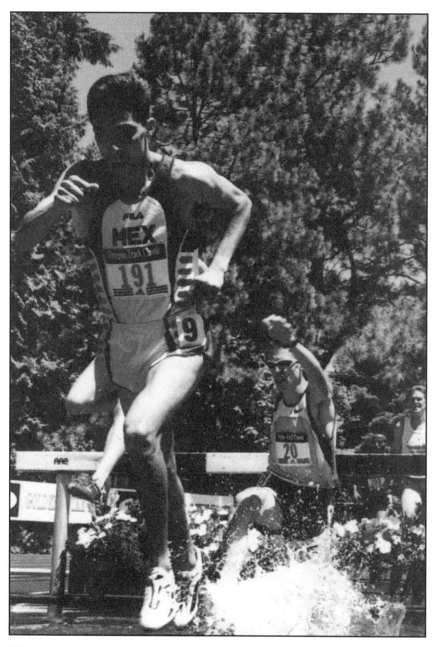

PHOTO 15.1—Steeplechase action at the 2000 Oregon Track Classic, Lewis & Clark College. Photo by the author.

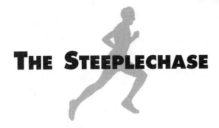

CHAPTER 15

THE STEEPLECHASE

The 1972 Olympic Champion in the Steeplechase, Kip Keino of Kenya, once referred to the steeplechase as a "race for animals." In fact, the steeplechase event originated in English horse races, which were run across the countryside, using church steeples to mark the start and finish. In 1850, faced with ground conditions unfit for settling a wager by means of a horse race, Halifax Wyatt proposed instead that the matter be settled by a human footrace. The first steeplechase was conducted on a two-mile course over 24 barriers composed of hedges and water-filled ditches. The steeplechase was contested in the 1900 Olympic Games, and in 1920, the distance was fixed at 3,000 meters. In 1952, Horace Ashenfelter, an FBI agent, defeated Vladimir Kazantsev of the Russian police for the Olympic Gold Medal. Ashenfelter's success and George Young's Bronze Medal in the 1968 Olympic Games stand as the best performances by American athletes in this event at the international level (Hartwick, 1981).

The Need for Introduction at the High School Level

In part, the lack of American success is due to the fact that high school athletes seldom compete in the steeplechase. Occasionally, the event will be contested in an invitational meet at a facility that has a water jump. It would be beneficial for state high school championships nationwide to include a modified 2,000 meters steeplechase event. This hypothetical high school event could be run over barriers, but perhaps not include the water jump hazard. These changes would make the event easy to stage from a logistical and economic standpoint.

Prospects for the Steeplechase

Collegiate coaches will often make steeplechasers out of athletes who do not appear to be talented enough to excel at either 1,500 or 5,000 meters. However, the best steeplechasers are those with the aerobic ability to compete at 5,000 meters, but who then sharpen themselves to attain peak condition in the 1,500 and 3,000-meter events. Ideally, a male steeplechaser should be long legged, with at least a 34-inch inseam. However, others should not be prematurely ruled out, as some relatively short athletes have excelled in this event. To effectively negotiate the steeplechase barriers, the athlete must also be well coordinated, flexible, and physically stronger than the average distance runner. So rather than being a mediocre athlete, the true steeplechaser will likely be the most talented distance runner on any given athletic team.

The Steeplechase Barriers

The 3,000-meter steeplechase event requires athletes to negotiate 28 barriers and 7 water jumps. The height of the men's barriers is 36 inches, whereas the height of the women's is presently 30 inches. So the steeplechaser needs to be an excellent hurdler and capable of leading with either leg. Some runners will step on the first barrier, or otherwise step on barriers when caught in traffic and being jostled. It is far better to be safe than sorry. Athletes who hit a barrier will often have to retire from the race with an injury. The barriers weigh between 80-100 kg and do not move or deflect in the least when hit. This being said, it is normally most efficient to hurdle all of the barriers, with the exception of the water jumps.

The Steeplechase Water Jump

The men's water jump hazard is 30 inches (70 cm) deep adjacent to the barrier, and gradually decreases as it extends 12 feet beyond. The water jump hazard should be taken with a quick step. The athletes then push off from the barrier so as to land while still one to two feet from the far end of the water hazard, thus in slightly less than 12 inches of water. This cushions their landing and facilitates recovery of their running rhythm. Generally, if athletes land too far from the barrier in too shallow water, they will greatly flex at the knee and dramatically lean forwards, thus unduly lowering their center of gravity. This can cause a considerable loss of momentum, rhythm, and demonstrable speed when exiting the water jump. On the other hand, if they land too deep in the water, this will also reduce their exit speed.

Some athletes will hurdle the water hazard on the last one or two laps of the steeplechase event. Done properly, this technique can be worth five to 10 yards, depending on the quality of the field. However, if they bobble, they will be fortunate to come out even—or worse, could finish the competition sitting in the water hazard. This technique needs to be well rehearsed when athletes are fresh, but it should also be practiced occasionally when they are fatigued. However, this technique can increase the risk of injury, and is not prudent for every individual. Nevertheless, when steeplechasers are able to run the last one or two laps at 64 seconds/400 meters pace or faster, it becomes a viable option and potent competitive weapon. At this speed, the act of stepping and pushing off the barrier can be difficult to do, and can unduly slow athletes. This can prevent runners from attaining the success they might otherwise enjoy at the national and international levels. When running at a 64-second pace or faster, athletes hurdling the water hazard will actually land in nearly the same position in the water as when stepping and pushing off the barrier when running at only 70-second pace.

When teaching athletes to negotiate the water jump it can help to start with a six-by-six-inch barrier affixed to the ground in a grass field or at the head of a long jump pit. The landing area can then be marked to indicate the 12-foot line and the target landing point at about 10 feet. Over a period of weeks, this barrier can be raised to 24, 30, and finally to 36 inches (Dellinger, 1978). Alternatively, athletes can work off a 36-inch barrier from the beginning, and initially land only six feet beyond the barrier, but then gradually work their way out to 10 feet. Athletes need

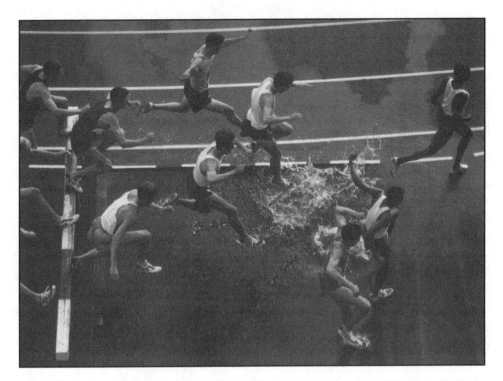

PHOTO 15.2—Athletes pushing off from the water jump barrier, 1996 Penn Relays.
Photo from Victah Sailer / Photorun.

to learn to step the barrier with the toe of the shoe hanging over so they can make a quick transition as they push off and extend horizontally. When stepping the barrier, the heel should not be lower than the barrier, or steeplechasers will block themselves before they are on top of the barrier (Hislop, 1999). The University of Oregon uses a resilient plywood cover on the water jump pit to allow athletes to practice a dry landing before actually attempting the water hazard.

If steeplechasers do not have access to a facility with a water hazard, they can take a makeshift six-by-six-inch barrier to a shallow body of water, and then set it up near the waterline. Athletes can then practice hurdling over the barrier and into water. If they trip on the barrier they are not likely to become injured, rather, will fall into the water and land on the underlying sand surface. As an alternative, coaches and athletes can use a six-by-six-inch beam and two carpenter horses to make a portable barrier for use in conjunction with a long jump pit.

Prerequisite Conditioning

Again, the steeplechaser needs to be an excellent hurdler. The athlete should be taught from the start to be able to lead with either leg, and this entails being able to trail with either leg as well. It sometimes helps to do some preliminary screening of prospective steeplechasers with the use of hurdles and simple hurdle drills. However, once a group of prospective steeplechasers has been identified, they should first be given a foundation of at least one month of specific strength and flexibility work before beginning lead-leg or trailing-leg drills, or attempting to hurdle.

As discussed in Chapter 7, there is a logical progression to stretching and flexibility work. Athletes should be able to perform the basic static stretches and PNF exercises before attempting any dynamic flexibility exercises. And the latter should be mastered before they begin to practice hurdling. For the novice hurdler or steeplechaser, the hamstring stretch, the hurdler's stretch (or L7), and those stretches directed towards the adductors of the leg will normally require the most work.

The L7 position is perhaps the single most beneficial stretching exercise for the steeplechaser, both novice and master. The lead leg should extend straight out in front of the athlete's torso, and the trail leg should project at a 90-degree angle from the lead leg to form an "L" shape—a straight line drawn through the hips should intersect the knee of the trail leg. The toe of the trail leg should be dorsiflexed, and a straight line drawn between the end of the toe and the knee of the trail leg should be approximately parallel to the lead leg. Athletes should be able to sit comfortably and study in this position. It helps to lean forward and hold the stretch for 10 to 30 seconds while keeping the back straight and head up— thus leading with the chin as opposed to the forehead. Athletes should also grasp the knee of their trail leg and similarly hold this stretch position for 10 to 30 seconds and repeat. Steeplechasers can then practice leaning forward, breathing naturally, and moving their arms as when hurdling. They should alternate stretches and work on both legs so as to be able to lead with either leg in competition (Hislop, 1995). When athletes are able to sit comfortably on the floor in the L7 position and perform these exercises well, then they are ready to begin dynamic flexibility exercises.

Dynamic flexibility exercises should always progress from simple, slow movements to more complex, rapid movements. Athletes should be able to do the 100-up routine—that is, from a standing position, raise one knee above the waist while simultaneously dorsiflexing the elevated foot, then return it near to the floor without touching down for 100 reps. When they master this, athletes can begin practicing lead leg drills by positioning a hurdle against a wall, or by making a target on a wall three to six inches above a mark at 36 inches. Athletes should stand five to seven feet from the wall, advance a step with their trail leg, then raise and lead with the knee, extending their foot in a slow-motion kicking action. The lead foot should rotate approximately 45° from vertical as the knee is extended, because this will permit less clearance height of the barrier, but the knee should never fully extend or lock. When they master this, they can accelerate the action and the foot of the lead leg can perform "wall attacks"—that is, touching and rebounding from an opposing wall. If athletes fail to dorsiflex their lead foot, or leads with the foot as opposed to the knee, a box or other obstacle can be placed in front of them so that they will hit it unless the correct technique is used. Sometimes it helps to use a kicking technique when teaching athletes to lead with the knee, and the appropriate verbal cue would then be to "knee-kick." This kicking action will cause the leg to recoil, and the lead foot then returns to the track surface faster. It will also cause a so-called "delayed rear leg action," characterized by greater extension. It thus brings the torso closer to the barrier, causing a greater proportion of the stride to be in front of the barrier. All of this

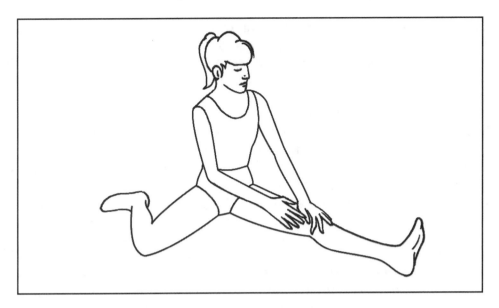

Figure 15.1—The L7 position

helps to speed and facilitate the clearance of the athletes over the barrier. The steeplechaser should also focus on cultivating balance and plantarflexion during this exercise.

A variety of exercises or devices can be used to specifically condition the lead leg, including: L-sit pull-ups, inverted sit-ups, sit-ups in which athletes raise torso and legs simultaneously and clap hands behind their legs, Anisimova drills, as well as the use of surgical tubing, ankle weights, and weighted shoes. Further, athletes should be capable of the "50-ups" routine with the trailing leg. In this regard, athletes should form a window with the trailing arm while raising the trailing leg up and out to the side at approximately 90° as if clearing a hurdle. As they raise the trailing leg, the foot should be dorsiflexed and cocked to the side, but kept as close as possible to the buttocks. The knee of the trailing leg should remain slightly higher than the trailing foot. The trailing leg should not get behind the hip, since that can induce rotation. When sufficient levels of flexibility and strength have been acquired, continuous trail leg exercises over the edge of a hurdle can then be done to good effect, and the exercise can become more vigorous with improved skill levels. For example, athletes can place a 36-inch hurdle three to four feet from a wall, and stand beside it facing the wall with the heel of the trailing leg slightly forward of the plane of the hurdle barrier. They can lean forward and put their hands on the wall, extend the trail leg behind as if completing their stride, then bring the trailing leg forward over the hurdle in the L7 position. The athletes should be up on the ball of the lead foot while bringing the trail leg over the hurdle. They should then work to increase the accuracy and speed at which the trail leg encircles the hurdle. Steeplechasers will eventually be able to stand next to a hurdle without substantially bracing themselves and perform trail leg drills.

In training abduction of the trail leg, variations of the following exercise can be useful: Athletes may lie on their sides upon the floor, or assume the hands and knees position, then extend from the hip and perform reps in relatively straight or circular movements with the trail leg to the side or behind. If more resistance is needed, weights or surgical tubing can be used. The use of a fixed weight and pulley system at floor level is particularly helpful in strengthening the adductors and abductors. An athlete can then move in a semicircle around the fixed position of the apparatus—that is, from a 12 o'clock to a 6 o'clock position and vice-versa. This can be done by taking one step, then performing a flexion or extension movement with the leg affixed to the pulley apparatus, then continuing by taking another step and repeating the exercise. Strength endurance activities such as running in sand, cross-country skiing, bicycling, and running in up to one foot of water along a beach can also benefit steeplechasers. Swimming the breast-stroke, or performing lead-leg, trail-leg, and other hurdle exercises in a pool can also provide a positive training effect (McFarlane, 1996). It can be advantageous for athletes to learn how to tread water, possibly with the use of a floatation belt, while incorporating a running motion—and to use this exercise on recovery days as a form of prehabilitation. Most importantly, before ever attempting to hurdle, would-be steeplechasers should first acquire the requisite range of motion, flexibility, strength, coordination and balance through general conditioning work.

The steeplechaser's technique carries the torso closer to vertical than when clearing a barrier in the 110 meters hurdles. The angle of the athlete's head while hurdling a barrier can largely determine the angle of the torso and position of the center of gravity. Normally, it is best to keep your head up and your vision focused about 15 yards ahead on the track, and for the torso to recover to a more vertical position almost immediately after you clear a barrier. Like the hurdler, the steeplechaser should get the lead foot down on the track surface as quickly as possible, but then stay high on the lead foot by first making contact with the ball of the foot. The steeplechaser can then be characterized as a midfoot or forefoot striker when hurdling a barrier.

Steeplechasers require strong and nimble feet. They also need to be able to balance and maneuver well when up on the balls of their feet. Steeplechasers benefit from auxiliary exercises such as barefoot running, plyometric exercises, jumping rope, burpies, jumping jacks, trampoline work, and weight training exercises such as curls, military press, and the snatch while balancing on the balls of their feet. Climbing in a rock gym (using proper safety equipment) can also strengthen the hands and feet. It also requires the same focus and level of concentration as hurdling. Athletes can also greatly strengthen their feet by climbing ten stadium steps barefoot, carrying dumbbells or five-gallon buckets of water in each hand, then slowly stepping down backwards. Buckets are inexpensive and can be filled with more water as the athletes progress. And in the event they lose their balance, the water will spill but no damage will be done. Many are shocked at the difference between what athletes can do while wearing shoes, versus performing this exercise barefoot.

Lead Leg and Trail Leg Hurdling Drills

When teaching lead leg and trail leg drills over hurdles, it can help to practice over three to five hurdles spaced less than 10 to 12 feet apart. The athletes can then turn and repeat the desired drill by negotiating a second flight of hurdles set two lanes to the outside, facing in the opposite direction. They can use the open lane between two opposing hurdles to alternately practice these drills with either leg. To practice alternating lead legs, a flight of three to five hurdles can be set up to require four instead of three or five steps between them. When proficiency has been demonstrated with hurdles set at 30 inches, athletes can then move up to 36 inches. At this time, the athletes would be working off the left or right side, but not the entire hurdle.

When athletes begin running hurdle drills, attention should be given to optimizing their arm action. The lead hand should be turned thumb-side-up, and the elbow should drive vigorously backwards and flex to create a "window" for the trail leg to pass through. Nevertheless, the arm action is not so rapid or wide as that for specialists in the 110 meters hurdles event due to the much slower speeds associated with barrier clearance in the steeplechase.

Women's Nylons

When first teaching hurdling to young or inexperienced athletes, there is an invaluable piece of equipment that every coach should have—namely, a half dozen women's nylons. Take a pair of nylons and cut the leg portions off. Set up two flights of hurdles, leaving an open lane between them. Then, stretch and tie each of the nylons between two hurdles. Use the same knot that you start with when tying shoelaces—that is, before you form the loops. The nylons are resilient enough to take a moderate blow and remain in place, yet athletes will know when they have made contact. If athletes miss badly, the knot will slip and they will not trip. The nylons are almost indestructible, and it only takes a second to re-tie the free ends back into place. This "secret weapon" can save novice hurdlers many battered knees, shins, ankles, toes, and several spread eagle landings on the track. Novices will be able to experiment and get closer to the hurdles—that is, they can be more aggressive and progress more rapidly toward mastering sound technique. However, once athletes master good hurdle technique, abandon the nylons and assign a high penalty for hitting a barrier during practice.

Hurdling and The Ritual

When athletes are finally learning to negotiate a full hurdle, it can help to use only a single hurdle and to place another hurdle right alongside, facing the opposite direction. This is the practice of Coach Chick Hislop of Weber State University, who many consider to be the finest steeplechase coach in the United States. Hislop has helped many athletes, and the author is indebted to him for generously providing his own writings and constructive criticism to enhance this treatment of the steeplechase.

Given two adjacent hurdles facing opposite directions, the athletes can then focus on a single target, and the act of turning about requires them to make a conscious effort to re-focus on the next hurdle. If they negotiate a flight of hurdles, athletes might shift from a more cognitive mode to automatism. While automatism is advantageous if not required for the 110 meters hurdles, this is not so for steeplechase, since the athletes move more freely about the track and then assume random positions relative to the barriers. Accordingly, random practice is needed to develop the requisite set of skills. In this drill, athletes move down the track at varying distances to randomly change their approach and lead leg. When this drill is performed, the coach may wish to stand about 15 feet from the hurdles so that brief comments on technique can be given as the athletes wheel around. Hislop commonly has athletes take 100 hurdles in this manner, and refers to this training session as "the ritual." Prior to a competition, after warming up, the athletes can then engage in the ritual and take about 20 hurdles. Since the penalty for hitting a barrier in competition can be catastrophic, it is prudent for athletes to assign themselves with a 100-hurdle penalty if they happen to hit a hurdle during training. However, there can also be times and circumstances when hitting a hurdle might signal the end of a training session (Hislop, 1984, and 1999).

Hitting a Barrier

The imagination does not really prepare athletes for the stark reality of what can happen when they hit a barrier. It does not move or deflect in the least, rather, it is like running into a brick wall. It is probably better for athletes to first experience hitting a barrier in training, rather than in competition. And if there is such a thing as a best time for this, it is probably after they have mastered conventional hurdles, but prior to hurdling over barriers. A steeplechase barrier can be set up on the infield grass and padded with an old wrestling mat or futon to reduce the risk of injury when athletes begin to hurdle the barriers. Pads can also be placed on the ground on either side of their line of approach and exit. If and when they do hit the barrier, the risk of injury will be low and they can then walk away with the benefit of a sobering lesson.

Sometimes athletes will develop a mental block, fixate on a barrier, or some other aspect of hurdling technique, thereby suffering both a break in concentration and movement. In this case, the coach can sit or kneel about 15 yards down the track and suggest that the athletes focus on the coach's eyes as they clear the barrier or water jump hazard.

> *If I plan to enter this particular young man in a steeplechase again, I owe it to his parents to make sure he knows how to fall without killing himself. I made him take swimming last year...*
>
> —Bill Bowerman, on why he made Kenny Moore take gymnastics

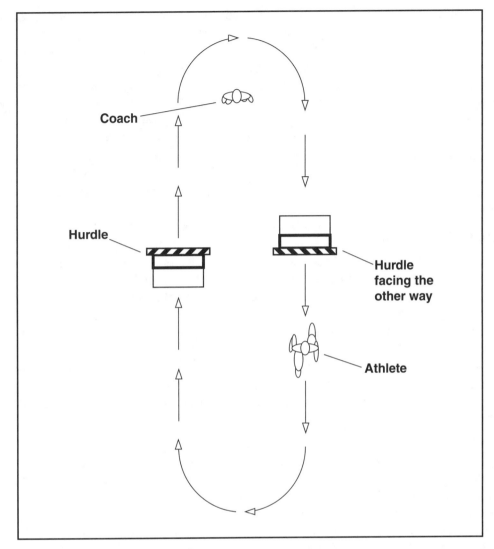

Figure 15.2—Top plan view, "the ritual"

Breathing and the Steeplechase

Steeplechasers need to be aware of their breathing, and should train their breath control. Often, steeplechasers inhale while leading with the knee and pause their breathing momentarily until their trail leg comes up. They then exhale forcefully, simultaneously thrusting the elbow of their lead arm back as they drive their lead foot towards the surface and descend over the hurdle or barrier. It is normal for a quick inhale to accompany actions that raise one's center of gravity. However, a markedly interrupted breathing technique is undesirable in the steeplechase. And generally, the slower and poorer the athletes' technique, the longer this breathing interruption will be. This can pose a problem, since steeplechasers need all the oxygen they can get to race well over 3,000 meters. For every fraction of a second that athletes interrupt their ventilation, they likely lose at least twice that much time in the race. Steeplechasers need to learn how to breathe while bending forward from the waist, and can practice this from the sitting L7 position. It can also help for steeplechasers to practice some hypoxic training—that is, to occasionally run or swim a short distance while holding their breath. Puffing your cheeks and exhaling forcefully while coming off a barrier can also place some backpressure on the lungs and aid in oxygenation of the blood. With improved technique, the amount of time spent over the barriers will decrease and this will reduce disturbance to the breathing and running rhythm of the athletes. As a result, when the pace approaches 70 seconds/400 meters there is less of a performance difference between a two-mile run on the flat and the 3,000 meters steeplechase. In this regard, a performance differential of 20 seconds or less becomes possible.

Steeplechase Footwear

It is difficult to find suitable footwear for the steeplechase. For a number of years, Nike, Inc. has manufactured a limited quantity of track spikes exclusively for the steeplechase, but the availability of the product fluctuates. Often, only the top collegiate athletes and promotional athletes have been able to obtain a pair. Further, the extremely lightweight construction of the shoe does not lend itself to prolonged use. Often, only one or two races can be run in the shoes before they need to be retired. Few other shoe manufacturers have even considered making a specialty shoe for this event. Historically, Adidas, AG has produced fine specialty shoes for many sport activities, and a good product for the steeplechase called the "Adistar Steeplechase" is presently available.

In general terms, the steeplechase spike needs to be lightweight, even after being immersed in water. It requires ventilation means for shedding water. And it should elevate the heel by about a centimeter. It can help for the forefoot spike plate to be covered with a layer of synthetic rubber, or thermoplastic material with good adhesive properties *vis-á-vis* the wet and often painted surface of the water jump barrier. In order to better push off and extend over the water hazard, the forefoot area of the track spikes should be able to flatten, and even plantarflex, when athletes step and extend from the water jump barrier. Accordingly, it is sometimes advantageous to cut flex grooves into the forefoot area of the track spike plate so that it will be capable of articulating in the desired manner.

Warm-Up Routine

A proper warm-up routine for steeplechasers includes preliminary and light flexibility work to attain full range of motion in the major joints. This should be followed by a warm-up to break a sweat and attain a pulse rate of 120 bpm. Whenever possible, it is beneficial to warm-up and warm-down by running barefoot, but with hurdlers or steeplechasers this is almost an imperative. If grass is not available, a rubberized track surface can be preferable to not running barefoot at all. Barefoot running does a great deal to enhance proprioception and plantarflexion. After running barefoot, athletes experience a heightened awareness regarding their feet and will be up on their toes instead of down on their heels. Whenever possible, they should complete their warm-up by running 10 x 100 meters diagonally across the infield, then jog a fast 50 meters to the opposite side in a continuous fashion. Athletes should then stretch in earnest and focus on the major muscle groups by conducting the following in sequence: static stretching, PNF, and then dynamic flexibility exercises, including the continuous Yoga-like routine presented in Chapter 7. Having accomplished this, steeplechasers will be ready for hurdle exercises such as "the ritual," described previously.

Integrating Running and Technique Work

The 3,000-meter steeplechaser's background conditioning and sharpening work generally corresponds to that of a 1,500-meter sided 5,000-meter runner. The conditioning requirements have been addressed in Chapters 1-6. During the base and hill periods, steeplechasers should practice their hurdle technique two or three times each week, whereas during the sharpening period they should actually be hurdling over obstacles once a week. Nevertheless, athletes should guard against conducting too much work over obstacles, since the associated shock loading can take a toll and result in injury. Accordingly, strive to integrate the required technique work with the general conditioning and sharpening work approximately three times a week in a sensible manner.

When working with novice steeplechasers, it is best to teach and practice new hurdle techniques when they are fresh. This would suggest doing technique work in a morning session, or prior to the primary afternoon training session. It can also help to conduct technique work on easy recovery days after the more demanding conditioning work performed the day before. However, once athletes have acquired the necessary technique, they also need to condition themselves to hurdling and taking barriers while in a state of fatigue, since that is what they will experience in actual competition. To do this, barriers can be placed next to an open lane, thus enabling the athletes to run on the flat or over obstacles during the sharpening workouts or time trials. In particular, when they are running distances longer than 400 meters, such as 800, 1,000, 1,200 or 1,600 meters, the athletes can then run alternating laps on the flat and over obstacles. In contrast with novice athletes, experienced steeplechasers can sometimes practice lead-leg and trail-leg drills, or hurdle obstacles after a demanding training session.

Determining Correct Split Times When Competing At Various Facilities

Track and field facilities differ in their geometry and positioning of the water jump, hence both the starting line position and the split times given can vary greatly. Coaches and athletes should then familiarize themselves with the projected split times for each particular track and field facility. Hislop calculates split times at various facilities by using the information provided in Table 15.1 (Hislop, 1984). For example, if an athlete wants to run 8:40 for the steeplechase at a facility with an outside water jump and the starting line is 50 meters from the finish line, then the calculations would appear as follows:

- 8:40 = 520 seconds = 1.73 seconds per 10 meters
- 5 X (1.73 seconds, from Table 15.1) = 8.65 seconds
- 520 seconds - 8.65 seconds = 511.35 seconds
- 511.35 seconds divided equally into 7 laps = 73 seconds/400 meters pace

In the case of a facility having an inside water jump and a starting line 230 meters from the finish line—then the calculations would appear as follows:

- 8:40 = 520 seconds = 1.73 seconds per 10 meters
- 23 X (1.73 seconds, from Table 15.1) = 39.8 seconds.
- 520 seconds - 39.8 seconds = 480.2 seconds.
- 480.2 seconds divided equally into 7 laps = 68.5 seconds/400 meters pace.

Racing

Athletes are wise to take the precaution of stepping the first barrier, since in the first lap the field is normally bunched-up and there can be a lot of jostling. In the abstract, there are only three good positions when running the first 2,400 meters of the steeplechase: in a lead group of no more than three or four athletes and positioned right off someone's shoulder, in lane two or three outside of the pack, or within striking distance behind the pack. If athletes are tangled up in the pack or boxed in along the rail, then they are simply in danger of hitting a barrier or crashing at the water jump. Prudent athletes will stay out of trouble because in the steeplechase that translates into hitting a barrier, or having a disaster at the water jump. Athletes with a superior fitness level can sometimes run clear of the field and avoid the problem. Other athletes can adopt the tactic of sitting behind the pack, and later make a deliberate move past the group to attain a favorable position. Sometimes an athlete can move from behind the pack and make a breakaway in the space of 100 meters.

Many athletes will greatly accelerate as they approach the barriers, since this facilitates hurdling. However, this common practice can also be a substitute for poor hurdling technique and inferior conditioning. And it is an expensive substitute, because these changes in pace represent an inefficient use of limited energy reserves. Better to have well conditioned specific muscle groups and a more efficient hurdling technique. Sometimes steeplechasers can make significant gains by improving the speed of their immediate attack and hurdling technique, rather than by accelerating greatly over the 15 meters preceding each obstacle.

Even pacing in the early laps of a steeplechase can be crucial to a successful performance. If athletes go out too fast, they can slow greatly in the middle or late portions of a race and this will make hurdling that much more difficult. In the steeplechase, there are enough disturbances of rhythm and pace due to hurdling the obstacles, and so the novice should not compound matters with uneven pacing. However, the race tactics of elite American athletes are sometimes far too predictable. In the United States, the steeplechase event has been dominated by a handful of individuals over the past 20 years. These athletes generally pace

8:00 = 480 seconds = 1.60 seconds per 10 meters

8:05 = 485 seconds = 1.61 seconds per 10 meters

8:10 = 490 seconds = 1.63 seconds per 10 meters

8:15 = 495 seconds = 1.65 seconds per 10 meters

8:20 = 500 seconds = 1.66 seconds per 10 meters

8:25 = 505 seconds = 1.68 seconds per 10 meters

8:30 = 510 seconds = 1.70 seconds per 10 meters

8:35 = 515 seconds = 1.71 seconds per 10 meters

8:40 = 520 seconds = 1.73 seconds per 10 meters

8:45 = 525 seconds = 1.75 seconds per 10 meters

8:50 = 530 seconds = 1.76 seconds per 10 meters

8:55 = 535 seconds = 1.78 seconds per 10 meters

9:00 = 540 seconds = 1.80 seconds per 10 meters

9:05 = 545 seconds = 1.81 seconds per 10 meters

9:10 = 550 seconds = 1.83 seconds per 10 meters

9:15 = 555 seconds = 1.85 seconds per 10 meters

9:20 = 560 seconds = 1.86 seconds per 10 meters

9:25 = 565 seconds = 1.88 seconds per 10 meters

9:30 = 570 seconds = 1.90 seconds per 10 meters

9:35 = 575 seconds = 1.91 seconds per 10 meters

9:40 = 580 seconds = 1.93 seconds per 10 meters

9:45 = 585 seconds = 1.95 seconds per 10 meters

9:50 = 590 seconds = 1.97 seconds per 10 meters

9:55 = 595 seconds = 1.98 seconds per 10 meters

TABLE 15.1—Times for the 3,000-Meter Steeplechase (Hislop, 1984, reproduced with permission)

themselves evenly and then attack with less than two laps remaining, or simply run away from the field. Not often do we see dramatic surging, or a hard breakaway attempt in the fourth or fifth lap, or even someone hurdling the water jump. Athletes need to be prepared for these tactics when competing in a field that includes the Kenyans.

The steeplechase is a highly technical event, but athletes should not over-intellectualize during competition. Rather, the goal is to become so proficient that the execution of proper technique will not interfere with the ability to concentrate and focus.

> *In possession of infallible technique, the individual places himself at the mercy of inspiration.*
> —Daisetz Suzuki

References

Adams, William, "Steeplechasing," *Track and Field Quarterly Review*, Volume 79, Number 3, 1979, pages 50-52.

Alford, Jim, "Steeplechase," *Track and Field Quarterly Review*, Volume 79, Number 3, 1979, pages 57-59.

Amery, Richard, "Australia's Kerry O'Brien," *Track and Field Quarterly Review*, Volume 72, Number 2, page 98.

Benson, Tony, "Steeplechasing: The Art of Interrupted Running," *Track and Field Quarterly Review*, Volume 93, Number 2, 1993, pages 27-29.

Bowerman, Bill, "Steeple Chase Training," *Proceedings of the International Track & Field Coaches Association, IX Congress*, George Dales, Editor, Santa Monica, California, July 30-August 2, 1984, pages 41-43.

Bowerman, Bill, *Coaching Track and Field*, William H. Freeman, Editor, Boston, Massachusetts: Houghton Mifflin Co., 1974.

Buehler, Al, and Roger Beardmore, "The 3000 meter Steeplechase," *Scholastic Coach*, Volume 44, Number 7, March, 1975, page 16, pages 116-117.

Bush, Jim, "Hurdles-Technique and Training," *Proceedings of the International Track & Field Coaches Association, IX Congress*, George Dales, Editor, Santa Monica, California, July 30-August 2, 1984, pages 29-31.

Cerutty, Percy, *Success: In Sport and Life*, London: Pelham Books Ltd., 1967.

Dellinger, Bill, and George Beres, *Winning Running*, Chicago, Illinois: Contemporary Books, Inc., 1978.

Dyson, Geoffrey, *The Mechanics of Athletics*, London: University of London Press, 1962.

Elder, A.C., and A.H. Thompson, "Water Jump Clearance Analysis," *Track Technique*, Number 29, September 1967, pages 923-925.

Elliott, Charles, "Steeplechase: Technical Analysis," *Track and Field Quarterly Review*, Volume 72, Number 2, 1972, pages 96-97.

Fisher, Bill, "The Steeplechase," *Track and Field Quarterly Review*, Volume 82, Number 3, 1982, pages 39-40.

Fix, David, and Nancy Smith, "Analysis Chart for Steeplechase Water Jumping," *Track and Field Quarterly Review*, Volume 84, Number 3, 1984, pages 23-25.

Gambetta, Vern, *Hurdling and Steeplechasing*, Mountain View, California: World Publications, August Runner's World Booklet of the month, Number 35, 1974.

Gartland, John, and Phil Henson, "A Comparison of the Hurdle SC Water Barrier Technique with the Conventional Water Barrier Technique," *Track and Field Quarterly Review*, Volume 84, Number 3, 1984, pages 26-28.

Griak, Roy, "Steeplechase—Points to Remember," *Track and Field Quarterly Review*, Volume 82, Number 3, 1982, page 41.

Hartwick, Barry, "The 3,000m Steeplechase," *Track and Field Quarterly Review*, Volume 81, Number 3, 1981, pages 43-56.

Hessel, Del G., "The Steeplechase - A Unique Event," *Track and Field Quarterly Review*, Volume 81, Number 3, 1981, pages 41-42.

Hislop, Chick, *Conversation on the Steeplechase*, Eugene, Oregon, 1999.

Hislop, Chick, "Distance Hurdle Technique," *Distance Running Elite Clinic for Steeplechasers*, Ogden, Utah, 1995.

Hislop, Chick, "Flexibility And Wall Drills For The Distance Hurdler," *Distance Running Elite Clinic for Steeplechasers*, Ogden, Utah, 1995.

Hislop, Chick, "Steeplechase Technique," *Proceedings of the International Track & Field Coaches Association, IX Congress*, George Dales, Editor, Santa Monica, California, July 30-August 2, 1984, pages 44-47.

Huntsman, Stan, "The Distance Training of Doug Brown," *Track and Field Quarterly Review*, Volume 73, Number 3, 1973, pages 178-179.

Jarver, Jess, Editor, "The Hurdles: Contemporary Theory," *Technique and Training*, Los Altos, California: TAFnews Press, 1981.

Kressler, Raymond, "Rider College Steeplechase Clinic," *Track and Field Quarterly Review*, Volume 71, Number 1, 1971, pages 35-38.

Lindeman, Ralph, "400 Meter Hurdle Theory," *Track and Field Coaches Review*, Volume 95, Number 1, 1995, pages 33-36.

McFarlane, Brent, "Pool Training... It Works!," *Proceedings of the International Track & Field Coaches Association, XIV Congress*, George Dales, Editor, Atlanta, Georgia: July 22-25, 1996, pages 196-198.

McFarlane, Brent, *The Science of Hurdling*, Ottawa, Canada: The Canadian Track and Field Association, 1999.

Nehemiah, Renaldo, "Mechanics of High Hurdles," *Track and Field Coaches Review*, Volume 95, Number 1, 1995, pages 39-41.

Popov, T., "3000 meter Steeplechase Hurdle Clearance," *Track and Field Quarterly Review*, Volume 79, Number 3, 1979, page 60.

Ross, Wilber L., *The Hurdler's Bible*, 2nd Edition, Arlington, Virginia: Yates Printing Company, 1969.

Saunders, Tony, "Steeplechase Technique and Training," *Track Technique*, Number 35, March 1969, pages 1102-1103.

Suzuki, Daisetz, *Zen and Japanese Culture*, Princeton, New Jersey: Bollinger Foundation, Inc., Princeton University Press, 1973.

Warhurst, Ron, "Training for Distance Running and the Steeplechase," *Track and Field Quarterly Review*, Volume 85, Number 3, 1985, pages 13-14.

Watts, Denis, "Hints on Steeplechasing," *Track Technique*, Number 41, September 1970, pages 1306-1307.

Werner, Chick, "The Steeplechase," *Track in Theory and Technique*, Richmond, California: Worldwide Publishing Co., 1962.

Wiger, Chick, "The 3000 meter Steeplechase," *Track and Field Quarterly Review*, Volume 79, Number 3, 1979, pages 53-56.

Will-Weber, Mark, Editor, *The Quotable Runner*, Halcottsville, New York: Breakaway Books, 2001.

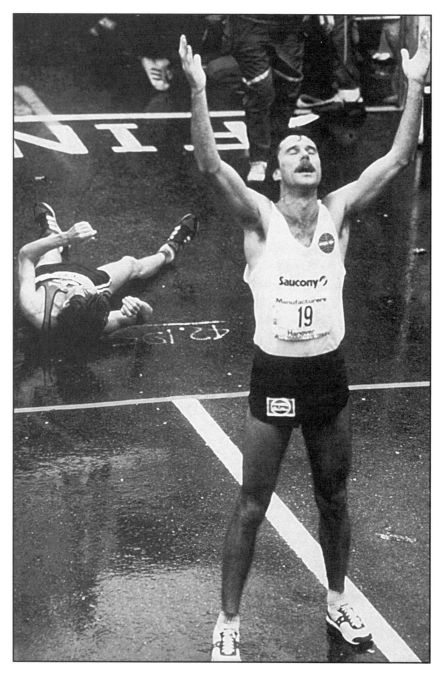

PHOTO 16.1—The agony and ecstasy of the marathon. Rod Dixon with arms outstretched in victory and Geoff Smith lying exhausted at the finish of the 1983 New York Marathon. Photo by Barbara Kinney. Copyright USA TODAY, 1983. Reprinted with permission.

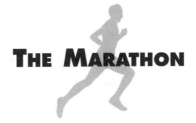

CHAPTER 16

THE MARATHON

Legend has it that Pheidippides, the ancient Greek messenger who ran to Athens to announce the defeat of the Persians in the battle of Marathon, died after completing his mission. However, this is likely the "Hollywood" version of events, since he was actually one of the highly conditioned *hemerodromoi*, or intercity messengers of ancient Greece, and he had already covered a much longer distance of about 140 miles the previous day, in a vain attempt to solicit the help of the Spartans (Newsholme, Leech, Duester, 1994). In conjunction with the 1908 London Olympic games, the distance of the marathon event was fixed at 26 miles 365 yards, since that was the distance required to finish before the King and Queen's booth. The marathon tends to conjure up images of dreaming the impossible dream and beating the unbeatable foe, but the truth is, there is nothing especially sacred or noble about this distance.

Recreational Runners and the Marathon

Thirty years ago, only a few hundred people would participate in marathon events, but today the contestants number in the tens of thousands. The question is whether this is truly a positive development with respect to the health and welfare of the participants? The author believes that it would have been better for today's participants if the distance between Marathon and Athens had been half as long, and if the position of the Royal booth had cut the course even shorter. Why? For the answer, we need only to look at the effects of running the marathon on both elite athletes and recreational runners.

> *Why couldn't Pheidippides have died here?*
>
> —Frank Shorter, upon reaching the 16 mile mark in one of his first marathons

Elite Runner Marathon Casualties

Given the present national and world marks, an elite athlete will have to cover upwards of 100 miles per week in their training to be competitive at this distance. If you survey the top twenty marathon runners in the world, the average weekly mileage during the base period now exceeds 120 miles per week, and a few even cover over 160 miles per week—more mileage than some put on their cars. And in this country, most of the training will be conducted on asphalt roads and in athletic shoes. The horse can cover such distances naturally and normally, but humans are configured to do so by walking rather than running. The amount of work that athletes must put forth to be competitive at this distance imposes chronic training over-loads. Many marathon athletes retire after suffering a debilitating injury or poor health, rather than because of the allure of more attractive prospects outside the sport. If one follows the history of elite marathon runners into retirement, there exist clear indications of premature arthritis and lingering soft tissue injury. In some cases, athletes who have over-trained suffer endocrine problems (Barron, Noakes, Levy, Smith, Millar, 1985).

Recreational Runner Marathon Casualties

Often the recreational runner assumes a considerable training over-load merely by attempting to complete the marathon distance. Some attempt as much in one day as they might normally cover in almost a week. It is not a sound training practice to increase the training load in a workout by over 10% in a single session. However, many recreational runners assume many times that by competing in a marathon. The results are predictable. Too many runners suffer injuries from dramatically increasing their training in preparation for this event, but also as the direct result of having completed a marathon. Unfortunately, individuals with relatively little training are sometimes encouraged to participate in a marathon, and numerous books exist which include advice for novice runners who wish to make the attempt.

The author wishes to de-bunk and deflate some of the current mystique surrounding the marathon, since he does not believe that it constitutes the best focus for recreational distance runners who are truly interested in cultivating their long-term physical and mental health. Of course, many distance runners want to run a marathon at least once in their lifetime, and for some individuals, once will be enough. In this case, the athlete will likely have three to five years of training background, and a solid foundation upon which to base an effort in the marathon. Even so, recreational and even elite distance runners generally should not compete in more than one or two marathons during a calendar year. And the vast majority of recreational distance runners are perhaps best advised to forego the marathon. Instead, it can be far healthier for them to focus their training and racing efforts on shorter distances in the range between the mile and 10,000 meters.

> *To describe the agony of a marathon to someone who's never run it is like trying to explain color to someone who was born blind.*
>
> —Jerome Drayton

Down And Out For A Month

Following a full effort in the marathon, both elite and recreational runners are normally hobbled for several days. This is due in part to injury from shock loading and eccentric muscle contractions, but also the consumption of muscle protein during the event (Janssen, 1987). A great deal depends upon how well athletes prepare for the marathon, and how they subsequently manage their recovery. It generally takes about a month for individuals to feel they have recovered. This puts the activity into proper perspective—ask yourself what other trauma or physical activities require such an extended recovery period. Many broken bones mend in five to six weeks, and following a blood donation, an individual's blood profile restores to normal in approximately the same amount of time. Accordingly, you might do well to weigh the decision to run a marathon at full effort as you would an injury or a minor surgery that requires at least a month of recuperation.

The Marathon As Mental Therapy

So why do it? The main character in the film *Forrest Gump* started running across the continent because he suffered a broken heart. Perhaps the historical inspiration for this character was Arthur Newton, who started running long distances after his wife left their African plantation. He subsequently traversed nearly every continent, but with the exception of Antarctica. It might have been a lot easier to find another woman. Running is sometimes a physical manifestation of psychological denial—a way to run away from something. And it can lend itself to obsessive and compulsive behavior. Preparing for and running a marathon seldom provides a viable solution for an individual's personal and emotional problems. It is far better to face those problems directly, and constructively address the demons that sometimes arise. Life is short. Do not take the path of Forrest Gump, or similarly, spend several years following telephone poles and train tracks like the character Travis in the film *Paris Texas*. As clinical psychologist Dr. Scott Pengelly sometimes says to athletes or patients: "De-nial... is not the name of a river in Egypt" (Pengelly, 1988-1997).

Sometimes uttering the phrase, "I'm doing a marathon," is a cry for attention. It can be a plea for help from an individual suffering from low self-esteem, who is seeking external remedy and support via kind words, love, and peer group acceptance. However, the remedy for low self-esteem does not lie in externals, but rather, in an internal process of self-cultivation. If you really want to develop internal power and self-respect, then run the marathon distance alone in practice, take a long drink of water, and don't say a word about it to anyone.

Distance running can be a form of moving meditation, but it's not a religion, nor is it a unique, mystical, transcendental experience. Indeed, it can have mystical and transcendental moments, but no more so than any other activity in which an individual cultivates excellence. Activities such as writing a novel, or volunteering to help others in need, normally exceed the social value of running a marathon. Accordingly, it is good to keep these things in perspective.

The Mile Versus The Marathon

If you are a recreational distance runner and concerned with cultivating long-term physical and mental health, then you would be best advised to train and compete at shorter distances in the range between the mile and 10,000 meters. It is possible to prepare for these events by training as little as 20 to 40 miles per week, thus greatly reduce the risk of suffering an over-use injury. This is a more manageable training load for individuals of any age, particularly when the recreational athlete has other more important priorities and responsibilities in life. Further, an event like the mile requires a balance of aerobic and anaerobic abilities, and is a healthier distance both for which to train and compete. It is also a truer test of an athlete's overall fitness and running ability. That is why the 1,500 meters and mile remains the glamour event of track and field.

Training for the mile or 5,000 meters also makes more sense from the standpoint of how our bodies age. As we become older, our metabolism tends to shift from anabolism towards catabolism. For example, a man does not normally have as much testosterone going at age 45 as he did at 20. So to maintain health and fitness, it is generally advisable to place a greater emphasis on strength training as we age. It is now widely accepted that the elderly can often benefit greatly from a sensible strength-training program, and in part, due to the youthful response thereby solicited from the endocrine system (Campbell, Crim, Young, and Evans, 1994). Preparing for and competing in longer events (15 kilometers to the marathon) tends to render an individual's metabolism more catabolic, and that is not what most middle-aged or elderly people having a normal body weight really want or need in order to enhance their general health (Kuoppasalmi, et al., 1980, Tanaka, et al., 1986, Bonen, et al, 1987, Hackney, et al., 1988, Arce, et al., 1993, Jensen, et al., 1995, Urhausen, et al., 1995).

So You Still Want to Run a Marathon?

If you are a recreational distance runner with positive physical and mental reasons for running a marathon, then you might consider the following advice: Run the event at only 1/4 or 1/2-effort, and do not attempt to run any harder. If the difference between a full effort and a 1/2-effort is a marathon run in 2:36 versus 2:48, or 3:00 versus 3:18, what does the time really matter? If you finish still feeling relatively well in 3:18 when you can actually run about 3:00, are you a lesser individual by 18 minutes? One thing is certain, at 1/2-effort you will normally feel recovered within a few days or a week, but if you race full out, a month later you might still be feeling injured and exhausted. Start the marathon running easily, and slower than your approximate target pace. If you have need to travel to find a marathon event, then pick one with pleasant weather and a beautiful course. Stop and smell the roses along the way. If near the ocean, perhaps attempt to go surfing afterwards. Make the experience a small part of your larger vacation plans. People sometimes make the process of preparing and competing in a marathon the center of their lives, and behave as though it were the quest for the Holy Grail. In truth, the marathon is three hours of your life, more or less, on a Saturday or Sunday morning.

> *If you feel bad at 10 miles, you're in trouble. If you feel bad at 20 miles you're normal. If you don't feel bad at 26 miles, you're abnormal.*
>
> —Rob de Castella

A Marathon Training Schedule for Recreational Distance Runners

Let's say you are training about 40 miles per week and cultivating your fitness for the mile and 5,000 meters, but then decide you want to run a marathon. How should you train for it? In brief, you should hardly change anything at all. Simply, gradually extend the duration of the easy long run you normally undertake on the weekend. If 60 to 80 minutes has been the habit, then slowly build up to 90, and then to 100 minutes. On the last weekend of a given training meso-cycle in the base and hill periods, attempt to run for a full 110 to 120 minutes, but not beyond 120 minutes unless the spirit moves you. And during this run, do not be afraid to stop for a drink of water, a bathroom break, or to view the scenery. During the course of the athletic season, race anywhere between 1,500 meters to 15 kilometers in the usual manner by placing competitions at the end of a worthwhile break. Plan to race a distance no longer than 8,000 meters or five miles, somewhere between 10 to 14 days prior to the marathon event. Recover from this race over the next four to six days, then time trial—that is, run a distance between 1,500 and 3,000 meters at 3/4-effort on the fifth or sixth day before the Marathon. Recover over the next two or three days and then run a few relaxed stride-outs at 200 meters, no faster than 1,500 meters goal pace, on the third day before the marathon.

Given this approach, if you are fit enough to run a five-minute mile while only covering 40 miles per week, you will likely be far better off on race day than someone else who can only turn a mile in 5:30 as the result of so-called "marathon training." On race day, remember not to run the marathon at greater than 1/2-effort. An abstract schedule which could be suitable for a distance runner for the last 14 days preceding the marathon is provided:

14 Race 8,000 meters
13 Active Recovery
12 Easy Effort, Long Run, but not longer than 100 minutes.
11 Passive Recovery
10 1/2-Effort, Fartlek + 2-3(4 x 200m) at 1,500m goal pace
 9 Active Recovery
 8 Easy Effort, Long Run, but not longer than 80 minutes
 7 Passive Recovery
 6 3/4-Effort, Time Trial 1,500m-3,000m, or conduct the same distance in the uneven pace manner of the 30-40 drill
 5 Active Recovery
 4 Finishing Speed 6-8 x 200m at 1,500m goal pace
 3 Active Recovery
 2 Easy Recovery
 1 Day Before Race Routine
 0 Marathon

Ultras and Ironman Triathlon Events

Some individuals might wonder about participating in "Ultra" events such as 50-mile, 100-mile, or Ironman Triathlon events. From a long-term perspective, the benefit of these activities for athletes is questionable, since severe trials of this kind can threaten their subsequent motivation, fitness, and health. If you want to participate in ultra events, make sure your reasons for doing so are positive. The body with which you have been blessed is the only one that you will ever have.

Advice for Elite Distance Runners Attempting the Marathon

What about the elite athlete who desires to compete in the marathon? Appendix I provides an example of a marathon schedule for an elite athlete. However, it is important to address a number of common questions and mistakes regarding marathon preparation.

Perhaps the first great mistake for an elite athlete is to "become a marathoner," since to many this unfortunately means:

- Running high mileage in excess of 120 miles per week
- Conducting frequent interval or repetition workouts at marathon goal pace, such as sessions covering 15 kilometers including repetitions between one and five miles in distance
- Running predominantly road races and distances exceeding 8,000 meters

Within a year or two of engaging in this type of training most would-be marathoners have been reduced to economical shufflers. Their performances at 1,500 meters, 5,000 meters and 10,000 meters can regress significantly. In truth, they have lost some of the tools necessary to succeed at the highest level, even in the marathon event.

Elite athletes who desire to succeed in the marathon should only compete in this event once a year. Other than the possible need to qualify for a major international competition, there is only one reason for elite athletes to compete in more than one marathon a year—money. And if athletes are not in great need of money, the reason can sometimes be traced to vanity. Greed is the great killer of athletic careers.

If elite athletes desire to preserve the longevity of their careers and ability to perform in the marathon, they need to maintain their ability to compete on the track at the national and international levels in the 5,000 and 10,000 meters. For this reason, they should occasionally compete in off-distances, such as 1,500 and 3,000 meters, during the track season. One of the two athletic seasons conducted each year should then be directed towards the track, and the other to the marathon. This strikes a healthy balance and can permit improvement during both seasons. Training for the marathon then becomes preparation for the track season, and vice-versa.

For example, when Emil Zatopek won the marathon in the 1952 Olympic Games, it was after first winning the 5,000 and 10,000 meters. That was before the Olympic Games grew to such an extent that the 5,000 and 10,000 meters required numerous qualifying rounds. Frank Shorter and Kenny Moore placed first and fourth in the 1972 Olympic Marathon, and to date, this remains the best finish by the United States. At that time, both men were fit to run quality performances at 5,000 and 10,000 meters. Moore recalls running 13:44 for 5,000 meters in Scandinavia prior to the marathon, and being disqualified after having been shoved off the track by Jos Hermans and forced to make a detour through the long jump pit (Moore, 1999). In the 1972 Olympic Games, Frank Shorter placed fifth in the 10,000 meters final, and then eight days later won the Gold Medal in the marathon. In 1976, Shorter had won the 10,000 meters event in the Olympic Trials, but did not risk running the event in the Olympic Games, since he had developed a stress fracture in his foot. He then placed second in the Olympic marathon behind Valdemar Cierpinski (Shorter, 1999). Lasse Viren still managed to place fifth in the 1976 Olympic marathon after weathering numerous preliminary rounds en route to winning the 5,000 and 10,000 meters. Carlos Lopes ran 27:17.48 behind Fernando Mamede's 10,000 meters world record of 27:13.81 on July 2, then won the marathon in a time of 2:09.21 on August 12 in the 1984 Olympic Games. This makes the point that athletes should not move up to the marathon simply because their marks at 5,000 or 10,000 meters are not what they would like. In truth, if athletes cannot perform well in these events, they are not going to be competitive in the marathon against national or world-class performers. In this regard, recognize that an athlete who can run 10,000 meters at 4:30 per mile pace is likely to be just as efficient as one who can only run 10,000 meters at 4:45 per mile pace. When they meet and race in the range of 4:50 to 5:00-mile pace in the marathon, and the former athlete increases the pace to 4:40 at the 22-mile mark or makes a break with less than a kilometer to go, the outcome will normally be determined in his favor.

Accordingly, during the base and hill periods elite marathon runners should conduct the 3/4-effort anaerobic threshold and steady state training sessions between 10,000 meters and marathon goal pace. To maintain a high level of efficiency and running economy, they should once a week conduct an interval session consisting of something like 4 (4 x 200m), or 3 (4 x 300m) at 1,500 meters date pace, or 3-4 (4 x 400m) at 3,000 meters date pace. The quality of this session will then improve to goal pace during the sharpening period. This interval session can also serve to counteract the tendency of high mileage work to shift the blood pH too far towards the base side, particularly when athletes are training at altitude. During the sharpening period, athletes should essentially train as if preparing to compete in the 10,000 meters, except that they will need a longer than normal long run and higher overall mileage. Marathon runners need to be conditioned to run in excess of two hours. For this reason elite marathon runners should conduct a long run once every seven to 10 days. The maximum duration of the long run should gradually increase from two hours to over three hours by the end of the base and hill periods. In this regard, do not increase the duration of the long run every seven to 10 days, but rather only once every second or third week.

However, elite athletes should reduce the duration of the long run to less than or equal to two hours during the sharpening period, and then to less than 1:40 minutes during their taper or ascent to peak performance.

The Carbohydrate / Fatty Acid Threshold

To be successful in the marathon and even longer distances, athletes need to be able to efficiently use fatty acids as an energy source. At one time, many thought that carbohydrates were used almost exclusively for the first 90 minutes of the marathon, and when they were depleted, the runner would "hit the wall" and start using fatty acids as the primary energy source. What actually happens is a bit more complicated. When athletes are at rest or engaged in light exercise such as walking or easy running, most of their energy comes from fatty acids, particularly those in their blood plasma, and also their intramuscular triglycerides. In contrast to the adipose tissue you might find in the area of your "love handles" or thighs, which is essentially a useless form of fat unless you are facing starvation, the intramuscular triglycerides are stored in your muscle tissue. And a relatively small amount of fatty acids can provide a lot of energy—in particular, 35 kJ/ gram, as opposed to only 16 kJ/ gram for carbohydrates (Newsholme, Leech, and Duester, 1994). Think of the fatty acids as diesel fuel. It is not the best substrate for high-speed performance, but you can run economically for a long time while burning fatty acids. Aerobic lipolytic metabolism, or simply "fat metabolism," requires oxygen, whereas carbohydrates can be used both with oxygen (aerobic glycolysis) and without oxygen (anaerobic glycolysis) (Hawley, 1995). The energy demand of untrained athletes can largely be met by using fatty acids until they approach approximately 35% of their VO_2 maximum, but highly trained athletes can continue to use this substrate when performing at up to 65 to 70% of their VO_2 maximum (Hurley, 1986, Janssen, 1987, Sleamaker, 1989, Coyle, 1995, 1997).

Obviously, it is important for marathon runners to enhance their ability to use fat metabolism. The simple answer is quantity. Athletes need to assume relatively high mileage and distance runs having a long duration. This stimulates the creation of numerous mitochondria, capillaries, and large stores of intramuscular triglycerides. Figure 2.7 illustrates this training adaptation, and for convenience it is reproduced in this chapter as Figure 16.1.

Figure 16.1 suggests that fatty acid substrate use can be elevated to supply a substantial portion of the energy needed when functioning at 80% of VO_2 maximum. This may be pushing it with respect to distance runners, but the point is that an athlete's relative use of fatty acids as a substrate during exercise can be trained. As the body's total carbohydrate stores can only provide for about 90 minutes work in the marathon, greater relative use of fatty acids early on can spare the limited carbohydrate stores for later use. This can also help prevent or delay the more dramatic shift towards the use of fatty acids, commonly known as "hitting the wall," in the later stages of the marathon.

However, when athletes exercise at a rate or intensity that exceeds the ability of fat metabolism to provide the required energy, then carbohydrates must be

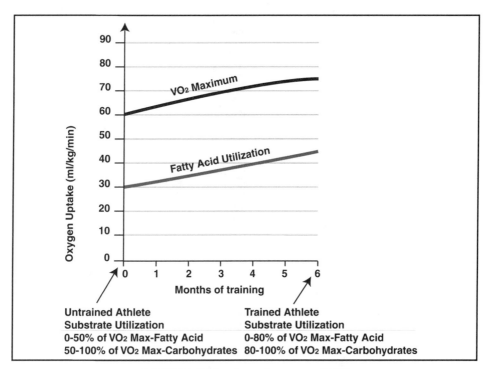

FIGURE 16.1—from Janssen, 1987

used to meet the energy demand. The primary limitation of fat metabolism is that it can only provide energy half as fast as aerobic glycolysis using carbohydrates. Further, the intramuscular triglycerides burn rather like diesel fuel, whereas carbohydrates burn like high-octane premium and provide more power. The process of aerobic glycolysis (i.e., burning carbohydrates in the presence of oxygen) produces twice the amount of ATP per unit time and 11% more energy than triglycerides (Newsholme and Leech, 1983, Janssen, 1987, Newsholme, Leech, and Duester, 1994, Coyle, 1995, 1997, and Autio, 2000). These carbohydrates are present in the form of blood glucose and are stored in the form of muscle glycogen and hepatic (liver) glycogen. When running a marathon, the approximate total energy that can be derived from *blood* glucose provides for 4 minutes, *muscle* glycogen 71 minutes, and *hepatic* glycogen 18 minutes of exercise (Newsholme and Leech, 1983). Some portion of fatty acids must then be used to cover the marathon distance. In truth, fatty acids and carbohydrates are both being used from the start of the marathon. But somewhere in the range between 35 to 70% of VO_2 maximum, the relative ratio of consumption shifts more dramatically towards carbohydrates whenever athletes exceed their carbohydrate/fatty-acid threshold (Sahlin, 1986, and, Brooks et al, 1994).

The point at which this transition takes place can be identified by both the respiratory quotient (RQ) and the onset of lactic acid accumulation. An RQ of .707 indicates that 100% of fatty acids are being used as substrates, whereas an RQ of 1.0 indicates that 100% of carbohydrates are being used as substrates. The point at which the total energy contribution comes equally from carbohydrates

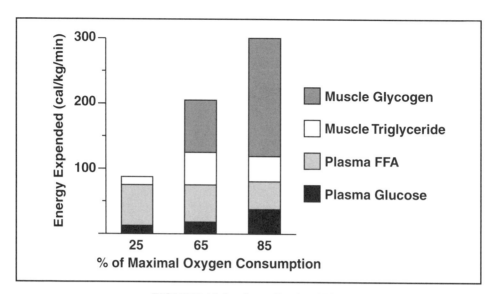

FIGURE 16.2—from Coyle, 1995

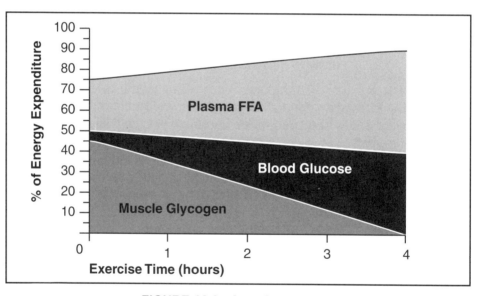

FIGURE 16.3—from Coyle, 1995

and fatty acids corresponds to a RQ of .85 (Brooks et al., 1994). One researcher investigated the relative amount of carbohydrates and fatty acids used when the amount of oxygen made available to runners was changed. The athletes exercised at 65% of VO_2 maximum and were provided with air containing 14%, 21%, and 30% oxygen. As a point of reference, air normally consists of about 21% oxygen at sea level. Given only 14% oxygen, the RQ was .965 and only 11.2% fatty acids were used. Given 21% oxygen, the RQ was .889 and 35.8% fatty acids were used. And given 30% oxygen, the RQ was .874 and 41.2% fatty acids were used (Linnarsson, 1974). The more oxygen that is available, the more that fatty acids can be used. Accordingly, when athletes are not acclimatized to altitude, or when they face hot and humid conditions, they will metabolize more

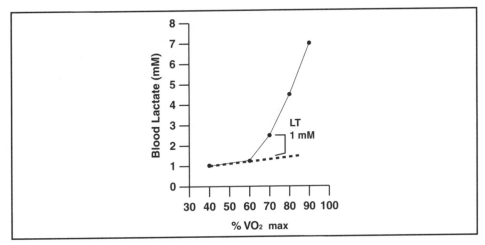

FIGURE 16.4—From Coyle, 1995

carbohydrates. Another researcher, studied the relative use of fatty acids when athletes exercised at various percentages of their VO_2 maximum. Fatty acids were found to provide 60% of the energy at 20% of VO_2 maximum, 53% of the energy at 50% of VO_2 maximum, 36% of the energy at 70% of VO_2 maximum, and three to 13% of the energy at 85 to 90% of VO_2 maximum (Pruett, 1970).

Figure 16.2 shows the relative use of fatty acids in the form of intramuscular triglycerides and plasma free fatty acids, and also that of carbohydrates in the form of muscle glycogen and plasma glucose, at various levels of exercise intensity. Figure 16.3 shows the percentage of energy produced by various substrates over time when exercising at 65 to 75% of VO_2 maximum.

Figures 16.2 and 16.3 are especially relevant to this discussion since it has been found that lactate accumulation typically begins in marathoners at about 70% of VO_2 maximum—and they maintain approximately 75% of VO_2 maximum during the event (Costill and Fox, 1969, Costill et al., 1973, Coyle, 1995). Coyle defines the lactate threshold as the intensity of exercise at which blood lactate concentration is 1mM above baseline (Coyle, 1995). Figure 16.4, adapted from Coyle, depicts a typical blood lactate accumulation curve for trained runners working at various percentages of their VO_2 maximum.

The blood lactate level in an individual at rest is normally approximately 1.0 mM. As indicated in Figure 16.4, the lactate threshold is at about 70% of VO_2 maximum and a blood lactate of 2.5 mM. This value may correspond with the carbohydrate/fatty-acid threshold of a highly trained athlete, which is different and lower than the anaerobic threshold corresponding to the heart-rate deflection point. The onset of lactate accumulation provides a concrete reference point for when the metabolism begins to shift from the use of fatty acids to carbohydrates, since fat metabolism is not associated with the production of blood lactate. The rate of blood lactate accumulation can vary considerably from one person to another, and also in the same individual, depending upon the nature of their training program and fitness level. Hence, there is nothing determinate about the particular lactate curve shown in Figure 16.4. Jack Daniels has found that well trained athletes consistently work at approximately 86 to 88% of their VO_2 maximum when conducting a one-hour steady state run (Daniels, 1999). This concrete result can then be used as a benchmark to assess and predict an athlete's performance potential at various distances. Moreover, this level of intensity closely corresponds to the anaerobic threshold and heart-rate deflection point of well-trained athletes. The blood lactate value associated with the anaerobic threshold most often seen in the literature is 4 mM. However, the actual blood lactate levels exhibited by distance runners commonly varies between 4 and 8 mM during a one hour steady state run (Daniels, 1999, Coyle, 1999, Costill, 1999).

Athletes can raise their carbohydrate/fatty-acid threshold by adopting a training protocol analogous to how the anaerobic threshold can be raised. But neither the anaerobic threshold steady state nor the evenly paced steady-state runs emphasized during the base and hill periods best accomplish this task. Both of these training activities have high intensities and require the predominant use of carbohydrates as fuel. Instead, the long run achieves this result. However, rather than conducting an easy long run at less than or equal to 1/4-effort, the competitive marathon runner should perform the long run at 1/2-effort, or slighter better—that is, between approximately 60 to 70% of their VO_2 maximum, right along the carbohydrate/fatty-acid threshold. By the end of the base and hill periods, the elite marathon athlete running at sea level does not then conduct the long run at 6:30 to 7:00 minutes pace, but rather at 6:00 minutes pace or even better, and for a duration in the range between two to three-and-a-half hours.

Kenny Moore, the fourth place finisher in the 1972 Olympic Marathon, confided that he built himself up to such a degree that he eventually covered 38 miles at 6:00 minute pace in his long run. Moore felt he needed to conduct an extremely long run to compensate for the fact that he did not and could not regularly exceed 90 miles a week in his training and remain injury free, whereas he knew that Frank Shorter would sometimes log 140 miles per week in preparation for the marathon (Moore, 1999). Shorter's long run lasted two hours and he ran it on paved roads. He would begin at about 6:00 minute pace, but then would increase the pace over the second half of the training session according to how well he felt (Shorter, 1999). However, you must also appreciate and factor in that this training session was sometimes being conducted on demanding terrain and at an altitude between 5,400 and 8,000 feet in Boulder, Colorado.

Therefore, the long run conducted at 1/2-effort, or slightly better, can be regarded as an essential ingredient for marathon success. Nevertheless, exercise physiologists do not fully understand how the body becomes more efficient at using fatty acids, or why otherwise comparable individuals exhibit such different blood lactate responses during exercise. However, a number of things provide us with some clues. Elite athletes with similar VO_2 maximums and anaerobic thresholds do not always have the same level of success at the marathon as they do at 5,000 and 10,000 meters. All other things being equal, the 80-to-90-mile per week athlete is not competitive with the 100-to-120-mile per week athlete when they line up in the marathon. And the latter tends to have difficulty competing with the 120-to-140-mile per week athlete. Generally, the talented 80-to-90-mile per week athlete will be a 2:14 to 2:20 marathoner, the 100-to-120-mile per week athlete a 2:10 to 2:12 marathoner, and the athlete running 120 to 140 miles per week a sub 2:10 marathoner. When training for the marathon, more than in any other running event, quantity does matter.

Elite athletes with many years of training might be able to slightly elevate their VO_2 maximum, anaerobic threshold, stroke volume, and both their muscle mitochondria and capillary density by taking on higher mileage and a long run lasting between two to three-and-a-half hours. However, the author does not believe that most of their subsequent improvement can be traced to these variables. Another possibility is optimization with respect to muscle fiber type, in particular, the Type I and Type IIc muscle fibers, and their related aerobic enzyme activity. Nevertheless, probably the greatest single variable influenced by taking on higher mileage and the two-to-three-and-a-half-hour run is running economy. To run 120 miles per week on a regular basis, athletes have to become extremely efficient, otherwise they soon beat themselves up and become injured. Frank Shorter had a VO_2 maximum of 71.3 ml/kg/min and Derek Clayton, a VO_2 maximum of 69.7 ml/kg/min, which are not especially high values for elite athletes, but both men had excellent running economy.

So far, this discussion of running economy has focused an athlete's gross mechanical efficiency. However, a more subtle aspect of running economy concerns an athlete's technique and application of force. It has been found with cyclists that athletes with a higher anaerobic threshold sometimes accomplish this task by distributing the power output over greater muscle mass (Coyle, 1995). This lowers the intensity of local muscle contractions, and can thereby result in less occlusion of blood supply. Further, this allows specific muscle fibers to be less frequently activated, permitting them more recovery time. And this probably also means they can use a greater proportion of fatty acids as a substrate and spare the use of carbohydrates while the athlete functions at a higher percentage of VO_2 maximum. This is important in helping to maintain elevated blood glucose levels in the latter stages of a marathon, thus avoid central fatigue and the dramatic shift towards using fatty acids that results in athletes "hitting the wall." It is also important for clearing blood lactate, which is produced when carbohydrates are being used as the primary substrate. Recognize that blood lactate and VO_2 maximum tests are gross indicators with respect to input and output, but they do not really tell us much about the actual use of oxygen and production of lactate within specific muscle groups.

Geoff Hollister at Nike, Inc. once commented that he had observed the wear pattern of Frank Shorter's shoes and remarked that Shorter used his entire foot—that is, he distributed the load and forces over a large surface area. Shorter estimates that he probably did about half of his training on natural surfaces, and he alternated periods of training at altitude in Boulder, Colorado with brief stays at sea level (Shorter, 1999). His running technique also stands out in the minds of many observers as both economic and graceful. The great Australian distance runners of the 1950's and 1960's conducted a significant portion of their training on natural surfaces, as do the African runners whenever training in their home country. Certainly, the amount of hip extension exhibited by the African runners is not found in athletes who do most of their running on asphalt. Further, when athletes run on natural terrain there is a constant, subtle variation and improvisation of their footplant, stride, arm carriage, hand gestures, and overall running technique. Their running tempo dictates the primary rhythm or melody, and to borrow two other words from the realm of music, they also have *Rubato* or *Descant*. As opposed to being robotic, the movements of these athletes appear relaxed, fluid, and artistic, as in dance. The introduction of spontaneous subtle variations and improvisations in running movements distributes the workload over more muscle mass. Unfortunately, this aspect of running economy is often overlooked. Emil Zatopek, the 1952 Olympic Champion at 5,000 meters, 10,000 meters and the marathon, was known for spontaneous variations in his running technique and facial expressions. When cornered by a reporter and asked about his unaesthetic technique, he simply replied that running was not like ice skating—it was not necessary to smile and please the judges, it was only necessary to run fast (Mader, 1979).

The Australian coach Percy Cerutty well understood this phenomenon, as evinced in the following excerpts (Cerutty, 1961):

> *Everything pulses in Nature; there is ebb and flow, a wave system is found in all or most things; nothing is static; nothing fixed or permanent; nothing without oscillation of some kind, yet athletes run as if their energy poured out in a steady stream... Running is movement, but variety in those movements is the essence of it...*
>
> *These cyclic wave motions are not necessarily very obvious, but the athlete must have them: must be conscious of them: able to vary and use them at will.*
>
> *Even the forward progression should be in a series of moving waves or cycle beats. Not necessarily obvious, but there, all the same. Everything in Nature conforms to a pulse or rhythm, to wave motions, surges and rest periods. The athlete must seek the means to use these things, to feel them in his own experience, if he would achieve the ends that lead to superlative performance.*
>
> —Percy Cerutty

Depletion of Muscle Glycogen during sustained exercise		
Duration of exercise (min.)	Content of glycogen ($\mu mol.g^{-1}$ fresh muscle)[†]	
	Untrained	Trained
0	94	100
20	39	55
40	22	39
60	11	14
80	0.6 (exhaustion)	11
90	—	0.16 (exhaustion)

*Data from Hermansen et al. (1967)
[†]Glycogen measured in quadriceps muscle after removal of biopsy sample

TABLE 16.1—from Newsholme, 1983

Some might interpret Cerutty's remarks as poetic, but the case can be made that he accurately described aspects of running economy and performance that have not yet received enough attention by exercise physiologists. Now with the advent of portable VO_2 maximum and lactate equipment, researchers might consider getting out into the field and observing what takes place when running on asphalt, grass, woodchips, and barefoot along the beach and over sand dunes. There may be something worthwhile to be learned from such field experiments.

Central Versus Peripheral Fatigue

Part of the phenomenon of "hitting the wall" has to do with the brain's reaction to the lowering of blood sugar and diminished reserves of carbohydrates. The brain can only use carbohydrates as a source of fuel. When blood sugar levels drop beyond a certain point, signaling that carbohydrate stores are approaching total depletion, the brain suddenly steps in as if to say: "Sorry muscles, but I have to save the rest here for me. You will have to burn mostly fatty acids and some proteins now." It is a matter of the central nervous system protecting itself, in contrast to peripheral fatigue. As shown in Table 16.1, a trained athlete can deplete muscle glycogen levels to a significantly lower level than an untrained individual before reaching exhaustion.

However, it does not appear that well trained athletes can actually change their characteristic concentration of blood glucose that triggers central fatigue. There are differences between individuals, but a highly trained an individual's central fatigue "magic number" for low blood glucose remains substantially the same over many years. Edward F. Coyle stated that he tested one subject over a period of 15 years in various states of fitness. Whenever the individual would hit a low glucose level of 2.5 mM, central fatigue would set in and the individual could invariably tell him when it happened (Coyle, 1999). Note that hypoglycemia can cause temporary mental impairment, loss of consciousness and coma, so do not take it lightly.

Low blood glucose is not the only contributor to central fatigue. The action of a number of neurotransmitters is also involved. Of the 20 amino acids, three branched-chain amino acids are oxidized in muscle as opposed to the liver. If the concentration of branched-chain amino acids in the blood decreases, then more tryptophan will enter the brain and cause more 5-HT (5-hydroxytryptamine, a neurotransmitter) to be produced. This substance acts as a depressant, inducing feelings of fatigue, decreased aggressiveness, and drowsiness (Newsholme, Leech and Duester, 1994).

Humans and other predatory animals tend to protect brain function by shutting down mechanical function so as to maintain blood glucose levels and sufficient carbohydrate stores. Some animals that rely solely on flight as a survival mechanism may not have the same safeguards or biochemical inhibitions. A horse or an antelope either outruns the bear or cheetah or it dies. These animals are then capable of literally running themselves to death. However, humans have survived in their struggle against other predators with the use of superior intelligence.

Altitude Training Is Essential

Elite athletes will also need to train at altitude to increase their red blood cell count and thereby enhance their aerobic ability. In 1972 and 1976 Frank Shorter lived in Boulder, Colorado, and alternated training at altitude with brief stays at sea level prior to his successful Olympic marathons. In contrast, Eastern Block athletes were then being drugged and doped. A study by Melvin Williams, published in 1981, showed an average increase in performance from blood re-infusion of about 10 seconds per mile for men running five miles in approximately 30 minutes (Williams, Wesseldine, Somma, and Schuster, 1981). This is slightly over a two-percent increase in performance and approximates the USATF's allowance of three percent for the outdoor championship qualifying standards in events 1,500 meters or longer, and performances delivered at facilities at 4,000 feet or more altitude. An honest athlete simply cannot afford to give that much of an advantage to a competitor who might be training at sea level but engaging in these practices. Neither can an athlete living at sea level expect to compete on equal footing in the marathon against those who live at altitude and run on demanding terrain, such as the Kenyans. Athletes wanting to compete at the international level in the marathon need, at least occasionally, to train at altitude (See Chapter 13).

Marathon Equipment

As discussed in Chapter 10, the selection of athletic footwear can significantly affect competitive results. Sometimes it is possible to achieve a two-ounce reduction in shoe weight over a stock commercial racing flat, and this is worth at least a full minute in the marathon. There is also the question of whether the spring stiffness of a given shoe is tuned to the individual's biomechanics and running technique. Again, Ned Frederick was able to demonstrate a change in oxygen uptake of approximately 1.3% in subjects running at racing speeds in NIKE AIR® racing flats, and such an improvement in running economy can be worth between one and three minutes in the marathon (Frederick, Clarke, Larsen, and Cooper, 1983). Adidas-Salomon AG introduced track spikes for the 2000 Olympic Games that claimed to provide an average improvement of 1.8% in running economy, and perhaps even as much as 4% (Nielsen, 2000). The author has also invented athletic shoes including carbon fiber spring elements that provide substantial improvement in running economy (U.S. 6,449,878). In brief, athletic shoes are undergoing a major transformation, but even the differences between any two conventional articles of footwear can be substantial. Athletes should select a lightweight shoe that provides optimal stiffness for their body mass and running technique, but also good heat dissipating qualities, traction, and overall performance for the anticipated environmental conditions.

As discussed in Chapter 12, athletes should test the apparel they would think to use or might be given as team issue. Despite the commercial claims, many so-called high technology fibers and materials do not perform well in the practical application: Buyer beware. Test the singlet both wet and dry in various environmental conditions to see how it behaves. A white singlet is generally best, and if direct sunlight and hot conditions are anticipated, athletes might wish to fashion a singlet with protection over the top of their shoulders, since this will reduce dehydration. Likewise, a white cap made of a material which does not retain heat, rather, includes vents, a visor, and an extension for covering the back of the neck can be helpful. The former Ironman Triathlon Champion Mark Allen made custom modifications to his apparel along these lines (Allen and Babbit, 1998). The right socks also need to be figured out well before a marathon. And given the various insoles used on racing flats, athletes should test their shoe and sock combination to really know if it works well. As discussed earlier, conventional athletic shorts with a restrictive inner liner may not help with heat dissipation and thermoregulation. And unless you expect to begin by running straight into the sun, do not use sunglasses, since they block the air stream from making contact with the area around your eyes. The head and face dissipate a significant amount of heat due to the high degree of vascularization in this area, and athletes are unwise to compromise this potential cooling effect.

Pre-Race Diet is Important

Athletes should make sure that their intramuscular triglyceride stores are not depleted going into a marathon. If athletes have been in hard training for several months, and do not sufficiently reduce their mileage two weeks prior to the marathon, then they may end up "hitting the wall." However, those who consume an adequate proportion of fatty acids from vegetable sources in their diet will less likely become depleted. Obviously, the use of intramuscular triglycerides as a substrate is even more important in competitive events having a longer duration, such as the Ironman Triathlon, or Tour de France. Accordingly, the intramuscular

Effect of diet on muscle glycogen content and duration of exercise*		
Diet and conditions	Muscle glycogen content before exercise (μmol.g^{-1})	Duration of exercise (min.)
1. Normal mixed diet	97	116
2. Low carbohydrate diet for three days	36	57
3. High carbohydrate diet for three days	183	166

*Data from Bergström, et al. (1967)

TABLE 16.2—from Newsholme, 1983

triglyceride stores need to be maintained during training, and should be topped off starting about two weeks before the marathon event. In part, athletes accomplish this by easing their workloads during the worthwhile break associated with the ascent to peak performance. However, they also require a balanced diet, including approximately 70% carbohydrates, 20% fat, and 10% protein. Athletes should not consume an ultra high carbohydrate, low fat, low protein diet of pasta, including starch derived from wheat. Instead, they should consume adequate amounts of "hunter gatherer" foods, including fruits, vegetables and nuts. For example, athletes might also consume berries, grapes, cantaloupe, bananas, oranges, peaches, apricots, pears, apples, pineapple, dates, raisins, sunflower seeds, almonds, pistachios, avocados, beans, lentils, yams, whole grain rice, oats, and corn. When preparing food, use sunflower, safflower, or olive oil, which consist of monounsaturated or polyunsaturated fats. Humans are by nature omnivores, thus benefit from consuming meat occasionally, and also require the Omega 3 oils found fish (Cerutty, 1961 and 1967, Newsholme, Leech, and Duester, 1994, Autio, 2000, Coyle, Jeukendrup, Oseto, Hodgkinson, Zderic, 2000).

After the last time trial or so-called "depletion effort" three to five days before the competition, the primary dietary focus should be to successfully accomplish carbohydrate loading. An individual's available carbohydrate stores in the form of stored muscle and liver glycogen can dramatically affect his or her performance in the marathon. Table 16.2 illustrates the effect of various carbohydrate diets on athletic performance.

In this regard, athletes should not undertake the severe, so-called "depletion diet"—that is, a three-day carbohydrate depletion followed by a three-day high carbohydrate diet. This places a stressor on athletes at a time when the primary aim of the training program is to remove the same and facilitate peak performance. Athletes should simply "carbohydrate load" by maintaining a high carbohydrate diet, particularly during the last three to five days before the marathon. They should also make sure to stay well hydrated during this period. Do not make the mistake of waiting until the day before the event to start drinking and eating adequately. The evening before a marathon, athletes should eat a large carbohydrate meal with a moderate glycemic index, such as spaghetti (For more information on the glycemic index, see Podell and Proctor, *The G-Index Diet*, 1993).

Fluid Replacement and Diet on Race Day

The morning of the marathon, athletes should awake and rise at least four hours before the event. It helps to be fully carbohydrate loaded, but athletes should also have relatively stable blood glucose levels. For example, athletes should beware of consuming simple sugars too close to start time, and beginning the race with a much elevated or suppressed blood sugar level, since this is known to hinder performance in the marathon (Costill, 1986, Montain, Hopper, Coggan, Coyle, 1991). In this regard, the body processes different foods at different characteristic rates, and every individual is unique. So it will be necessary to experiment and get the race day diet figured out in the months preceding the competition. Some athletes are able to eat a breakfast including foods with a moderate glycemic index such as pasta about four hours before the race. Others can eat a breakfast including foods with a higher glycemic index, such as pancakes with maple syrup and peaches, two to three hours before the event. And still others can have toast one-and-a-half to two hours before a competition. Milk or other foods with lactose should generally be avoided.

Some marathoners will take tea or coffee an hour or two prior to a race. The caffeine in tea, coffee, and some soft drinks can facilitate greater mobilization of fatty acids (Newsholme and Leech, 1983). There is now in place a positive urine-testing threshold for caffeine of 12 mcg/ml. Please see the USATF rulebook, doping rule 67. However, a normal cup of tea, coffee or a can of Coca-Cola® with the fizz out of it will not trip the test, nor does it constitute drug abuse.

If an elite athlete has prepared well, often it is best to simply go with water during the marathon. However, it is extremely important to start drinking water in the early stages of the competition. Generally, the more water an athlete can ingest earlier in the race the better, since it is not possible to compensate for the amount of fluid that will be lost during the race. If necessary, lose a few seconds at the water stations early on, in order to get down as much fluid as possible, because it will pay the time back double in the latter stages of the race. Athletes should also practice how to grab a cup or bottle and drink on the run, because it is harder than it looks. Alternately, some bottles are now available which have a valve on the top or bottom to permit rapid delivery of fluid.

However, realize that the needs of recreational runners who will be on the course for three or more hours are different than those of the elite runners. From a physiological standpoint, there is a big difference between running for a little more than two hours at 75% VO_2 maximum, versus four hours at 50% VO_2 maximum. It may help to prepare a replacement drink including electrolytes, particularly when competing in heat and humidity. Nevertheless, it is generally a big mistake for athletes to take fluid replacement drinks that are not under their control, including many of those commercially available. Most commercial products are far too concentrated and need to be substantially diluted to be ingested and properly absorbed. Otherwise, athletes have a good chance of throwing up the drink and further dehydrating themselves.

Some athletes might even want to take energy supplements during the marathon. Many runners have had success with a weak mixture of tea with honey. The closest thing to the hepatic and muscle glycogen that athletes will exhaust during the course of a marathon is glucose, a simple monosaccharide sugar. Glucose tablets are commercially available, and are normally used to rapidly stabilize low blood sugar levels in diabetics. Since the glycogen stores of runners will be nearly exhausted, and blood sugar levels can be significantly depressed, they essentially have the same need in the latter stages of a marathon, and immediately afterwards. However, recognize that different forms of sugar are absorbed at different rates. So the particular form of sugar most suitable for use would depend on the runner's condition, and also the remaining duration of the event. Athletes will also consume protein during the marathon. A large number of suitable commercial products having different formulations are available. And so, after experimenting in training sessions and perfecting the "formula" to be used, those runners who will be out on the course for three or more hours might consider taking an energy supplement (Coyle, 1992).

Aerodynamic Drag

Again, the marathon is a race of efficiency, thus the effects of aerodynamic drag and drafting can be substantial. As previously discussed in Chapter 14, closely following an individual or pack of runners in calm conditions can provide an energy savings corresponding to approximately one second/400 meters—that is, about 105 seconds or 1:45 in the marathon. And whenever headwinds are present, the energy savings can increase markedly, thus be doubled or tripled. Further, drafting can also reduce the rate of evaporation and dehydration. If and when an athlete takes the lead at 18 miles, leaving behind a pack of trailing runners, then they need to be at least 32 seconds fitter than the rest of the field to hold off a possible late charge from someone drafting in the trailing group. Accordingly, it is sometimes wise to be patient in the marathon.

Warm Up and Race Conduct

Because fatty-acid metabolism has such a relatively slow rate of mobilization and is so significant to the marathon, athletes should perform 20 minutes of easy walking or jogging at least an hour prior to the race. After the start, they should run as evenly and easily as possible through the first five miles. If they set too fast an early pace, they will force their metabolisms into using a higher percentage of carbohydrates for fuel and deplete that source far earlier than if they had instead gone out "as fast as necessary but slow as possible."

The marathon is a mirror that can reflect and magnify an individual's physical or mental imperfections tenfold. Once the race begins, nothing needs to be said to athletes about their mental state or specific race tactics. Shorter revealed his understanding when he watched Kenyan Douglas Wakiihuri win the 1987 World

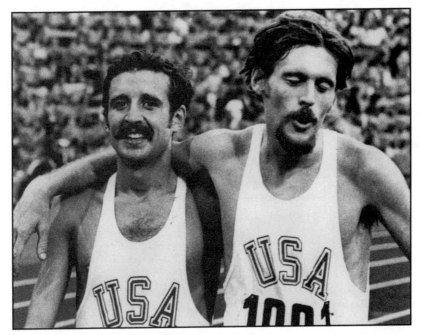

PHOTO 16.2—Frank Shorter (left) and Kenny Moore (right) after the marathon, 1972 Olympic Games. Photo from AP/ Wide World Photos.

Championships marathon and used the word "unconscious." He stated that in a marathon, "you don't want to be thinking about anything in particular." The Japanese Coach Kiyoshi Nakamura, who had trained Wakiihuri, would have used the word *mushin*, which translates roughly as "no mind." Shorter's former Olympic teammate Kenny Moore also knew the "right stuff" when he saw it—and wrote a gracious article on Wakiihuri and Nakamura entitled "A Man of Two Worlds," in *Sports Illustrated* (Moore, 1987).

There is a story about the legendary Japanese *kensei*, or "sword saint," Miyamoto Musashi. It is said that he was once approached by a student who desired to learn the art of swordsmanship. Musashi took the student on, but after months of merely doing boring housework the student asked to be "trained." And so Musashi demonstrated the proper posture and technique, and then instructed him to practice swordsmanship while walking around the house. After several months, the student became bored, and so Musashi told him to continue to practice while walking around the house in the other direction. When the student finally tired of this he again approached his master. But this time, Musashi surprised him by feigning an attack. The student passed the test and Musashi exclaimed: "Great, you can concentrate—you're already a master!" In many ways, training and successfully competing in the marathon is a lot like this story.

In conclusion, the marathon is an event that humbles and exalts, agonizes and exhilarates, injures and strengthens body, mind and spirit. Sometimes this 26.2-mile metaphor for life transcends the individual.

> *To believe this story you must believe that the human race can be one joyous family, working together, laughing together, achieving the impossible. I believe it because I saw it happen. Last Sunday, in one of the most trouble-striken cities in the world, 11,532 men and women from 40 countries in the world, assisted by over a million black, white, and yellow people, Protestants and Catholics, Jews and Muslims, Buddhists and Confusians, laughed, cheered, and suffered during the greatest folk festival the world has seen.*

—Chris Brasher, in celebration of the 1979 New York Marathon

References

Allen, Mark and Bob Babbit, *Mark Allen's Total Triathlete*, Chicago, Illinois: Contemporary Books, Inc., 1998, page 138.

Arce, J., and M.J. De Souza, L.S. Pescatello, A.A. Luciano, "Subclinical Alterations in Hormone and Semen Profile in Athletes," *Fertility and Sterility*, Volume 59, Number 2, February 1993, pages 398-404.

Autio, James, *The Digital Mantrap*, eBola Communications: Del Mar, California, 2000.

Bergström, J., and L. Hermansen, E. Hultman, B. Saltin, "Diet, Muscle Glycogen and Physical Performance," *Acta Physiologica Scandinavica*, Volume 71, Number 2, October-November 1967, pages 140-150.

Barron, J.L., and T.D. Noakes, W. Levy, C. Smith, R.P. Millar, "Hypothalamic Dysfunction in Overtrained Athletes," *Journal of Clinical Endocrinology and Metabolism*, Volume 60, Number 4, April, 1985, pages 803-806.

Bonen, A., and H.A. Keizer, "Pituitary, Ovarian, and Adrenal Hormone Responses to Marathon Running," *International Journal of Sports Medicine*, Volume 8, Supplement 3, December, 1987, pages 161-167.

Brand-Miller, Jennie, and Kay Foster-Powell, Stephen Colagiuri, Thomas M.S. Wolever, Anthony Leeds, *The Glucose Revolution: The Authoritative Guide to the Glycaemic Index-The Groundbreaking Medical Discovery*, New York: Marlowe & Co., 1999.

Brooks, G.A., and J. Mercier, "Balance of Carbohydrate and Lipid Utilization During Exercise: The "Crossover" Concept," *Journal of Applied Physiology*, Volume 76, Number 6, 1994, pages 2253-2261.

Campbell, W.W., and W.C. Crim, V.R.Young, W.J. Evans, "Increased Energy Requirements and Changes in Body Composition With Resistance Training in Older Adults," *American Journal of Clinical Nutrition*, Volume 60, Number 2, August, 1994, pages 167-175.

Cerutty, Percy, *Athletics: How To Become A Champion*, London: The Sportman's Book Club, 1961, pages 148 and 155.

Cerutty, Percy, *Success: In Sport and Life*, London: Pelham Books, Ltd., 1967.

Costill, David L., *Conversation on Exercise Physiology and Metabolism*, Muncie, Indiana, 1999.

Costill, David L., *Inside Running: Basics of Sports Physiology*, Carmel, Indiana: Cooper Publishing Group, LLC, 1986.

Costill, David L., and E.L. Fox, "Energetics of Marathon Running," *Medicine in Science and Sports*, Volume 1, 1969, pages 81-86.

Costill, David L., and L.H. Thomason, E. Roberts, "Fractional Utilization of the Aerobic Capacity During Distance Running," *Medicine in Science and Sports*, Volume 5, 1973, pages 248-252.

Coyle, E.F., "Carbohydrate Feeding During Exercise," *International Journal of Sports Medicine*, Supplement 1, Volume 13, October, 1992, pages S126-128.

Coyle, E.F., *Conversation on Exercise and Metabolism*, Austin, Texas, 1999.

Coyle, E.F., "Fatty Acid Oxidation Is Directly Regulated By Carbohydrate Metabolism During Exercise," *American Journal of Physiology*, Volume 273, 1997, pages E 268-275.

Coyle, E.F., "Integration of the Physiological Factors Determining Endurance Performance Ability," *Exercise Sport Science Review*, Volume 23, 1995, pages 25-63.

Coyle, E.F., "Substrate Utilization During Exercise In Active People," *American Journal of Clinical Nutrition*, Volume 61, 4th Supplement, 1995, pages 968S-979S.

Coyle, E.F., and A.E. Jeukendrup, M.C. Oseto, B.J. Hodgkinson, T. Zderic, "A Low Fat Diet Alters Intramuscular Substrates And Reduces Lipolysis And Fat Oxidation During Exercise," Submitted to the *American Journal of Physiology*, 2000.

Daniels, Jack, *Conversation on VO$_2$ Maximum and Lactate Threshold*, Cortland, New York, 1999.

Frederick, E.C., and T.E. Clarke, J.L. Larsen, L.B. Cooper, "The Effects of Shoe Cushioning on the Oxygen demands of Running," in *Biomechanical Aspects of Sports Shoes and Playing Surfaces*, B.M. Nigg and B.A. Kerr, Editors, Calgary, Alberta: University of Calgary, 1983, pages 107-114.

Hackney, A., and W.E. Sinning, B.C. Bruot, "Reproductive Hormonal Profiles of Endurance-Trained and Untrained Males," *Medicine and Science in Sports Exercise*, Volume 20, Number 1, February, 1988, pages 60-65.

Hawley, J.A., and W.G. Hopkins, "Aerobic Glycolytic And Aerobic Lipolytic Power Systems: A New Paradigm With Implications For Endurance and Ultra-Endurance Events," *Sports Medicine*, Volume 19, Number 4, 1995, pages 240-250.

Hermansen, L., and E. Hultman, B. Saltin, "Muscle Glycogen During Prolonged Sever Exercise," *Acta Physiologica Scandinavica*, Volume 71, Number 2, October-November 1967, pages 129-139.

Hurley, B.F., and P.M. Nemeth, W.H. Martin II, J.M. Hagberg, G.P. Dalsky, J.O. Holloszy, "Muscle Triglyceride Utilization During Exercise: Effect of Training," *Journal of Applied Physiology*, Volume 60, Number 2, 1986, pages 562-567.

Janssen, Peter G.J.M., *Training Lactate Pulse Rate*, Oulu, Finland: Polar Electro Oy, 1987.

Jensen, C., et al., "Prospective Study of Hormonal and Semen Profiles in Marathon Runners," *Fertility and Sterility*, Volume 64, Number 6, December, 1995, pages 1189-1196.

Kuoppasalmi, K., and H. Naveri, M. Harkonen, H. Adlercreutz, "Plasma Cortisol, Androstenedione, Testosterone and Luteinizing Hormone in Running Exercise of Different Intensities," *Scandinavian Journal of Clinical Laboratory Investigation*, Volume 40, Number 4, September, 1980, pages 403-409.

Linnarsson, D., "Dynamics of Pulmonary Gas Exchange And Heart Rate Changes At Start And End Of Exercise," *Acta Phsysiologica Scandanavica*, Volume 1, Supplement 415, 1974, pages 1-68.

Lyden, Robert, U.S. Patent 6,449,878, *Article of Footwear Having a Spring Element and Selectively Removable Components*, 2002.

Mader, Milan, Conversation with Milan Mader, former Czech National Team Member and Finalist, 1964 Olympic 10,000 meters, Minneapolis, Minnesota, 1979.

Montain, S.J., and M.K. Hopper, A.R. Coggan, E.F. Coyle, "Exercise Metabolism At Different Time Intervals After A Meal," *Journal of Applied Physiology*, Volume 70, Number 2, February 1991, pages 882-888.

Moore, Kenny, *Conversation on Athletic Training*, Kailua, Hawaii, 1999.

Moore, Kenny, "A Man of Two Worlds," *Sports Illustrated*, September, 1987.

Musashi, Miyamoto, *A Book Of Five Rings*, Translated by Victor Harris, New York: The Overlook Press, 1982, page 66.

Newsholme, E.A., and A.R. Leech, *Biochemistry for the Medical Sciences*, Chichester, England: John Wiley & Sons Ltd., 1983, page 376.

Newsholme, E.A, and A.R. Leech, Glenda Duester, *Keep On Running*, Chichester, England: John Wiley & Sons Ltd., 1994.

Nielsen, Peter, "Tuned Shoes May Help Runners Break Olympic Records," *Reuters*, *http://reuters.com*, August 9, 2000.

Pengelly, Scott, Conversations on Arousal Addiction in Athletes, Eugene, Oregon, 1988-1997.

Podell, Richard, and William Proctor, *The G-Index Diet*, New York: Warner Books, 1993.

Pruett, E.D.R., "FFA Mobilization During And After Prolonged Severe Muscular Work In Men," *Journal of Applied Physiology*, Volume 29, Number 6, 1970, pages 809-815.

Sahlin, K., "Metabolic Changes Limiting Muscle Performance," *Biochemistry of Exercise VI*, Saltin, B., Editor, Champaign, Illinois: Human Kinetics, 1986.

Shorter, Frank, *Conversation on Athletic Training*, Boulder, Colorado, 1999.

Sleamaker, R.H., Serious Training For *Serious Athletes: Comprehensive Training Plans For Endurance Sports*, Champaign, Illinois: Human Kinetics, 1989.

Tanaka, H., and J. Cleroux, J. de Champlain, J.R. Ducharme, R. Collu, "Persistent Effects of a Marathon Run on the Pituitary-Testicular Axis," *Journal of Endocrinological Investigation*, Volume 9, Number 2, April, 1986, pages 97-101.

Urhausen, A., and H. Gabriel, W. Kindermann, "Blood Hormones as Markers of Training Stress and Overtraining," *Sports Medicine*, Volume 20, Number 4, October 1995, pages 251-276.

Williams, Melvin H., and Sid Wesseldine, Thomas Somma, Rudolf Schuster, "The Effect of Induced Erythrocythemia Upon 5-Mile Treadmill Run Time," *Medicine And Science In Sports And Exercise*, Volume 13, Number 3, 1981, pages 169-175.

Will-Weber, Mark, Editor, *The Quotable Runner*, Halcottsville, New York: Breakaway Books, 2001.

APPENDICES

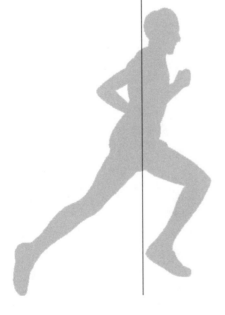

High School Training Schedule for 800 Meters

Base Period
Last 21 Day Training Meso-Cycle

Monday	Passive Recovery
Tuesday	3/4 Effort, Anaerobic Threshold Steady State
Wednesday	Active Recovery
Thursday	1/2 Effort, Fartlek + Date Pace
Friday	Active Recovery
Saturday	3/4 Effort, Steady State
Sunday	Easy Effort, Long Run, 50-80 minutes
Monday	Passive Recovery
Tuesday	3/4 Effort, Anaerobic Threshold Steady State
Wednesday	Active Recovery
Thursday	1/2 Effort, Fartlek + Date Pace
Friday	Active Recovery
Saturday	3/4 Effort, Steady State
Sunday	Easy Effort, Long Run, 50-80 minutes

Worthwhile Break

Monday	Passive Recovery
Tuesday	1/2 Effort, Fartlek + Date Pace
Wednesday	Active Recovery
Thursday	Easy Recovery
Friday	Day Before Race Routine
Saturday	Time Trial or Race
Sunday	Easy Effort, Long Run, 50-80 minutes

Hill Period
21-Day Training Meso-Cycle

Monday	Passive Recovery
Tuesday	3/4 Effort, Hill Circuit
Wednesday	Active Recovery
Thursday	1/2 Effort, Fartlek + Date Pace
Friday	Active Recovery
Saturday	3/4 Effort, Hill Workout
Sunday	Easy Effort, Long Run, 50-80 minutes
Monday	Passive Recovery
Tuesday	3/4 Effort, Hill Circuit
Wednesday	Active Recovery
Thursday	1/2 Effort, Fartlek + Date Pace
Friday	Active Recovery
Saturday	3/4 Effort, Hill Workout
Sunday	Easy Effort, Long Run, 50-80 minutes

Worthwhile Break

Monday	Passive Recovery
Tuesday	Time Trial or Race 800m, and 400m
Wednesday	Active Recovery + 4 x 100m at Finishing Speed
Thursday	Easy Recovery
Friday	Day Before Race Routine
Saturday	Race 1,500m
Sunday	Easy Effort, Long Run, 50-80 minutes

Sharpening Period
First Meso-Cycle

Monday	Passive Recovery
Tuesday	3/4 Effort, 3(4 x 300m) at 800m Goal Pace
Wednesday	Active Recovery
Thursday	1/2 Effort, Fartlek + 4 x 100m at Finishing Speed
Friday	Active Recovery
Saturday	3/4 Effort, 2(4 x 400m) at 1,500m Goal Pace
Sunday	Easy Effort, Long Run, 40-60 minutes

Worthwhile Break

Monday	Passive Recovery
Tuesday	Time Trial or Race 400m, and 200m
Wednesday	Active Recovery + 4 x 100m at Finishing Speed
Thursday	Easy Recovery
Friday	Day Before Race Routine
Saturday	Race 800m
Sunday	Easy Effort, Long Run, 40-60 minutes

Second Meso-Cycle

Monday	Passive Recovery
Tuesday	3/4 Effort, 4 x 400m at 800m Goal Pace
Wednesday	Active Recovery
Thursday	1/2 Effort, Fartlek + 4 x 100m at Finishing Speed
Friday	Active Recovery
Saturday	3/4 Effort, 3 x 500m at 800m Goal Pace, or Race 2 x 400m
Sunday	Easy Effort, Long Run, 40-60 minutes
Monday	Passive Recovery
Tuesday	1/2 Effort, Fartlek + 4 x 60m Starts
Wednesday	Active Recovery
Thursday	Time Trial(s) 600m, full recovery, then 300m

Worthwhile Break
9-10 Day Ascent to Plateau of Peak Performance

Friday	Active Recovery
Saturday	1/2 Effort, Fartlek + 3 x 60m Starts
Sunday	Easy Recovery
Monday	Day Before Race Routine
Tuesday	CONFERENCE PRELIM, Race 400m
Wednesday	Active Recovery
Thursday	CONFERENCE FINAL, Race 2 x 400m
Friday	Active Recovery
Saturday	Easy Effort, Long Run, 40-60 minutes
Sunday	Passive Recovery

14-to-21-Day Plateau of Peak Performance

Monday	Time Trial 300m slow-fast, full recovery, then 3 x 150m with Accelerations and full walk recovery
Tuesday	Active Recovery
Wednesday	Day Before Race Routine
Thursday	REGION PRELIM, Race 800m
Friday	Active Recovery
Saturday	REGION FINAL, Race 800m
Sunday	Easy Effort, Long Run, 40-60 minutes
Monday	Passive Recovery
Tuesday	Time Trial, 300m slow-fast, full recovery, then 3 x 150m with Accelerations and full walk recovery
Wednesday	Active Recovery
Thursday	Day Before Race Routine
Friday	STATE MEET PRELIM, Race 800m
Saturday	STATE MEET FINAL, Race 800m

High School Training Schedule for 1,500 Meters

Base Period
Last 21 Day Training Meso-Cycle

Monday	Passive Recovery
Tuesday	3/4-Effort, Anaerobic Threshold Steady State
Wednesday	Active Recovery
Thursday	1/2-Effort, Fartlek + Date Pace
Friday	Active Recovery
Saturday	3/4-Effort, Steady State
Sunday	Easy Effort, Long Run, 60-90 minutes

Monday	Passive Recovery
Tuesday	3/4-Effort, Anaerobic Threshold Steady State
Wednesday	Active Recovery
Thursday	1/2-Effort, Fartlek + Date Pace
Friday	Active Recovery
Saturday	3/4-Effort, Steady State
Sunday	Easy Effort, Long Run, 60-90 minutes

Worthwhile Break

Monday	Passive Recovery
Tuesday	1/2-Effort, Fartlek + Date Pace
Wednesday	Active Recovery
Thursday	Easy Recovery
Friday	Day Before Race Routine
Saturday	Time Trial or Race
Sunday	Easy Effort, Long Run, 60-90 minutes

Hill Period
21 Day Training Meso-Cycle

Monday	Passive Recovery
Tuesday	3/4-Effort, Hill Circuit
Wednesday	Active Recovery
Thursday	1/2-Effort, Fartlek + Date Pace
Friday	Active Recovery
Saturday	3/4-Effort, Hill Workout
Sunday	Easy Effort, Long Run, 60-90 minutes

Monday	Passive Recovery
Tuesday	3/4-Effort, Hill Circuit
Wednesday	Active Recovery
Thursday	1/2-Effort, Fartlek + Date Pace
Friday	Active Recovery
Saturday	3/4-Effort, Hill Workout
Sunday	Easy Effort, Long Run, 60-90 minutes

Worthwhile Break

Monday	Passive Recovery
Tuesday	Time Trial or Race 800m and 400m
Wednesday	Active Recovery + 5 x 150m at Finishing Speed
Thursday	Easy Recovery
Friday	Day Before Race Routine
Saturday	Race 3,000m
Sunday	Easy Effort, Long Run, 60-90 minutes

Sharpening Period
First Meso-Cycle

Monday	Passive Recovery
Tuesday	3/4-Effort, 3(4 x 300m) at 1,500m Goal Pace
Wednesday	Active Recovery
Thursday	1/2-Effort, Fartlek + 4 x 150m at Finishing Speed
Friday	Active Recovery
Saturday	3/4-Effort, 6 x 800m at 3,000m Goal Pace
Sunday	Easy Effort, Long Run, 60-80 minutes

Worthwhile Break

Monday	Passive Recovery
Tuesday	Time Trial or Race 800m and 400m
Wednesday	Active Recovery + 4 x 150m at Finishing Speed
Thursday	Easy Recovery
Friday	Day Before Race Routine
Saturday	Race 1,500m
Sunday	Easy Effort, Long Run, 60-80 minutes

Second Meso-Cycle

Monday	Passive Recovery
Tuesday	3/4-Effort, 2(4 x 400m) at 1,500m Goal Pace
Wednesday	Active Recovery
Thursday	1/2-Effort, Fartlek + 4 x 100m at Finishing Speed
Friday	Active Recovery
Saturday	Time Trial or Race 2 x 800m
Sunday	Easy Effort, Long Run, 60-80 minutes
Monday	Passive Recovery
Tuesday	1/2-Effort, Fartlek + 4 x 100m at Finishing Speed
Wednesday	Active Recovery
Thursday	3/4-Effort, 4 x 1,000m at 3,000m Goal Pace

Worthwhile Break
9-to-10-Day Ascent to Plateau of Peak Performance

Friday	Active Recovery
Saturday	1/2-Effort, Fartlek + 3 x 100m at Finishing Speed
Sunday	Easy Effort, Long Run, 40-60 minutes
Monday	Day Before Race Routine
Tuesday	CONFERENCE FINAL, Race 3,000m
Wednesday	Easy Effort, Long Run, 60-80 minutes
Thursday	Passive Recovery
Friday	Day Before Race Routine
Saturday	Time Trial, 1,000m, then 300m
Sunday	Active Recovery

14-21 Day Plateau of Peak Performance

Monday	1/4 Effort, Fartlek + 3 x 150m at Finishing Speed
Tuesday	Easy Recovery
Wednesday	Day Before Race Routine
Thursday	REGION FINAL, Race 3,000m
Friday	Active Recovery
Saturday	REGION FINAL, Race 1,500m
Sunday	Easy Effort, Long Run, 60-80 minutes
Monday	Passive Recovery
Tuesday	Time Trial, 800m of 50-60 drill, then 300m
Wednesday	Active Recovery + 3 x 150m with Accelerations
Thursday	Day Before Race Routine
Friday	STATE MEET FINAL, Race 3,000m
Saturday	STATE MEET FINAL, Race 1,500m

High School Training Schedule for 3,000 Meters

Base Period
Last 21 Day Training Meso-Cycle

Monday	Passive Recovery
Tuesday	3/4-Effort, Anaerobic Threshold Steady State
Wednesday	Active Recovery
Thursday	1/2-Effort, Fartlek + Date Pace
Friday	Active Recovery
Saturday	3/4-Effort, Steady State
Sunday	Easy Effort, Long Run, 70-100 minutes

Monday	Passive Recovery
Tuesday	3/4-Effort, Anaerobic Threshold Steady State
Wednesday	Active Recovery
Thursday	1/2-Effort, Fartlek + Date Pace
Friday	Active Recovery
Saturday	3/4-Effort, Steady State
Sunday	Easy Effort, Long Run, 70-100 minutes

Worthwhile Break

Monday	Passive Recovery
Tuesday	1/2-Effort, Fartlek + Date Pace
Wednesday	Active Recovery
Thursday	Easy Recovery
Friday	Day Before Race Routine
Saturday	Time Trial or Race
Sunday	Easy Effort, Long Run, 70-100 minutes

Hill Period
21 Day Training Meso-Cycle

Monday	Passive Recovery
Tuesday	3/4-Effort, Hill Circuit
Wednesday	Active Recovery
Thursday	1/2-Effort, Fartlek + Date Pace
Friday	Active Recovery
Saturday	3/4-Effort, Hill Workout
Sunday	Easy Effort, Long Run, 70-100 minutes

Monday	Passive Recovery
Tuesday	3/4-Effort, Hill Circuit
Wednesday	Active Recovery
Thursday	1/2-Effort, Fartlek + Date Pace
Friday	Active Recovery
Saturday	3/4-Effort, Hill Workout
Sunday	Easy Effort, Long Run, 70-100 minutes

Worthwhile Break

Monday   Passive Recovery
Tuesday   Time Trial or Race 800m, 400m
Wednesday   Active Recovery + 4 x 200m at Finishing Speed
Thursday   Easy Recovery
Friday   Day Before Race Routine
Saturday   Race 1,500m
Sunday   Easy Effort, Long Run, 70-100 minutes

Sharpening Period
First Meso-Cycle

Monday   Passive Recovery
Tuesday   3/4-Effort, 3(4 x 300m) at 1,500m Goal Pace
Wednesday   Active Recovery
Thursday   1/2-Effort, Fartlek + 4 x 200m at Finishing Speed
Friday   Active Recovery
Saturday   3/4-Effort, 6 x 800m at 3,000m Goal Pace
Sunday   Easy Effort, Long Run, 60-80 minutes

Worthwhile Break

Monday   Passive Recovery
Tuesday   Time Trial or Race 800m, 400m
Wednesday   Active Recovery + 4 x 150m at Finishing Speed
Thursday   Easy Recovery
Friday   Day Before Race Routine
Saturday   Race 3,000m
Sunday   Easy Effort, Long Run, 60-80 minutes

Second Meso-Cycle

Monday   Passive Recovery
Tuesday   3/4-Effort, 2(4 x 400m) at 1,500m Goal Pace
Wednesday   Active Recovery
Thursday   1/2-Effort, Fartlek + 4 x 150m at Finishing Speed
Friday   Active Recovery
Saturday   Time Trial or Race 2 x 800m
Sunday   Easy Effort, Long Run, 60-80 minutes
Monday   Passive Recovery
Tuesday   1/2-Effort, Fartlek + 4 x 150m at Finishing Speed
Wednesday   Active Recovery
Thursday   3/4-Effort, 4 x 1,000m at 3,000m Goal Pace

Worthwhile Break
9-10 Day Ascent to Plateau of Peak Performance

Friday	Easy Effort, Long Run, 60-80 minutes
Saturday	Active Recovery + 3 x 150 at Finishing Speed
Sunday	Easy Recovery
Monday	Day Before Race Routine
Tuesday	CONFERENCE FINAL, Race 3,000m
Wednesday	Easy Effort, Long Run, 60-80 minutes
Thursday	Passive Recovery
Friday	Day Before Race Routine
Saturday	Time Trial, 1,000m, then 300m
Sunday	Active Recovery

14-21 Day Plateau of Peak Performance

Monday	1/4 Effort, Fartlek + 3 x 150m at Finishing Speed
Tuesday	Easy Recovery
Wednesday	Day Before Race Routine
Thursday	REGION FINAL, Race 3,000m
Friday	Active Recovery
Saturday	REGION FINAL, Race 1,500m
Sunday	Easy Effort, Long Run, 60-80 minutes
Monday	Passive Recovery
Tuesday	Time Trial, 800m of 50-60 drill, then 300m
Wednesday	Active Recovery + 3 x 150m with Accelerations
Thursday	Day Before Race Routine
Friday	STATE MEET FINAL, Race 3,000m
Saturday	STATE MEET FINAL, Race 1,500m

High School Cross-Country Training Schedule For 5,000 Meters

Base Period
Last 21-Day Training Meso-Cycle

Monday	Passive Recovery
Tuesday	3/4-Effort, Anaerobic Threshold Steady State
Wednesday	Active Recovery
Thursday	1/2-Effort, Fartlek + Date Pace
Friday	Active Recovery
Saturday	3/4-Effort, Steady State
Sunday	Easy Effort, Long Run, 70-100 minutes

Monday	Passive Recovery
Tuesday	3/4-Effort, Anaerobic Threshold Steady State
Wednesday	Active Recovery
Thursday	1/2-Effort, Fartlek + Date Pace
Friday	Active Recovery
Saturday	3/4-Effort, Steady State
Sunday	Easy Effort, Long Run, 70-100 minutes

Worthwhile Break

Monday	Passive Recovery
Tuesday	1/2-Effort, Fartlek + Date Pace
Wednesday	Active Recovery
Thursday	Easy Recovery
Friday	Day Before Race Routine
Saturday	Race 5,000m
Sunday	Easy Effort, Long Run, 70-100 minutes

Hill Period
21-Day Training Meso-Cycle

Monday	Passive Recovery
Tuesday	3/4-Effort, Hill Circuit
Wednesday	Active Recovery
Thursday	1/2-Effort, Fartlek + Date Pace
Friday	Active Recovery
Saturday	3/4-Effort, Hill Workout
Sunday	Easy Effort, Long Run, 70-100 minutes

Monday	Passive Recovery
Tuesday	3/4-Effort, Hill Circuit
Wednesday	Active Recovery
Thursday	1/2-Effort, Fartlek + Date Pace
Friday	Active Recovery
Saturday	3/4-Effort, Hill Workout
Sunday	Easy Effort, Long Run, 70-100 minutes

Worthwhile Break

Monday	Passive Recovery
Tuesday	Time Trial 1,600m, then 300m
Wednesday	Active Recovery + 5 x 200m at Finishing Speed
Thursday	Easy Recovery
Friday	Day Before Race Routine
Saturday	Race 5,000m
Sunday	Easy Effort, Long Run, 70-100 minutes

Sharpening Period
First Meso-cycle

Monday	Passive Recovery
Tuesday	1/2-Effort, 3 (4 x 300m) at 1500m Goal Pace
Wednesday	Active Recovery
Thursday	1/2-Effort, Fartlek + 4 x 200m at Finishing Speed
Friday	Active Recovery
Saturday	3/4-Effort, 6 x 800m at 3,000m Goal Pace
Sunday	Easy Effort, Long Run, 60-90 minutes

Worthwhile Break

Monday	Passive Recovery
Tuesday	Time Trial 1,200m, then 300m
Wednesday	Active Recovery + 4 x 200m at Finishing Speed
Thursday	Easy Recovery
Friday	Day Before Race Routine
Saturday	Race 5,000m
Sunday	Easy Effort, Long Run, 60-90 minutes

Second Meso-Cycle

Monday	Passive Recovery
Tuesday	1/2-Effort, Fartlek + 4 x 200m at Finishing Speed
Wednesday	Active Recovery
Thursday	3/4-Effort, 2(4 x 400m) at 1,500m Goal Pace
Friday	Active Recovery
Saturday	1/2-Effort, Fartlek + 4 x 200m at Finishing Speed
Sunday	Easy Effort, Long Run, 60-90 minutes
Monday	Passive Recovery
Tuesday	3/4-Effort, 4 x 1,200m at 5,000m Goal Pace

Worthwhile Break
9-to-10-Day Ascent to Plateau of Peak Performance

Wednesday	Active Recovery
Thursday	1/2-Effort, Fartlek + 3 x 200m at Finishing Speed
Friday	Easy Recovery
Saturday	Time Trial 1,600m
Sunday	Active Recovery + 4 x 150m with Accelerations
Monday	Easy Recovery
Tuesday	Day Before Race Routine
Wednesday	CONFERENCE FINAL, Race 5,000m
Thursday	Easy Effort, Long Run, 60-80 minutes
Friday	Passive Recovery

14-to-21-Day Plateau of Peak Performance

Saturday	Day Before Race Routine
Sunday	Time Trial 1,200m, then 300m
Monday	Active Recovery + 3 x 150m at Finishing Speed
Tuesday	Easy Recovery
Wednesday	Day Before Race Routine
Thursday	REGION FINAL, Race 5,000m
Friday	Easy Effort, Long Run, 60-80 minutes
Saturday	Passive Recovery
Sunday	Active Recovery + 6 x 200m at 1,500m Goal Pace
Monday	Day Before Race Routine
Tuesday	Time Trial, 1,000m, then 300m
Wednesday	Active Recovery + 3 x 150m with Accelerations
Thursday	Easy Recovery
Friday	Day Before Race Routine
Saturday	STATE MEET FINAL, Race 5,000m

Senior Men's Training Schedule for 10,000 Meters

Base Period
Last 21-Day Training Meso-Cycle

Monday	Passive Recovery
Tuesday	3/4-Effort, Anaerobic Threshold Steady State
Wednesday	Active Recovery
Thursday	1/2-Effort, Fartlek + Date Pace
Friday	Active Recovery
Saturday	3/4-Effort, Steady State
Sunday	Easy Effort, Long Run, 80-110 minutes
Monday	Passive Recovery
Tuesday	3/4-Effort, Anaerobic Threshold Steady State
Wednesday	Active Recovery
Thursday	1/2-Effort, Fartlek + Date Pace
Friday	Active Recovery
Saturday	3/4-Effort, Steady State
Sunday	Easy Effort, Long Run, 80-110 minutes

Worthwhile Break

Monday	Passive Recovery
Tuesday	1/2-Effort, Fartlek + Date Pace
Wednesday	Active Recovery
Thursday	Easy Recovery
Friday	Day Before Race Routine
Saturday	Race 5k or 8k on the Road
Sunday	Easy Effort, Long Run, 80-100 minutes

Hill Period
21-Day Training Meso-Cycle

Monday	Passive Recovery
Tuesday	1/2-Effort, Hill Circuit
Wednesday	Active Recovery
Thursday	1/2-Effort, Fartlek + Date Pace
Friday	Active Recovery
Saturday	3/4-Effort, Hill Workout
Sunday	Easy Effort, Long Run, 80-110 minutes
Monday	Passive Recovery
Tuesday	3/4-Effort, Hill Circuit
Wednesday	Active Recovery
Thursday	1/2-Effort, Fartlek + Date Pace
Friday	Active Recovery
Saturday	3/4-Effort, Hill Workout
Sunday	Easy Effort, Long Run, 80-110 minutes

Worthwhile Break

Monday	Passive Recovery
Tuesday	Time Trial 1,600m, then 300m
Wednesday	Active Recovery + 5 x 200m at Finishing Speed
Thursday	Easy Recovery
Friday	Day Before Race Routine
Saturday	Race 3,000m
Sunday	Easy Effort, Long Run, 80-110 minutes

Sharpening Period
First Meso-Cycle

Monday	Passive Recovery
Tuesday	3/4-Effort, 2(5 x 400m) at 1,500m Goal Pace
Wednesday	Active Recovery
Thursday	1/2-Effort, Fartlek + 4 x 200m at Finishing Speed
Friday	Active Recovery
Saturday	3/4-Effort, 8 x 800m at 5,000m Goal Pace
Sunday	Easy Effort, Long Run, 80-100 minutes

Worthwhile Break

Monday	Passive Recovery
Tuesday	Time Trial 1,200m, then 300m
Wednesday	Active Recovery + 4 x 200m at Finishing Speed
Thursday	Easy Recovery
Friday	Day Before Race Routine
Saturday	Race 5,000m
Sunday	Easy Effort, Long Run, 80-100 minutes

Second Meso-Cycle

Monday	Passive Recovery
Tuesday	1/2-Effort, Fartlek + 3 x 200m at Finishing Speed
Wednesday	Active Recovery
Thursday	3/4-Effort, 4-5 x 1,600m at 10,000m Goal Pace
Friday	Active Recovery
Saturday	1/2-Effort, Fartlek + 3 x 200m at 1,500m Goal Pace

Worthwhile Break
9-to-10-Day Ascent to Plateau of Peak Performance

19	Sunday	Easy Effort, Long Run, 80-90 minutes
20	Monday	Passive Recovery
21	Tuesday	1/2-Effort, Fartlek + 3 x 200m at Finishing Speed
22	Wednesday	Active Recovery
23	Thursday	2/3-Effort, 5 x 1,000m at 5,000m Goal Pace
24	Friday	Easy Effort, Long Run, 80-100 minutes
25	Saturday	Passive Recovery
26	Sunday	Time Trial, 2,000m 30-40 drill, then 300m
27	Monday	Active Recovery + 4 x 150m at Finishing Speed

14-to-21-Day Plateau of Peak Performance

MARCH

28	Tuesday	Easy Recovery
29	Wednesday	Day Before Race Routine
30	Thursday	CHAMPIONSHIP PRELIM, Race 10,000m
31	Friday	Active Recovery
1	Saturday	Active Recovery
2	Sunday	CHAMPIONSHIP FINAL, Race 10,000m

APRIL

Senior Men's Training Schedule For The Marathon

Base Period
Last 21 Day Training Meso-Cycle

3	Monday	Passive Recovery
4	Tuesday	3/4-Effort, Anaerobic Threshold Steady State
5	Wednesday	Active Recovery
6	Thursday	1/2-Effort, Fartlek + Date Pace
7	Friday	Active Recovery
8	Saturday	3/4-Effort, Steady State
9	Sunday	Easy Effort, Long Run, 100-120 minutes
10	Monday	Passive Recovery
11	Tuesday	3/4-Effort, Anaerobic Threshold Steady State
12	Wednesday	Active Recovery
13	Thursday	1/2-Effort, Fartlek + Date Pace
14	Friday	Active Recovery
15	Saturday	3/4-Effort, Steady State
16	Sunday	Easy Effort, Long Run, 110-130 minutes

Worthwhile Break

17	Monday	Passive Recovery
18	Tuesday	1/2-Effort, Fartlek + Date Pace
19	Wednesday	Active Recovery
20	Thursday	Easy Recovery
21	Friday	Day Before Race Routine
22	Saturday	Time Trial or Race 15K on the Road
23	Sunday	Easy Effort, Long Run, 100-120 minutes

Hill Period
21 Day Training Meso-Cycle

24	Monday	Passive Recovery
25	Tuesday	1/2-Effort, Hill Circuit
26	Wednesday	Active Recovery
27	Thursday	1/2-Effort, Fartlek + Date Pace
28	Friday	Active Recovery
29	Saturday	3/4-Effort, Hill Workout
30	Sunday	Easy Effort, Long Run, 100-120 minutes
1	Monday	Passive Recovery
2	Tuesday	3/4-Effort, Hill Circuit
3	Wednesday	Active Recovery
4	Thursday	1/2-Effort, Fartlek + Date Pace
5	Friday	Active Recovery
6	Saturday	3/4-Effort, Hill Workout
7	Sunday	Easy Effort, Long Run, 100-120 minutes

Worthwhile Break

8	Monday	Passive Recovery
9	Tuesday	Time Trial 1,600m, 400m
10	Wednesday	Active Recovery + 5 x 200m at Finishing Speed
11	Thursday	Easy Recovery
12	Friday	Day Before Race Routine
13	Saturday	Race 5,000m
14	Sunday	Easy Effort, Long Run, 80-110 minutes

Sharpening Period
First Meso-Cycle

15	Monday	Passive Recovery
16	Tuesday	1/2-Effort, Fartlek + 8 x 200m at 3,000m Goal Pace
17	Wednesday	Active Recovery
18	Thursday	3/4-Effort, 2(5 x 400m) at 1,500m Goal Pace
19	Friday	Active Recovery
20	Saturday	1/2-Effort, Fartlek + 4 x 200m at Finishing Speed
21	Sunday	Easy Effort, Long Run, 90-110 minutes

Worthwhile Break

22	Monday	Passive Recovery
23	Tuesday	Time Trial 2,400m 30-40 drill, then 400m
24	Wednesday	Active Recovery + 4 x 200m at Finishing Speed
25	Thursday	Easy Recovery
26	Friday	Day Before Race Routine
27	Saturday	Race 10,000m
28	Sunday	Easy Effort, Long Run, 80-100 minutes

Second Meso-Cycle

29	Monday	Passive Recovery
30	Tuesday	1/2-Effort, Fartlek + 8 x 200m at 1,500m Goal Pace
31	Wednesday	Active Recovery
1	Thursday	3/4-Effort, 6-8 x 800m at 5,000m Goal Pace
2	Friday	Active Recovery
3	Saturday	1/2-Effort, Fartlek + 4 x 200m at Finishing Speed
4	Sunday	Active Recovery
5	Monday	3/4-Effort, 4-5 x 1,600m at 10,000m Goal Pace
6	Tuesday	Easy Effort, Long Run, 80-90 minutes

Worthwhile Break
9-to-10-Day Ascent to Plateau of Peak Performance

7	Wednesday	Passive Recovery
8	Thursday	1/2-Effort, Fartlek + 3 x 200m at Finishing Speed
9	Friday	Active Recovery
10	Saturday	2/3-Effort, 5 x 1,000m at 5,000m Goal Pace
11	Sunday	Active Recovery
12	Monday	Easy Effort, Long Run, 80-100 minutes
13	Tuesday	Passive Recovery
14	Wednesday	Time Trial, 2,400m 30-40 drill, then 400m
15	Thursday	Active Recovery + 6-8 x 200m at 1,500m Goal Pace

14-to-21-Day Plateau of Peak Performance

16	Friday	Easy Recovery
17	Saturday	Day Before Race Routine
18	Sunday	MARATHON FINAL

Abduct: To point or move a limb or other portion of the body away from the midline.

Acquisition: Adaption resulting in improvement of an individual's potential performance level. A stage of training in which athletes assume generally increasing and changing training loads to elevate their performance potential. This generally corresponds to the preparation phase, and activity conducted during the base, hill and sharpening periods.

Acquisitive: Training efforts with the goal of effecting acquisition.

Active Recovery: A training session conducted at less than or equal to a 1/4-effort, normally performed the day after a 1/2- or 3/4-effort. On a day of active recovery, mature athletes generally undertake an easy morning run of less than 25 minutes, and a longer afternoon or evening run. Easy swimming can be substituted for the morning run. In the course of the afternoon session, athletes should include a few easy accelerations, preferably on undulating natural terrain.

Adduct: To point or move a limb or other portion of the body towards the midline.

Actual Performance: The athlete's demonstrable athletic level at any given point in time. It is approximately equal to the athlete's performance potential at the end of a worthwhile break, and also during the peak period.

Aerobic Ability: The ability of an athlete's metabolism to extract and use oxygen when producing energy for useful work. It is commonly measured in ml/kg/min, and hence referred to as maximum oxygen uptake or VO_2 maximum.

Aerodynamic Drag: The sum of friction-induced drag and pressure-induced drag. Pressure-induced drag contributes most substantially to the aerodynamic drag experienced when running. See *Friction Induced Drag* and *Pressure Induced Drag*.

Anabolism: Constructive body-building metabolism.

Anaerobic Threshold: The point at which an athlete begins to more substantially use the ATP-Lactic energy system during exercise. In particular, the deviation point in the relatively linear heart-rate response when an athlete takes on a gradually increasing aerobic workload. The anaerobic threshold can also be determined by blood lactate measurement. In this case, it is the point where blood lactate deviates from the baseline level by 1mM as an individual performs a gradually increasing aerobic workload. It is commonly associated with a value of approximately 4mM.

Anaerobic Threshold Steady State (ATSS): A 3/4-effort distance run normally conducted during the base or hill periods. It is generally 70-80% of the distance of an even paced steady state (SS) run. Throughout an ATSS training session athletes run at slightly below their anaerobic threshold, then increase their effort while briefly crossing the threshold, then recover by running as close as possible to steady state pace. The ATSS workout can be conducted by simply undertaking an evenly paced steady state run over hilly terrain.

Ascent: The period of 7-14 days, and normally 9-10 days preceding the plateau of peak performance within the peak period. It consists of a worthwhile break in which training loads are normally reduced below 60% of maximum working capacity. The method of easing training loads at this time is sometimes also referred to as tapering.

Athletic Level: The highest standard of performance an athlete is expected to attain within the peak period of the current athletic season. Within a given athletic season, it is the athlete's estimated performance potential at a particular point in time, or demonstrated athletic performance.

ATP-Aerobic: The aerobic energy system that predominates in demanding efforts lasting over 3:00 minutes.

ATP-Lactic: The anaerobic energy system associated with substantial lactic acid production and use that predominates in exhausting efforts lasting between 45 seconds and 3:00 minutes. This energy system is used substantially in the 800-meter event.

ATP-PC: The Adenosine Triphosphate-Phosphocreatine anaerobic energy system that predominates in explosive efforts lasting up through 45 seconds. Sprinters rely substantially on this energy system.

Balance: An appropriate ratio of development between over-distance and under-distance events that enables optimal performance in the main race event. The presence of numerous preliminary heats in an anticipated competition can influence decisions made with respect to proper balance.

Bi-Annual: The conduct of two athletic seasons in a calendar year.

Biennial: A two-year developmental and peaking scenario.

Callusing: Training loads which are intended to condition an athlete to a specific physical or mental stressor.

Catabolism: Body-wasting metabolism. Transformation in which tissue is changed into energy and waste products of a simpler chemical composition.

Competitive Phase: A stage of athletic development characterized by performance in the peak period.

Concentric: A muscular contraction characterized by shortening.

Consolidation: Realization of performance potential by actual performance, and in particular, at the end of a meso-cycle during a worthwhile break or the peak period.

Date Pace: High quality work conducted during the base and hill periods to enable a gradual progression of physiological and biomechanical function with minimal risk of injury, and establish a sound foundation to support later work at goal pace during the sharpening period. Date pace is normally reduced from goal pace by 1 second per 400 meters for each meso-cycle preceding the start of the sharpening period. Date pace work can also be used to maintain or improve an athlete's running economy, and thus facilitates the conduct of quality base and hill work. Date pace work is normally performed once a week.

Day Before Race Routine (DBR): A training session required to place an athlete's cardiovascular system into a high state of readiness when three or more days separate a time trial or race from the primary competition, as is normally the case in the absence of preliminary heats. This workout normally includes a warm-up, several easy short accelerations with a full recovery, and then running a hollow 400 meters—that is, accelerating the first 100 meters, floating the next 200 meters, and then accelerating the last 100 meters, to solicit a pulse response slightly exceeding the athlete's heart rate deflection point and anaerobic threshold.

DBR: See *Day Before Race Routine*.

Decline: The stage of training associated with the transition phase, post-season recovery and complete absence of training loads. Because of the phenomenon of delayed transformation, this stage facilitates acquisition of the performance potential created during the preceding athletic season.

Deflection Point: The point at which the heart rate response deviates from a linear progression as an individual crosses the anaerobic threshold.

Delayed Transformation: The late arrival of improved performance potential observed in the early portion of a macro-cycle due to work undertaken in the previous athletic season. A period of post-season recovery following an athletic season can facilitate acquisition via delayed transformation.

Dorsal: The top side of the foot.

Dorsiflexion: Upward movement of the foot or toes about a joint.

Easy Recovery: A training session often conducted at less than or equal to a 1/4-effort, the day after an active recovery session and two days prior to a competition. It generally consists of a single easy run lasting less than 40 minutes, and includes a thorough stretching and flexibility session. Easy swimming can sometimes be substituted for the running session.

Eccentric: A muscular contraction characterized by lengthening.

Economy: See *Running Economy*.

Efficiency: Running technique associated with low oxygen consumption relative to an athlete's body weight and speed. See *Running Economy*.

Epiphysial Growth Plate: The region of long bones associated with growth.

Equilibrium: In the context of a steady-state run, a condition in which an adequate supply of oxygen meets the training-load demand such that an athlete functions aerobically.

Equilibrium (The Principle of): A training principle that suggests optimal acquisition of fitness and athletic performance is achieved by maintaining a balance between different aspects of fitness, such as endurance, strength and speed.

Equivalent Performances: The projected level of athletic performance in an over-distance or under-distance event based on an actual or projected performance in the main race event, and vice-versa.

Extended Peak Period: A peak period that begins with a short peak period, but which extends the plateau of peak performance beyond the normal 2-3 weeks by including stabilizing training efforts.

External Training Load: A training load or workout defined using a tangible medium of expression.

Fartlek: A Scandinavian word meaning "speed-play," and training technique invented by Coach Gosta Holmer. In the context of this treatment, Fartlek normally comprises a 1/2-effort training session conducted during the base or hill period. However, it is sometimes also conducted during the sharpening and peak period in order to help maintain the fitness acquired through preceding base and strength work. The early portion of a Fartlek workout is normally run on hilly or rolling terrain on a natural surface. Often date pace work can then be conducted and integrated with a Fartlek workout.

Finishing Speed (FS): Speed work generally similar to that conducted by sprinters intended to improve an athlete's closing speed over the last 400 meters of a race. This work normally consists of a brief series of controlled accelerations and reps, having a distance not greater than 400 meters. Between each rep, the athlete is permitted a full recovery period. Finishing speed work should always be progressed to enable optimal performance during the peak period. The desired maximum closing speed over 100 or 200 meters constitutes goal-finishing speed. Finishing speed work can be progressed so as to advance the quality and speed by .5 seconds/200 meters in each meso-cycle leading to the plateau of peak performance.

Friction-Induced drag: The work done when air (or a fluid) slows and produces heat by encountering a surface.

Goal Pace: The desired and selected pace for performance in the main race event during the peak period.

Habituation: The tendency of the human body to grow accustomed to a particular stimulus or training-load. The body will then cease to respond with as much supercompensation and acquisition, and thus not continue to realize steady improvement in performance potential.

Hard Day-Easy Day Rule: A training method in which a hard day of training is alternated with an easy day to facilitate recovery and supercompensation. This method is not always viable depending on the magnitude and type of training loads being assumed.

Internal Training Load: The level of effort imposed by an external training load on an athlete, as might be measured by subjective feedback, heart rate, oxygen uptake, respiratory quotient, or blood lactate.

Interval Workout: A series of running efforts conducted equal to or slower than goal pace in the main race event that utilize a continuous jog or running recovery period lasting less than 2:30 minutes. Intervals are often performed in a series characterized by 3-6 reps using a relatively short recovery period, but will often include a longer recovery period at the series break. Accordingly, intervals place a substantial venous preload on the heart, and also impose a relatively high workload on the diaphragm.

Inward Rotation: Rotation of the midfoot or forefoot towards the medial side.

Lateral Side: The side of a limb furthest from the midline of the body.

Load Waves: A visual representation of training loads and their effects. The proper integration of succeeding supercompensation effects is undulatory in nature. Training loads are conducted with optimal frequency when placed at the crest of each succeeding supercompensation effect.

Macro-Cycle: A large training cycle comprising numerous micro and meso-cycles corresponding to an entire athletic season. The aim of a properly constructed macro-cycle is to enable optimal performance during the peak period.

Main Race Event: The racing distance selected for optimal performance during the peak period.

Medial Side: This side of a limb closest to the midline of the body.

Mega-Cycle: The largest of the training cycles, comprising two or more athletic seasons, or years of athletic development. Multiple-year developmental and peaking scenarios always entail mega-cycle planning.

Meso-Cycle: A medium training cycle corresponding to the monthly view of athletic training, comprising several micro-cycles of varying work capacity.

Micro-Cycle: A small training cycle comprising a series of load waves corresponding to the interfacing of day-to-day training and weekly view of athletic training.

MRE: See *Main Race Event*.

Multiple Peak Period: A complex peak period including at least two relatively widely separated plateaus of peak performance within a single athletic season. The multiple peak period normally begins with a short or extended peak period and is followed by a period of regenerative work that enables an athlete to re-ascend and compete upon a second plateau of peak performance within the same athletic season.

Muscular Hypertrophy: Enlargement of muscle tissue in response to training.

Neuromuscular Stereotype: A pattern or dominant habit of movement instilled by repetition, conditioning and motor learning.

ODE: See *Over-Distance Event*.

Outward Rotation: Rotation of the midfoot or forefoot towards the lateral side.

Over-Distance Event: The racing distance immediately over the athlete's selected main race event.

Passive Recovery: A day off from demanding running. Alternately, easy swimming and light stretching can be performed.

Peak: The highest athletic level attained during an athletic season. Achieving optimal physical and mental fitness for athletic performance. The time and place at which a personal best performance in the main race event is planned or takes place.

Performance Potential: An athlete's capability or potential athletic level at any given point in time, determined by innate talent, previous acquisition, and the training loads being assumed.

Plantar: The bottom side of the foot.

Plantar Fasciitis: Injury or inflammation of connective tissue located in the sole of the foot.

Plantarflexion: Downward movement of the foot or toes about a joint.

Plateau of Peak Performance: The relatively brief segment of the peak period lasting approximately 14-21 days in which optimal athletic performances are possible. The plateau of peak performance follows an ascent or taper having a duration of 7-14 days, and most commonly, 9-10 days. The planning and schedule for the athletic season should place the major championship competitions upon the plateau.

Preparatory Phase: A stage of athletic development characterized by acquisitive training efforts, including the base, hill, and sharpening periods.

Pressure-Induced Drag: The work done in overcoming the build-up of high pressure in front of an object due to its pushing open a hole in the air (or a fluid) and creating a wake of low pressure behind it. The formula for calculating pressure-induced aerodynamic drag is: $D = .5(p) (Ap) (Cd) V^2$, where D = the force of drag in Newtons, p = air density(Kg/m^3), Ap = the projected frontal area normal to the air stream (m^2), Cd = the coefficient of drag expressing the aerodynamic efficiency of the object, and V = the velocity of the object in meters per second.

Pronation: Inward rotation of the calcaneus (or heel) associated with articulation of the sub-talar joint. Also sometimes called eversion.

Proprioceptor: A sensory organ located in muscles, tendons, or other connective tissue which senses force or movement.

Q Angle: The downward and inward angle of the femur and upper leg measured from the hip towards the knee.

Quadrennial: A four-year developmental and peaking scenario, such as between succeeding Olympic Games.

Regeneration: Rebuilding or restoring a previously attained performance potential and athletic level.

Regenerative: Training loads intended for effecting regeneration.

Repetitions / Repetition Workout: A series of two or more high quality running efforts conducted equal to or less than goal pace in the main race event utilizing a recovery period equal to or greater than 2:30 minutes. In contrast to interval workouts, the venous preload on the heart and workload on the diaphragm is much reduced during recovery periods. Repetition workouts are normally conducted late in the sharpening period and sometimes place heavy demands on the anaerobic ATP-PC and ATP-Lactic acid metabolisms.

Running Economy: The amount of oxygen consumed relative to an athlete's body weight and speed commonly expressed in milliliters (ml) per kilogram (kg) per minute (min). The protocol for testing running economy commonly includes treadmill running at several predetermined speeds while recording oxygen consumption. An often-used reference point is 268 meters/minute, corresponding to 6:00 minute mile pace. An athlete's oxygen consumption at various running speeds can then be expressed as a percentage of his or her VO_2 maximum, and the individual's relative economy can be subject to comparison.

Sharpening: High quality work conducted approximately equal to or faster than goal pace in the main race event, and in such a manner as to cause an athlete to progress rapidly towards attaining peak fitness.

Short Peak Period: A simple peak period consisting of a 7-14 day and most commonly, a 9-10 day worthwhile break and ascent to a plateau of peak performance lasting 2-3 weeks.

Speed Endurance: A term sometimes used to refer to the conduct of intervals or repetitions, normally at speeds equal to or less than goal pace, to train the ATP-Lactic acid anaerobic energy metabolism.

Stabilization: Training loads undertaken during a worthwhile break, extended peak period, or multiple peak period, with the intention of maintaining an athlete's performance potential.

Stabilizing: Training loads intended for stabilization.

Steady State (SS): An evenly paced 3/4-effort run performed near an athlete's anaerobic threshold, normally conducted during the base and hill periods. With mature distance runners, a common benchmark used to evaluate their performance potential is the steady state pace they can maintain for one hour, or ten miles.

Supercompensation: A temporary enhancement of an athlete's performance potential resulting from the conduct of a training load that has stimulated an overcompensation adaptation. The correct time to assume another training load is at the peak of a supercompensation response.

Supination: Outward rotation of the calcaneus (or heel) associated with articulation of the sub-talar joint. Also sometimes called inversion.

Taper: See *Ascent.*

Training Load: A physical or mental stimulus intended to cause a progression effect and elevate potential and actual performance levels. Physical training loads comprise some combination of quantity (volume and duration), and quality (intensity, frequency, and density).

Transition: See *Decline.*

Transitional Phase: A phase of athletic development characterized by dramatic reduction or elimination of training loads. A period of decline consisting of post-season recovery.

Tri-Annual: The conduct of three athletic seasons in a calendar year. Generally, this practice is not as conducive to long-term athletic development as a bi-annual configuration.

Triennial: A three-year developmental and peaking scenario.

Two Day Rule: A rule based upon common observation and experience suggesting that the degree of injury in a muscle, tendon or other connective tissue may not be fully apparent until the second day after the initial occurrence. It is generally accurate.

UDE: See *Under-Distance Event*.

Under-Distance Event: The racing distance immediately under the athlete's selected main race event.

Valgus: Orientated, angled, bent, or twisted outward.

Varus: Orientated, angled, bent, or twisted inward.

Vector: A means of showing mathematically and/or visually both direction and magnitude, in this case, athletic development over time.

VO$_2$ Maximum: A scientific measurement of an athlete's aerobic ability or maximum oxygen uptake, commonly expressed in units of ml/kg/min.

Worthwhile Break: An easing of training effort to less than 60% of maximum working capacity following a period of more demanding acquisitive work. It is inadvisable to continue acquisitive efforts without periodically including worthwhile breaks in which the training loads are reduced to avoid the onset of residual and chronic fatigue. A time trial or competition is normally placed at the end of a worthwhile break, when, due to recovery, an athlete's performance potential and actual performance capability are substantially the same.

BIBLIOGRAPHY

Abmayer, Walter, and Mike Kosgei. "Kenya Cross-Country Training." *Track & Field Quarterly Review.* Volume 91, Number 2, 1991, pages 43-44.

Adamik, Jaroslav. U.S. Patent 4,302,892, *Athletic Shoe and Sole Therefor.* 1981.

Adams, William. "Steeplechasing." *Track and Field Quarterly Review.* Volume 79, Number 3, 1979, pages 50-52.

Alexander, F. Matthias. *The Alexander Technique: The Essential Writings of F. Matthias Alexander.* Edward Maisel, Editor. New York: Carol Publishing Group. 1995.

Alford, Jim. "Steeplechase." *Track and Field Quarterly Review.* Volume 79, Number 3, 1979, pages 57-59.

Allen, Mark and Bob Babbit. *Mark Allen's Total Triathlete.* Chicago, Illinois: Contemporary Books, Inc. 1998, page 138.

Amery, Richard. "Australia's Kerry O'Brien." *Track and Field Quarterly Review.* Volume 72, Number 2, 1972, page 98.

Anderson, Owen. "Sleep—Don't Train—At Altitude: Son of Big Bang Theorist Develops Big Bag Theory And High Altitude Bed." *Running Research News.* Volume 8, Number 3, May-June, 1992.

Aquinas, St. Thomas. *An Introduction to St. Thomas Aquinas: The Summa Contra Gentiles* (excerpts). Anthony C. Pegis, Editor. New York: The Modern Library, Random House, Inc. 1948.

Arce, J., and M.J. De Souza, L.S. Pescatello, A.A. Luciano. "Subclinical Alterations in Hormone and Semen Profile in Athletes." *Fertility and Sterility.* Volume 59, Number 2, February, 1993, pages 398-404.

Arieti, Silvano. *Creativity: The Magic Synthesis.* New York: Basic Books, Inc. 1976.

Aristotle. *The Ethics of Aristotle: The Nichomachean Ethics.* Translated by J.A.K. Thompson. Introduction by Jonathan Barnes. London: Penguin Books. 1976.

Aristotle. *The Politics of Aristotle.* Translated, with an Introduction, Notes, and Appendices by Ernest Barker. Oxford: Clarendon Press. 1946.

Åstrand, Per Olaf, and Kaare Rodahl. *Textbook of Work Physiology.* 3rd Edition. New York: McGrawHill Book Company. 1986.

Augustine. *The City of God.* Garden City, New York: Image Books / Doubleday & Company, Inc. 1958.

Autio, James. *The Digital Mantrap.* eBola Communications: Del Mar, California. 2000.

Bannister, Roger. *The Four Minute Mile.* New York: Dodd, Mead, & Co. 1955.

Barker, Dennis, Editor. "Running with Lydiard." *Fitsport.* Volume 1, Number 11, March, 1984.

Barron, J.L., and T.D. Noakes, W. Levy, C. Smith, R.P. Millar. "Hypothalamic Dysfunction in Overtrained Athletes." *Journal of Clinical Endocrinology and Metabolism.* Volume 60, Number 4, April, 1985. pages 803-806.

Bassett, D.R., and C.R. Kyle, L. Passfield, J.P. Broker, E.R. Burke. "Comparing Cycling World Hour Records, 1967-1996: Modeling with Empirical Data." *Medicine and Science in Sports and Exercise.* Volume 31, Number 11, November, 1999, pages 1665-1676.

Bates, Barry. U.S. Patent 4,364,189, *Running Shoe with Differential Cushioning,* 1982.

Bates, Barry, and S.L. James, L.R. Osternig. "Foot Function During the Support Phase of Running." *American Journal of Sports Medicine.* Volume 7, 1979, page 328.

Becker, Robert. *The Body Electric: Electromagnetism and the Foundation of Life.* New York: William Morrow & Co. 1987.

Benoit Samuelson, Joan, and Gloria Averbuch. *Joan Samuelson's Running for Women.* Emmaus, Pennsylvania: Rodale Press, Inc. 1995.

Benson, Tony. "Steeplechasing: The Art of Interrupted Running." *Track and Field Quarterly Review*. Volume 93, Number 2, 1993, pages 27-29.

Berghold, Franz. "Sport Medical Aspects of Hiking and Mountain Climbing in the Alps." *Schweizerische Zeitschrift fur Sportmedizin*. Volume 30, Number 1, 1982, pages 5-12.

Berglund, Bo. "High Altitude Training." *Sports Medicine*. Volume 14, Number 5, 1992.

Bergström, J., and L. Hermansen, E. Hultman, B. Saltin. "Diet, Muscle Glycogen and Physical Performance." *Acta Physiologica Scandinavica*. Volume 71, Number 2, October-November, 1967, pages 140-150.

Bly, Robert. *A Little Book on the Human Shadow*. William Booth, Editor. San Francisco, California: HarperCollins Publishers. 1988.

Bompa, Tudor O. *Theory and Methodology of Training*. 3rd Edition. Dubuque, Iowa: Kendall / Hunt Publishing Company. 1994.

Bonen, A., and H.A. Keizer. "Pituitary, Ovarian, and Adrenal Hormone Responses to Marathon Running." *International Journal of Sports Medicine*. Volume 8, Supplement 3, December 1987, pages 161-167.

Bowerman, William. "The Bowerman Runner's World Series," (6 articles). *Runner's World*. October 1978 – March 1979.

Bowerman, William, *Coaching Track and Field*. William H. Freeman, Editor. Boston, Massachusetts: Houghton Mifflin Company. 1974.

Bowerman, William. "Steeple Chase Training." *Proceedings of the International Track & Field Coaches Association, IX Congress*. George Dales, Editor. Santa Monica, California, July 30-August 2, 1984, pages 41-43.

Bowerman, William, and William H. Freeman. *High Performance Training for Track and Field*. Champaign, Illinois: Human Kinetics. 1991.

Brand-Miller, Jennie, and Kay Foster-Powell, Stephen Colagiuri, Thomas M.S. Wolever, Anthony Leeds. *The Glucose Revolution: The Authoritative Guide to the Glycaemic Index-The Groundbreaking Medical Discovery*. New York: Marlowe & Co. 1999.

Brooks, G.A., and Mercier, J. "Balance of Carbohydrate and Lipid Utilization During Exercise: The Crossover Concept." *Journal of Applied Physiology*. Volume 76 Number 6, 1994, pages 2253-2261.

Brownlie, Leonard R. "High Performance Sports Apparel." *NIKE Sport Research Review*. May/June, 1989.

Brownlie, Leonard R. *Ph.D. Thesis, Aerodynamic Characteristics of Sports Apparel*. Simon Fraser University. November, 1992.

Brownlie, Leonard R., et al. "The Influence of Apparel on Aerodynamic Drag in Running." *Annals of Physiological Anthropology*. Volume 6, Number 3, 1987, page 133.

Buehler, Al, and Roger Beardmore. "The 3000 Meter Steeplechase." *Scholastic Coach*. Volume 44, Number 7, March, 1975, page 16, and pages 116-117.

Burke, Edmund. *Reflections on the Revolutions in France*. III, 1790.

Bush, Jim. "Hurdles— Technique and Training." *Proceedings of the International Track & Field Coaches Association, IX Congress*. George Dales, Editor. Santa Monica, California, July 30-August 2, 1984, pages 29-31.

Campbell, W.W., and W.C. Crim, V.R. Young, W.J. Evans. "Increased Energy Requirements and Changes in Body Composition With Resistance Training in Older Adults." *American Journal of Clinical Nutrition*. Volume 60, Number 2, August, 1994, pages 167-175.

Catlin, M.E., and R.H. Dressendorfer. "Effect of Shoe Weight on the Energy Cost of Running." *Medicine and Science in Sports*. Volume 11, Number 1, 1970, page 80.

Cavanagh, Peter. *The Running Shoe Book*. Mountain View, California: Anderson World, 1980.

Cavanagh, Peter. U.S. Patent 4,449,306, *Running Shoe Sole Construction*. 1984.

Cavanagh, Peter. U.S. Patent 4,506,462, *Running Shoe with Pronation Limiting Heel*. 1985.

Cavanagh, Peter. Editor. *Biomechanics of Distance Running*. Champaign, Illinois: Human Kinetics Books, 1990.

Cavanagh, Peter, and M.A. LaFortune. "Ground Reaction Forces in Distance Running." *Journal of Biomechanics*. Volume 13, 1980, pages 397-406.

Cavanagh, Peter, and M.L. Pollock, J. Landa. "A Biomechanical Comparison of Elite and Good Distance Runners." *Annals of the New York Academy of Sciences*. Volume 301, 1977, pages 328-345.

Cavanagh, Peter, and G.A. Valiant, K.W. Misevich. "Biological Aspects of Modeling Shoe / Foot Interaction During Running." *Sport Shoes and Playing Surfaces*. E. C. Frederick, Editor. Champaign, Illinois: Human Kinetics. 1984, pages 24-26.

Cecil Textbook of Medicine. 20th Edition. Philadelphia, Pennsylvania: W.B. Saunders, Co. 1996.

Cerutty, Percy. *Athletics: How to Become a Champion*. London: The Sportsman's Book Club. 1961.

Cerutty, Percy. *Audio Tape Recording*. 1970's.

Cerutty, Percy. *Middle Distance Running*. Great Britain: Pelham Books, Ltd. 1964.

Cerutty, Percy. *Sport Is My Life*. London: Stanley Paul and Company, Ltd. 1966.

Cerutty, Percy. *Success: In Sport and Life*. London: Pelham Books, Ltd. 1967.

Cheskin, Melvin, and K.J. Sherkin, B. Bates. *Athletic Footwear*. Fairchild Publications. 1989.

Chopra, Deepak. *The Seven Spiritual Laws of Success*. San Rafael, California: Amber-Allen Publishing. 1994.

Clarke, Ron, and Alan Trengove. *The Unforgiving Minute*. London: Pelham Books, Ltd. 1966.

Clarke, Ron, and Norman Harris. *The Lonely Breed*. London: Pelham Books, Ltd. 1967.

Clarke, T.E., and E.C. Frederick, L.B. Cooper. "Biomechanical Measurement of Running Shoe Cushioning Properties." in *Biomechanical Aspects of Sports Shoes and Playing Surfaces*. B.M. Nigg and B.A. Kerr, Editors. Calgary, Alberta: University of Calgary. 1983. pages 25-33.

Clarke, T.E., and E.C. Frederick, C.L. Hamill. "The Effect of Shoe Design Upon Rearfoot Control in Running." *Medicine and Science in Sports and Exercise*. Volume 15, Number 5, 1983. pages 376-381.

Clarke, T.E., and M.A. LaFortune, K.R. Williams, P. Cavanagh. "The Relationship between Center of Pressure and Rearfoot Movement in Running." *Medicine and Science in Sports and Exercise*. Volume 12, Number 2, 1980, page 192.

Clarke, T. E., et al. U.S. Patent 4,439,936, *Shock Attenuating Outer Sole*. 1984.

Clayton, Derek. *Running to the Top*. Mountain View, California: Anderson World, Inc. 1980.

Clement, D. B., and R. C. Asmundson, C. W. Medhurst. "Hemoglobin Values: Comparative Survey of the 1976 Canadian Olympic Team." *Journal of the Canadian Medical Association*. Volume 117, 1977, pages 614-616.

Clement, D. B., and J. Taunton, J. P. Wiley, G. Smart, K. McNicol. "The Effects of Corrective Orthotic Devices on Oxygen Uptake During Running." *Proceedings of the World Congress on Sports Medicine*. L. Prokop, Editor. Vienna: World Congress on Sports Medicine, 1984, pages 648-655.

Coe, Sebastian, and David Miller. *Running Free*. New York: St. Martin's Press. 1981.

Costill, David L. *Conversation on Exercise Physiology and Metabolism*. Muncie, Indiana. 1999.

Costill, David L. *Inside Running: Basics of Sports Physiology*. Carmel, Indiana: Cooper Publishing Group, LLC. 1986.

Costill, David L. *A Scientific Approach to Distance Running*. Los Altos, California: Tafnews Press. 1979.

Costill, David L., and J. Daniels, W. Evans, et al. "Skeletal Muscle Enzymes and Fiber Composition in Male and Female Track Athletes." *Journal of Applied Physiology*. Volume 40, 1976. pages 149-154.

Costill, David L., and E. L. Fox. "Energetics of Marathon Running." *Medicine in Science and Sports*. Volume 1, 1969, pages 81-86.

Costill, David L., and W.F. Kammer, A. Fisher. "Fluid Injestion During Distance Running." *Archives of Environmental Health*. Volume 21, 1970, pages 520-525.

Costill, David L., and L. H. Thomason, E. Roberts. "Fractional Utilization of the Aerobic Capacity During Distance Running." *Medicine in Science and Sports*. Volume 5, 1973. pages 248-252.

Couch, Jean. *The Runner's Yoga Book*. Berkeley, California: Rodmell Press. 1990.

Cowan, James. *Mysteries of the Dream-Time*. Dorset, England: Prism Press. 1989.

Cowen, Connell, and Melvyn Kinder. "Daddy's Little Girl." *Smart Women/Foolish Choices*. New York: Clarkson N. Potter, Inc. 1985.

Coyle, Edward F. "Carbohydrate Feeding During Exercise." *International Journal of Sports Medicine*. Volume 13, Suppliment 1, October, 1992, pages S 126-128.

Coyle, Edward F. *Conversation on Exercise Physiology and Metabolism*. Austin, Texas. 1999.

Coyle, Edward F. "Fatty Acid Oxidation Is Directly Regulated By Carbohydrate Metabolism During Exercise." *American Journal of Physiology*. Volume 273, 1997, pages E 268-275.

Coyle, Edward F. "Integration of the Physiological Factors Determining Endurance Performance Ability." *Exercise Sport Science Review*. Volume 23, 1995, pages 25-63.

Coyle, Edward F. "Substrate Utilization During Exercise In Active People." *American Journal of Clinical Nutrition*. Volume 61, 4th Suppliment, 1995, pages 968S-979S.

Coyle, Edward F., and Effie Coyle. "Carbohydrates That Speed Recovery From Training." *The Physician and Sportsmedicine*. Volume 21, Number 2, 1983, pages 111-123.

Coyle, Edward F., and Jeukendrup, A.E., Oseto, M.C., Hodgkinson, B.J., Zderic, T. "A Low Fat Diet Alters Intramuscular Substrates And Reduces Lipolysis And Fat Oxidation During Exercise." Submitted to the *American Journal of Physiology*. 2000.

Dales, George. *Conversations on Acclimatization to Altitude*. Kalamazoo, Michigan. 1997.

Daniels, Jack, "Altitude and Athletic Training and Performance," *American Journal of Sports Medicine*, Volume 7, 1979, pages 371-373.

Daniels, Jack. *Conversation on VO$_2$ maximum and Lactate Threshold*. 1999.

Daniels, Jack. *Conversations on Altitude Training*. 1984-1997.

Daniels, Jack. *Conversations on Iron Deficiency Anemia*. 1984-1997.

Daniels, Jack. *Daniel's Running Formula*. Champaign, Illinois: Human Kinetics Publishers. 1998.

Daniels, Jack. "Equating Sea Level and Altitude Distance Running Times." *Track & Field Quarterly Review*. Volume 75, Number 4, 1975, pages 38-39.

Daniels, Jack. "A Physiologists View of Running Economy." *Medicine and Science in Sports and Exercise*. Volume 17, Number 3, 1985, pages 1-23.

Daniels, Jack. "Training Where The Air is Rare." *Runner's World*. June, 1980.

Daniels, Jack, and Jimmy Gilbert. *Oxygen Power*. Tempe, Arizona: Published Privately. 1979.

Daniels, Jack, and Neil Oldridge. "The Effects of Alternate Exposure to Altitude and Sea Level On World-Class Middle-Distance Runners." *Medicine and Science in Sports*. Volume 2, Number 3, 1970, pages 107-112.

Daniels, Jack, and Nancy Scardina, John Hayes, Peter Foley. "Elite and Subelite Female Middle- and Long-Distance Runners." *Sport and Elite Performers*. Daniel M. Landers, Editor. Champaign, Illinois: Human Kinetics, 1986, pages 57-72.

Davies, C.T.M. "Effects of Wind Assistance and Resistance on the Forward Motion of a Runner." *Journal of Applied Physiology*. Volume 48, 1980, pages 702-709.

Deane, Herbert. *The Political and Social Ideals of St. Augustine*. New York: Columbia University Press. 1963.

DeClercq, D., and P. Aerts, M. Kunnen. "The Mechanical Characteristics of the Human Heel Pad During Footstrike in Running: An In Vivo Cinearadiographic Study." *Journal of Biomechanics*. Volume 27, Number 10, 1994, pages 1213-1222.

Dellinger, Bill. "The Dellinger Runner's World Series." (4 articles). *Runner's World*. January-April, 1981.

Dellinger, Bill. "Easy to Be Hard." *Runner's World*. June, 1980.

Dellinger, Bill. "A Runner's Philosophy." *Track & Field Quarterly Review*. Volume 79, Number 3, 1979, pages 13-16.

Dellinger, Bill. "University of Oregon Distance Training." *Track & Field Quarterly Review*. Volume 73, Number 3, 1973, pages 146-153.

Dellinger, Bill, and Georges Beres. *Winning Running*. Chicago, Illinois: Contemporary Books, Inc. 1978.

Deshimaru, Taisen. *The Zen Way to the Martial Arts*. Introduction by George Leonards. Translated by Nancy Amphoux. New York: E. P. Dutton. 1982.

Dick, F. W. *Training Theory*. London: British Amateur Athletic Board. 1984.

Dill, D.B., and K.Braithwaite, W.C. Adams, E.M. Bernauer. "Blood Volume or Middle-Distance Runners: Effect of 2300m Altitude and Comparison with Non-Athletes." *Medicine and Science in Sports and Exercise*. Volume 6, 1974, pages 1-7.

Dōgen. *A Primer of Sōtō Zen*. Translated by Reiho Masunaga. Honolulu: University of Hawaii Press. 1971.

Dōgen. *Moon in a Dewdrop: Writings of Zen Master Dōgen*. Kazuaki Tanahashi, Editor. San Francisco, California: North Point Press. 1985.

Doherty, Ken. *Modern Track & Field*. Boston: Houghton Mifflin Co. 1975.

Drake, Jonathan. *The Alexander Technique In Everyday Life*. Musselburgh, Scotland: Scotprint Ltd. 1996.

Dressendorfer, R. H., and C.E. Wade, E.C. Frederick. "Effect of Shoe Cushioning on the Development of Reticulocytosis in Distance Runners." *American Journal of Sports Medicine*. Volume 20, Number 2, 1992, pages 212-216.

Dufaux, B., and A. Hoederrath, I. Streitberg, W. Hollman, G. Assman. "Serum Ferritin, Transferrin, Haptoglobin, and Iron in Middle and Long Distance Runners, Elite Rowers, and Professional Racing Cyclists." *International Journal of Sports Medicine*. Volume 2, 1981. pages 43-46.

Dürckheim, Karlfried Graf. *The Call For The Master*. Translated by Vincent Nash. New York: E.P. Dutton. 1989.

Dürckheim, Karlfried Graf. *Hara: The Vital Center of Man*. Translated by S. von Kospoth and E. Healey. London: A Mandala Book. 1988.

Dyson, Geoffrey. *The Mechanics of Athletics*. 6th Edition. London: University of London Press. 1964.

Edington, C., and E. C. Frederick, Peter Cavanagh. "Rearfoot Motion in Distance Running." in *Biomechanics of Distance Running*. Peter Cavanagh, Editor. Champaign, Illinois: Human Kinetics Books. 1990.

Editors of Market House Books, Ltd. *The Bantam Medical Dictionary*. Revised Edition. New York: Bantam Books. 1990.

Elder, A.C., and A.H. Thompson. "Water Jump Clearance Analysis." *Track Technique*. Number 29, September, 1967, pages 923-925.

Elkind, David. "Erik Erikson's Eight Stages of Man." *New York Times Magazine*. April 5, 1970.

Elliott, Charles. "Steeplechase: Technical Analysis." *Track and Field Quarterly Review*. Volume 72, Number 2, 1972, pages 96-97.

Elliott, Herb, and Alan Trengove. *The Golden Mile*. London: Cassell & Co., Ltd. 1961.

Elliott, Richard. *The Competitive Edge*. New Jersey: Prentice/Hall, Inc. 1984.

Erikson, Erik. *Childhood and Society*. 2nd Edition. New York: W. W. Norton. 1963.

Erikson, Erik. *Identity: Youth & Crisis*. New York: W. W. Norton. 1968.

Erikson, Erik. *Life History and the Historical Moment*. New York: W. W. Norton. 1975.

Fagan, J., and I.L. Shepherd, Editors. *Gestalt Therapy Now*. Palo Alto, California: Science and Behavior Books. 1970. Harper Colophon. 1971.

Falsetti, H.L., and E.R. Burke, R. Feld, E.C. Frederick C. Ratering. "Hematological Variations after Endurance Running with Hard and Soft-Soled Running Shoes." *Physician and Sportsmedicine*. Volume 11, Number 8, 1983, pages 118-127.

Faulkner, J.A. "Training for Maximum Performance at Altitude." *The International Symposium on the Effects of Altitude on Physical Performance*. Albuquerque, New Mexico. March 3-6. 1966, pages 88-90.

Faulkner, J.A., and Jack Daniels, B. Balke. "The Effects of Training at Moderate Altitude on Physical Performance Capacity." *Journal of Applied Physiology*. Volume 23, 1967, pages 85-89.

Feldenkrais, Moshe. *Awareness Through Movement*. San Francisco, California: HarperCollins Publishers. 1990.

Ferstle, Jim. *The Dave Wottle Story*. Mountain View, California: World Publications. 1973.

Feynman, Richard. *The Feynman Lectures on Physics*. CIT: Addison Wesley Publishing Company. 1965.

Fišer, Ladislav. *Mílaři a Vytrvalshi*. Prague: Sportovní a Turistické Nakladatelství. 1965.

Fisher, Bill. "The Steeplechase." *Track and Field Quarterly Review*. Volume 82, Number 3, 1982, pages 39-40.

Fix, David, and Nancy Smith. "Analysis Chart for Steeplechase Water Jumping." *Track and Field Quarterly Review*. Volume 84, Number 3, 1984, pages 23-25.

Fox, Edward, and Donald Matthews. *The Physiological Basis of Physical Education and Athletics*. 3rd Edition. New York: Saunders College Publishing. 1981.

Frederick, E.C. "Measuring the Effects of Shoe and Surfaces on the Economy of Locomotion," *Biomechanical Aspects of Sports Shoes and Playing Surfaces*. B.M. Nigg, and B.A. Kerr, Editors. Calgary, Alberta: University of Calgary, 1983, pages 93-106.

Frederick, E.C. "Physiological and Ergonomics Factors in Running Shoe Design." *Applied Ergonomics*. Volume 15, Number 4, 1984, pages 281-287.

Frederick, E.C., and T.E. Clarke, J.L. Larsen, L.B. Cooper. "The Effects of Shoe Cushioning on the Oxygen demands of Running." *Biomechanical Aspects of Sports Shoes and Playing Surfaces*. B.M. Nigg, and B.A. Kerr, Editors. Calgary, Alberta: University of Calgary, 1983, pages 107-114.

Frederick, E.C., and Jack Daniels, J. Hayes. "The Effect of Shoe Weight on the Aerobic Demands of Running." *Current Topics in Sports Medicine: Proceedings of the World Congress of Sports Medicine*. N. Bachl, and L. Prokop, R. Suckert, Editors. Vienna: Urban & Schwartzenberg. 1983. pages 604-615.

Frederick, E. C., and E.T. Howley, and S. K. Powers. "Lower Oxygen Demands of Running in Soft-Soled Shoes." *Research Quarterly of Exercise and Sports*. Volume 57, Number 2, 1986. pages 174-177.

Frederick, E. C., et al. U.S. Patent 4,562,651, *Sole with V-Oriented Flex Grooves*. 1986.

Frederickson, Ray, et al. U.S. Patent 4,934,072. *Fluid Dynamic Shoe*. 1990.

Freeman, William H. *Peak When It Counts*. Mountain View, California: Track & Field News Press. 1989.

Freud, Sigmund. *The Standard Edition of the Complete Psychological Works of Sigmund Freud*. 24 Volumes. Translated and Edited by James Strackey, and Anna Freud. London: Hogarth Press. 1953-1974.

Galloway, Jeff. *Galloway's Book on Running*. Bolinas, California: Shelter Publications, Inc. 1984.

Gallway, Timothy. *The Inner Game of Tennis*. New York: Random House. 1974.

Gambetta, Vern. *Hurdling and Steeplechasing*. Runner's World Booklet of the Month, Number 35. Mountain View, California: World Publications, August, 1974.

Gamow, Rustem Igor, and Hugh Herr. U.S. Patent 5,367,790, *Shoe and Foot Prosthesis with a Coupled Spring System*. 1994.

Gandy, Georges. "Blueprinting the Perfect Runner." *Runner's World*. May-June, 1980.

Gardner, Howard. *Frames of Mind*. New York: Basic Books, Inc. 1983.

Gardner, James B., and J. Gerry Purdy. *Computerized Running Training Programs*. Los Altos, California: Tafnews Press. 1970.

Gartland, John, and Phil Henson. "A Comparison of the Hurdle SC Water Barrier Technique with the Conventional Water Barrier Technique." *Track and Field Quarterly Review*. Volume 84, Number 3, 1984, pages 26-28.

Gilmour, Garth H. *A Clean Pair of Heels: The Murray Halberg Story*. London: Herbert Jenkins, Ltd. 1963.

Gisolfi, C.V., and J. Cohen. "Relationships Among Training, Heat Acclimatization and Heat Tolerance in Men and Women: The Controversy Revisited." *Medicine and Science in Sports*. Volume 11, 1979, pages 56-59.

Gisolfi, C.V. Editor. "Symposium of the Thermal Effects of Exercise in the Heat." *Medicine and Science in Sports*. Volume 11, Number 1, 1979. pages 30-71.

Glover, Bob, and Pete Schuder. *The New Competitive Runner's Handbook*. New York: Penguin Books. 1988.

Goldman, Bob., et. al. *Death in the Lockeroom*. Tuscon, Arizona: The Body Press. 1987.

Goodall, Jane. *Through a Window*. Boston, Massachusetts: Houghton Mifflin Company. 1990.

Green, Lawrence, and Russell Pate. *Training For Young Distance Runners*. Champaign, Illinois: Human Kinetics. 1997.

Greene, Peter, and Thomas McMahon. "Reflex Stiffness of Man's Anti-Gravity Muscles During Kneebends While Carrying Extra Weights." *Journal of Biomechanics*. Volume 12, 1979, pages 881-891.

Griak, Roy. "Steeplechase—Points to Remember." *Track and Field Quarterly Review*. Volume 82, Number 3, 1982, page 41.

Gross, A., and C. Kyle, D. Malewicki. "The Aerodynamics of Human-Powered Land Vehicles." *Scientific American*. 1983, pages 142-152.

Groves, Harry. *Practical Coaching Techniques for Cross-Country and Distance Running*. Ames, Iowa: Championship Books. 1981.

Gutkowski, Larry, et al., U.S. Patent 5,729,912, *Article of Footwear Having Adjustable Widths, Footform and Cushioning*. 1998.

Gutkowski, Larry, et al., U.S. Patent 5,813,146, *Article of Footwear Having Adjustable Widths, Footform and Cushioning*. 1999.

Hackney, A., and W.E. Sinning, B.C. Bruot. "Reproductive Hormonal Profiles of Endurance-Trained and Untrained Males." *Medicine and Science in Sports Exercise*. Volume 20, Number 1, February, 1988, pages 60-65.

Hamill, C.L., and T.E. Clarke, E.C. Frederick, L.J. Goodyear, E.T. Howley. "Effects of Grade Running on Kinematics and Impact Force." *Medicine and Science in Sports and Exercise*. Volume 16, 1984, page 165.

Hanson, P.G. "Heat Injury in Runners." *Physician Sportsmedicine*. Volume 7, Number 6. 1979, pages 91-96.

Harre, Dietrich. Editor. *Principles of Sport Training*. Berlin: Sportverlag. 1982.

Harris, Cyril B. Editor. *Shock & Vibration Handbook*. 3rd Edition. New York: McGraw-Hill Book Company. 1988.

Hartwick, Barry. "The 3,000m Steeplechase." *Track and Field Quarterly Review*. Volume 81, Number 3, 1981, pages 43-56.

Hatcher, Chris, and Philip Himelstein. *The Handbook of Gestalt Therapy*. Northvale, New Jersey: Jason Aronson Inc. 1995.

Hatfield, Bradley., et. al. "Understanding Anxiety: Implications for Sport Performance." *NSCA Journal*. April-May, 1987.

Hawley, J.A., and W.G. Hopkins. "Aerobic Glycolytic And Aerobic Lipolytic Power Systems: A New Paradigm With Implications For Endurance and Ultra-Endurance Events." *Sports Medicine*. Volume 19, Number 4, 1995, pages 240-250.

Heads, Ian, and Geoff Armstrong, Editors. *Winning Attitudes*. Introduction by Herb Elliott. Sydney, Australia: Australian Olympic Committee, Mardie Grant Books. 2000.

Hendershott, Jon. Editor. *Ron Clarke Talks Track*. Los Altos, California: Tafnews Press. 1972.

Henderson, Joe. *Long Slow Distance: The Humane Way to Train*. Afterword by Amby Burfoot. Los Altos, California: Tafnews Press. 1969.

Henderson, Joe. Editor. *The Complete Marathoner*. Mountain View, California: World Publications. 1978.

Hendricks, Gay, and J. Carlson. *The Centered Athlete*. Englwood Cliffs, New Jersey: Prentice/Hall. 1982.

Hermansen, L., and E Hultman, B. Saltin. "Muscle Glycogen During Prolonged Severe Exercise." *Acta Physiologica Scandinavica*. Volume 71, Number 2, October-November, 1967, pages 129-139.

Herr Hugh, and G. Huang , N. Langman, R. Gamow. "A Mechanically Efficient Shoe Midsole Improves Running Economy, Stability, and Cushioning." *Journal of Applied Physiology*. 2003 (in press).

Herr, Hugh, et al. U.S. Patent 5,701,686, *Shoe and Foot Prosthesis with Bending Beam Spring Structures*. 1997.

Herr, Hugh, et al. U.S. Patent 6,029,374, *Shoe and Foot Prosthesis with Bending Beam Spring Structures*. 2000.

Herrigel, Eugen. *Zen in the Art of Archery*. Introduction by D. Suzuki. Translated by R. F. C. Hull. New York: Vintage Books/Random House. 1971.

Hessel, Del G. "The Steeplechase—A Unique Event." *Track and Field Quarterly Review*. Volume 81, Number 3, 1981, pages 41-42.

Hickson, R.C., and B.A. Dvorak, E.M. Gorostiaga, T.T. Kurowski, C. Foster. "Potential for Strength and Endurance Training to Amplify Endurance Performance." *Journal of Applied Physiology*. Volume 65, 1988, pages 2285-2290.

Higdon, Hal. *Run Fast*. Emmaus, Pennsylvania: Rodale Press. 1992.

Hill, A.V. "The Air Resistance to a Runner." *Proceedings of the Royal Society of London*. Series. B, pages 380-385.

Hislop, Chick. *Conversation on the Steeplechase*. Eugene, Oregon. 1999.

Hislop, Chick. "Distance Hurdle Technique." *Distance Running Elite Clinic for Steeplechasers*. Ogden, Utah. 1995.

Hislop, Chick. "Flexibility And Wall Drills For The Distance Hurdler." *Distance Running Elite Clinic for Steeplechasers*. Ogden, Utah. 1995.

Hislop, Chick. "Steeplechase Technique." *Proceedings of the International Track & Field Coaches Association, IX Congress*. George Dales, Editor. Santa Monica, California: July 30-August 2, 1984, pages 44-47.

Hoerner, S.F. *Fluid-Dynamic Drag*. Published by the author. 148 Busteed Drive, Midland Park, New Jersey. 1965.

Hoffman, P., M.D. "Conclusions Drawn From a Comparative Study of the Feet of Barefooted and Shoe-Wearing Peoples." *The American Journal of Orthopedic Surgery*. Volume III, Number 2, October, 1905, pages 105-136.

Hollister, Geoffrey, et al. U.S. Patent 4,043,058, *Athletic Training Shoe Having Foam Core and Apertured Sole Layers*. 1977.

Hoppenfeld, Stanley, M.D. *Physical Examination of the Spine & Extremities*. San Mateo, California: Appleton & Lange. 1976.

Houmard, J.A., and D.L. Costill, J.B. Mitchell, S.H. Park, T.C. Chenier. "The Role of Anaerobic Ability in Middle Distance Running Performance." *European Journal of Applied Physiology*. Volume 62, 1991, pages 40-43.

Humes, James C. *The Wit & Wisdom of Winston Churchill*. Forward by Richard M. Nixon. New York: HarperCollins Publishers. 1995.

Huntsman, Stan. "The Distance Training of Doug Brown." *Track and Field Quarterly Review*. 1973, pages 178-179.

Hurley, B.F., and P.M. Nemeth, W.H. Martin II, J.M. Hagberg, G.P. Dalsky, J.O. Holloszy. "Muscle Triglyceride Utilization During Exercise: Effect of Training." *Journal of Applied Physiology*, Volume 60, Number 2, 1986, pages 562-567.

Hyams, Joe. *Zen in the Martial Arts*. Los Angeles, California: J. P. Tarcher, Inc. 1979.

I Ching or Book of Changes. English translation by Cary F. Bynes from the German translation of Richard Wilhelm. Forward by C. G. Jung. Princeton, New Jersey: Princeton University Press. 1950.

Ivers, Tom. *The Fit Racehorse II*. Grand Prairie, Texas: Equine Research, Inc. 1994.

Jacob, Stanley W., and Clarice A. Francone. *Structure and Function in Man*. 3rd Edition, Philadelphia, Pennsylvania: W.B. Saunders Company. 1974.

James, Clifford. "Footprints and Feet of Natives of the Solomon Islands." *The Lancet*. December 30, 1939, pages 1390-1393.

James, S.L., and B.T. Bates, L.R. Osterning. "Injuries to Runners." *American Journal of Sports Medicine*. Volume 6, 1978, pages 40-50.

Janssen, Peter G.J.M. *Training Lactate Pulse-Rate*. 4th Edition. Oulu, Finland: Polar Electro Oy. 1987.

Jarver, Jess. Editor. *Middle Distances*. Los Altos, California: Tafnews Press. 1979.

Jarver, Jess. Editor. *Long Distances*. Los Altos, California: Tafnews Press. 1980.

Jarver, Jess. Editor. *The Hurdles: Contemporary Theory, Technique and Training*. Los Altos, California: TAFnews Press. 1981.

Jensen, C., et al. "Prospective Study of Hormonal and Semen Profiles in Marathon Runners." *Fertility and Sterility*. Volume 64, Number 6, December, 1995, pages 1189-1196.

Jordan, Tom. *Pre!*. Los Altos, California: Tafnews Press. 1977.

Jorgensen, U., and J. Ekstrand. "Significance of Heel Pad Confinement for the Shock Absorption at Heel Strike." *International Journal of Sports Medicine*. Volume 9, 1988, pages 468-473.

Jung, Carl. *The Collected Works of C. G. Jung*. Edited by Sir Herbert Read, et. al., 17 Volumes. Princeton New Jersey: Bollingen Foundation, Inc., Princeton University Press. 1966.

Jung, Carl. Editor. *Man and His Symbols*. New York: A Windfall Book / Doubleday & Company Inc. 1964.

Kammer, Reinhard. *The Way of the Sword. The Tengu-Geijutsu-Ron of Chozan Shissai*. Edited and with Introduction by Reinhard Kammer. Translated by Betty Fitzgerald. London: Arkana. 1986.

Kerdok, A., and A. Biewnere, T. McMahon, P. Weyand, H. Herr, Energetics and Mechanics of Human Running on Surfaces of Different Stiffness." *Journal of Applied Physiology*. Volume 92, 2001, pages 469-478.

Kerr, B.A., and L. Beauchamp, V. Fisher, R. Neil. "Footstrike Patterns in Distance Running." *Biomechanical Aspects of Sport Shoes and Playing Surfaces*. B. M. Nigg and B. A. Kerr, Editors. Calgary, Alberta: University of Calgary, 1983, pages 135-142.

Kersey, David. *Please Understand Me*. Del Mar, California: Prometheus Nemesis Books. 1978.

Kilgore, Bruce, et. al. U.S. Patent 5,046,267, *Athletic Shoe with Pronation Control Device*. 1991.

Kim, Hee-Jin. *Dōgen Kigen: Mystical Realist*. Tucson, Arizona: University of Arizona Press. 1987.

King, Winston. *Zen and the Way of the Sword*. New York: Oxford University Press. 1993.

Koch, Damien. *Conversation on Altitude Training and Racing at Sea Level*. Fort Collins, Colorado. 1999.

Koppel, Naomi. "IOC Approves EPO Tests For Sydney." *Associated Press*. August 1, 2000.

Kožík, František, *Zápotek the Marathon Victor*, Prague, Czechoslovakia: Artia, 1954.

Kraemer, William, and Steven J. Fleck. "Anaerobic Metabolism and Its Evaluation." *NSCA Journal*. April-May, 1982.

Kressler, Raymond. "Rider College Steeplechase Clinic." *Track and Field Quarterly Review*. Volume 71, Number 1, 1971, pages 35-38.

Kuoppasalmi, K., and H. Naveri, M. Harkonen, H. Adlercreutz. "Plasma Cortisol, Androstenedione, Testosterone and Luteinizing Hormone in Running Exercise of Different Intensities." *Scandinavian Journal of Clinical Laboratory Investigation*. Volume 40, Number 5, September, 1980, pages 403-409.

Kyle, Chester R. "Athletic Clothing." *Scientific American*. Volume 254, 1986, page 106.

Kyle, Chester R. *Conversations on Aerodynamic Drag*. Weed, California: 1989, and 1997.

Kyle, Chester R. "Reduction of Wind Resistance and Power Output of Racing Cyclists and Runners Travelling in Groups." *Ergonomics*. Volume 22, Number 4, 1979, page 387.

Kyle, Chester R., and Vincent J. Caiozzo. "The Effect of Athletic Clothing Aerodynamics Upon Running Speed." *Medicine and Science in Sports and Exercise*. Volume 18, Number 5, 1986, page 511.

Kyle, Chester R., and R. Walpert. "The Aerodynamic Drag of the Human Figure in Athletics." *Unpublished Report to the U.S. Olympic Committee*. Sports Science Division, Colorado Springs, Colorado.

LePak, Roy C. *A Theology of Christian Mystical Experience*. Washington D.C.: University Press of America. 1977.

Levine, B.D., and J. Stray-Gundersen, G. Duhaime, P.G. Schnell, D.B. Friedman. "Living High-Training Low: The Effect of Altitude Acclimatization/Normoxic Training in Trained Runners." *Medicine and Science in Sports and Exercise*. Volume 23, Supplement S25, 1991.

Liao, Waysun. *T'ai Chi Classics*. Boston: Shambhala. 1990.

Liddell-Hart, B. H. *Strategy*. New York: Frederick A. Praeger Publishers. 1967.

Lindeman, Ralph. "400 Meter Hurdle Theory." *Track and Field Coaches Review*. Volume 95, Number 1, 1995, pages 33-36.

Linnarsson, D. "Dynamics of Pulmonary Gas Exchange And Heart Rate Changes At Start And End Of Exercise." *Acta Phsysiologica Scandinivica*. Supplement 415, 1974, pages 1-68.

Liquori, Marty, and John L. Parker. *Marty Liquori's Guide for the Elite Runner*. Chicago, Illinois: Playboy Press Book. 1980.

Loehr, James. *Mental Toughness Training for Sports*. Lexington, Massachusetts: Stephen Greene Press. 1982.

Lyden, Robert. *Aerodynamic Apparel: Background for U.S. Patent Application, and/or Trademark Protection*. publicly disclosed, 1989.

Lyden, Robert. European Patent Application EP 0752216 A3, *Footwear with Differential Cushioning Regions*. published, 1997.

Lyden, Robert. *Ninety-Nine Questions: A Dialogue on the Nature of Just War with Francisco(s) De Vitoria and Suarez*. Plan B Paper, Hubert H. Humphrey Institute of Public Affairs. 1986.

Lyden, Robert. U.S. Patent D461,622, *Men's Underwear / Inner Liner for Athletic Shorts*. 2002.

Lyden, Robert. U.S. Patent D461,943, *Athletic Pants*. 2002.

Lyden, Robert. U.S. Patent D463,091, *Women's Underwear / Inner Liner for Athletic Shorts*. 2002.

Lyden, Robert. U.S. Patent D463,652, *Non-Stretch Front Waistband Portion for Wearing Apparel*. 2002.

Lyden, Robert. U.S. Patent D466,676, *Athletic Pants with Zippers*. 2002.

Lyden, Robert. U.S. Patent D467,055, *Athletic Shorts*. 2002.

Lyden, Robert. U.S. Patent D473,694, *Athletic Pants with Back Pocket*. 2003.

Lyden, Robert. U.S. Patent 4,674,206, *Midsole Construction / Shoe Insert*. 1987.

Lyden, Robert. U.S. Patent 5,101,580, *Personalized Footbed, Last, and Ankle Support*. 1991.

Lyden, Robert. U.S. Patent 5,203,793, *Conformable Cushioning and Stability Device for Articles of Footwear*. 1993.

Lyden, Robert. U.S. Patent 5,384,973, *Sole with Articulating Forefoot*. 1995.

Lyden, Robert. U.S. Patent 5,632,057, *Method of Making Light Cure Component for Articles of Footwear*. 1997.

Lyden, Robert. U.S. Patent 5,921,004, *Footwear with Stabilizers*. 1999.

Lyden, Robert. U.S. Patent 6,082,462, *Horseshoe Imparting Natural Conformance and Function Providing Adjustable Shape and Attenuation of Shock and Vibration*. 2001.

Lyden, Robert. U.S. Patent 6,243,879, *Anatomical and Shock Absorbing Athletic Pants*. 2001.

Lyden, Robert. U.S. Patent 6,243,880, *Athletic Shorts*. 2001.

Lyden, Robert. U.S. Patent 6,353,940, *Underwear*. 2002.

Lyden, Robert. U.S. Patent 6,449,878, *Article of Footwear Having Spring Element and Selectively Removable Components*. 2002.

Lyden, Robert. U.S. Patent 6,490,730, *Shin-Guard, Helmet, and Articles of Protective Equipment Including Light Cure Material*. 2002.

Lyden, Robert. U.S. Patent 6,523,835. *Blade for an Ice Skate*. 2003.

Lyden, Robert. U.S. Patent 6,601,042. *Customized Article of Footwear and Method of Conducting Retail and Internet Business*. 2003.

Lyden, Robert, and Mike Aveni. U.S. Patent 5,595,004, *Shoe Sole Including a Peripherally Disposed Cushioning Bladder*. 1997.

Lyden, Robert, and Mike Aveni. U.S. Patent 5,987,780, *Shoe Sole Including a Peripherally Disposed Cushioning Bladder*. 1999.

Lyden, Robert, and Souheng Wu, U.S. Patent 5,832,636, *Article of Footwear Having Non-Clogging Sole*. 1998.

Lyden, Robert, et. al. U.S. Patent 5,425,184, *Athletic Shoe with Rearfoot Strike Zone*. 1995.

Lyden, Robert, et. al. U.S. Patent 5,625,964, *Athletic Shoe with Rearfoot Strike Zone*. 1997.

Lyden, Robert, et. al. U.S. Patent 5,709,954, *Chemical Bonding of Rubber to Plastic in Articles of Footwear*. 1998.

Lyden, Robert, et. al. U.S. Patent 5,786,057, *Chemical Bonding of Rubber to Plastic in Articles of Footwear*. 1998.

Lyden, Robert, et. al. U.S. Patent 5,843,268, *Chemical Bonding of Rubber to Plastic in Articles of Footwear*. 1998.

Lyden, Robert, et. al. U.S. Patent 5,906,872, *Chemical Bonding of Rubber to Plastic in Articles of Footwear*. 1999.

Lyden, Robert, et. al. U.S. Patent 6,055,746, *Athletic Shoe with Rearfoot Strike Zone.* 2001.

Lydiard, Arthur. *Arthur Lydiard's Running Training Schedules.* 2nd Edition. Los Altos, California: Tafnews Press. 1970.

Lydiard, Arthur. *Distance Training For Masters.* Aachen: Meyer & Meyer Fachverlag und Buchhandel GmbH. 2000.

Lydiard, Arthur. *Distance Training For Women Athletes.* Aachen: Meyer & Meyer Fachverlag und Buchhandel GmbH. 1999.

Lydiard, Arthur. *Distance Training For Young Athletes.* Aachen: Meyer & Meyer Fachverlag und Buchhandel GmbH. 1999.

Lydiard, Arthur. *Running to the Top.* Aachen: Meyer & Meyer Fachverlag und Buchhandel GmbH. 1997.

Lydiard, Arthur. *Running With Lydiard.* Aachen: Meyer & Meyer Fachverlag und Buchhandel GmbH. 2000.

Lydiard, Arthur, and Garth Gilmour. *Run to the Top.* Auckland, New Zealand: Minerva, Ltd. 1962.

Lydiard, Arthur, and Garth Gilmour. *Running the Lydiard Way.* Mountain View, California: World Publications, Inc. 1978.

Lynch, Jerry. *The Total Runner.* New Jersey: PrenticeHall, Inc. 1987.

MacFarland, E. "How Olympic Records Depend on Location," *American Journal of Applied Physiology,* Volume 54, 1986, pages 513-519.

MacLellan, Gordon. "Skeletal Heel Strike Transcients, Measurement, Implications and Modifications." *Sport Shoes and Playing Surfaces.* E.C. Frederick, Editor. Champaign, Illinois: Human Kinetics, 1984, pages 76-86.

Mader, Milan. *Conversation with Milan Mader, former Czech National Team Member and 10,000 meters Finalist, 1964 Olympic Games.* Minneapolis, Minnesota. 1979.

Maier, Hanns. "Seko." *Runner's World.* June, 1981.

Maile, Florence, and Michael Selzer. *The Nuremberg Mind.* Introduction and Rorschach records by G. M. Gilbert, New York: Quadrangle Books / New York Times Book Company. 1975.

Maktoum, H.H. Sheikh Mohammed Bin Rashid Al. *Quotation from his Webpage.* http://www.sheikhmohammed.co.ae. 2000.

Malley, George. *Conversation on the Steeplechase.* Oregon. 1999.

Man-ch'ing, Cheng, and Robert W. Smith. *T'ai-Chi, The "Supreme Ultimate" Exercise for Health, Sport, and Self-Defense.* Rutland, Vermont: Charles E. Tuttle Co. 1994.

Marcinik, E.J., and G. Potts, S. Schlaback, P. Will, P. Dawson, B.F. Hurley, "Effects of Strength Training on Lactate Threshold and Endurance Performance." *Medical Science in Sports and Exercise.* Volume 23, 1991, pages 739-743.

Martin, David E. "The Challenge of Using Altitude to Improve Performance." *NSA by the IAAF.* Volume 9, Number 2, 1994, pages 51-57.

Martin, David E., and Peter Coe. *Better Training for Distance Runners.* Champaign, Illinois: Human Kinetics. 1997.

Martin, David E., and Donald F. May, Susan P. Pilbeam. "Ventilation Limitations to Performance Among Elite Male Distance Runners." *Sport and Elite Performers.* Daniel M. Landers, Editor. Champaign, Illinois: Human Kinetics, 1986, pages 121-131.

Martin, David T., and M. Ashenden, R. Parisotto, D. Pyne, A. Hahn. "Blood Testing for Professional Cyclists: What's a Fair Hematocrit Level?" *Sportsmedicine News.* March-April, 1997. http://www.sportsci.org/news/news9703/AISblood.html.

Maslow, A. H. "Cognition of Being in Peak Experiences." *Journal of Genetic Psychology.* Number 94, 1959, pages 43-66.

Maslow, A. H. "A Holistic Approach to Creativity." *Climate for Creativity*. C.W. Taylor, Editor. New York: Pergamon Press. 1972.

Maslow, A. H. *Motivation and Personality*. New York: Harper & Brothers. 1954.

Masters, Roy. "The Secrets Herb Believes Can Make You Run A Little Faster." *The Sydney Morning Herald*. June 25, 1999.

Matesic, Brian C., and Fred Cromartie. "Effects Music Has on Lap Pace, Heart Rate, and Perceived Exertion Rate During a 20-Minute Self-Paced Run." *The Sport Journal*. Daphne, Alabama: The United States Sport Academy. February, 2002. http://www.thesportjournal.org/2002Journal/Vol5-No1/music.htm

Matveyev, L. *Fundamentals of Sports Training*. Moscow: Progress Publishers. 1981.

McAtee, Robert E., and Jeff Charland. *Facilitated Stretching*. Champaign, Illinois: Human Kinetics Publishers. 1993.

McCraken, Grant. *Culture and Consumption: New Approaches to the Symbolic Character*. Indiana: Indiana University Press. 1988.

McFarlane, Brent. "Pool Training... It Works!" *Proceedings of the International Track & Field Coaches Association, XIV Congress*. George Dales, Editor. Atlanta, Georgia, July 22-25, 1996, pages 196-198.

McFarlane, Brent. *The Science of Hurdling*. Ottawa, Ontario, Canada: The Canadian Track and Field Association. 1999.

McKenzie, John. "Physical Preparation for Middle Distance and Distance Running." North Texas University. Unpublished Manuscript.

McMahon, T.A. "Muscles, Reflexes, and Locomotion." Princeton, New Jersey: Princeton University Press. 1984.

McMahon, T.A. "Spring-Like Properties of Muscles and Reflexes in Running." *Multiple Muscle Systems: Biomechanics and Movement Organization*. J.M. Winters, and S.L-Y. Woo, Editors. Springer-Verlag, 1990, pages 578-590.

McMahon, T.A., and George Cheng. "The Mechanics of Running: How Does Stiffness Couple with Speed." *Journal of Biomechanics*. Volume 23, Supplement 1, 1990, pages 65-78.

McMahon, T.A., and P.R. Green. "The Influence of Track Compliance on Running." *Journal of Biomechanics*. Volume 12, 1979, pages 893-904.

Minard, D. "Prevention of Heat Casualties in Marine Corps Recruits." *Military Medicine*. Volume 126, 1961, pages 261-265.

Misevich, Kenneth. U.S. Patent 4,557,059, *Athletic Running Shoe*. 1985.

Montain, S.J., and M.K. Hopper, A.R. Coggan, E.F. Coyle, "Exercise Metabolism At Different Time Intervals After A Meal." *Journal of Applied Physiology*. Volume 70, Number 2, February, 1991, pages 882-888.

Moore, Kenny. *Best Efforts*. Florida: Cedarwinds Press. 1992.

Moore, Kenny. *Conversation on Athletic Training*. Kailua, Hawaii. 1999.

Moore, Kenny. "A Man of Two Worlds." *Sports Illustrated*. 1988.

Morris, A.F., et. al. "Energy Source Utilization." *Middle Distances*. Edited by Jess Jarver. Los Altos: Tafnews Press. 1979.

Murphy, Michael. *The Psychic Side of Sports*. New York: Addison Wesley. 1978.

Musashi, Miyamoto. *A Book of Five Rings*. Translated by Victor Harris. New York: Overlook Press. 1982.

NSCA Journal. "Roundtable: Cardiovascular Effects of Weight Training." April-May, 1987.

Nehemiah, Renaldo. "Mechanics of High Hurdles." *Track and Field Coaches Review*. Volume 95, Number 1, 1995, pages 39-41.

Nelson, Cordner. *The Jim Ryun Story*. Los Altos, California: Tafnews Press. 1971.

Nelson, Cordner. *Track & Field: The Great Ones*. London: Pelham Books, Ltd. 1970.

Newhouse, I.J., and D.B. Clement. "Iron Status in Athletes: An Update." *Sports Medicine*. Volume 5, 1988, pages 337-352.

Newsholme, E.A., and A.R. Leech. *Biochemistry for the Medical Sciences*. Chichester, England: John Wiley & Sons Ltd. 1983.

Newsholme, E.A, and A.R. Leech, Glenda Duester. *Keep On Running*. Chichester, England: John Wiley & Sons Ltd., 1994.

Nicol, C.W. *Moving Zen*. New York: William Morrow & Company, Inc. 1975.

Nielsen, Peter. "Tuned Shoes May Help Runners Break Olympic Records." *Reuters*. http://reuters.com, August 9, 2000.

Nigg, B. M. "Biomechanical Aspects of Running." *Biomechanics of Running Shoes*. B. M. Nigg, Editor. Champaign, Illinois: Human Kinetics Publishers, 1984, pages 1-26.

Nigg, B.M., and M. Morlock. "The Influence of Lateral Heel Flare of Running Shoes on Pronation and Impact Forces." *Medicine and Science in Sports and Exercise*. Volume 19, 1987, pages 294-302.

Noakes, Tim. *Lore of Running*. 3rd Edition. Champaign, Illinois: Human Kinetics. 1991.

Norkin, Cynthia C., and Pamela K. Levangie. *Joint Structure and Function*. 2nd Edition. Philadelphia, Pennsylvania: F.A. Davis Company. 1992.

Noronha, Francis. *Kipchoge of Kenya*. Elimu Publishers, 1970. Distributed in the United States by Tafnews Press: Los Altos, California.

Norton, Edward. U.S. Patent 4,288,929, *Motion Control Device for Athletic Shoe*. 1981.

O'Neil, Jim. "Leader of the Pack," (Lydiard). *The Runner*. October, 1982.

Ovett, Steve. *Ovett: An Autobiography*. Great Britain: Collins/Glasgow. 1984.

Paavolainen, L., and K. Hakkinen, I. Hamalainen, A. Nummela, H. Rusko, "Explosive-Strength Training Improves 5-km Running Time by Improving Running Economy and Muscle Power." *Journal of Applied Physiology*. Volume 98, Issue 5, May, 1999, pages 1527-1533.

Pandolf, K.B., and R. L. Burse, R. F. Goldman. "Role of Physical Fitness in Heat Acclimatization, Decay and Reinduction." *Ergonomics*, Volume 20, 1977, pages 399-408.

Parker, John. *The Frank Shorter Story*. Mountain View, California: Runner's World Magazine. 1972.

Parker, John. *Once a Runner*. Florida: Cedarwinds Publishing Company. 1978.

Parker, Mark, et al. U.S. Patent 4,817,304, *Footwear with Adjustable Viseolastic Unit*. 1989.

Parracho, Rui, et al. U.S. Patent 4,731,939, *Athletic Shoe with External Counter and Cushion Assembly*. 1988.

Paske, et al. U.S. Patent D370,116. *Peripheral Bladder for a Shoe Sole*. 1996.

Paske, et al. U.S. Patent D374,341. *Element for a Shoe Sole*. 1996.

Patton, George S. *The Patton Papers*. Martin Blumenson, Editor. 2 Volumes. Boston, Massachusetts: Houghton Mifflin Company. 1972.

Pavlov, Ivan P. *Conditioned Reflexes: An Investigation of the Physiological*. New York: Dover Publications Inc. 1927.

Pedemonte, Jimmy. "Updated Acquisitions About Training Periodization." *NSCA Journal*. October - November, 1982.

Pengelly, Scott. *Conversations on Arousal Addiction in Athletes*. Eugene, Oregon. 1988-1997.

Peters, Keith. "Conversation with Steve Scott and Herb Elliott." *Running*. May-June, 1981.

Peterson, Kirtland. *Mind of the Ninja*. New York: Contemporary Books, Inc. 1986.

Piaget, Jean. *The Child's Conception of Time*. Translated by A. P. Pomerans. New York: Basic Books. 1970.

Piaget, Jean. *The Construction of Reality in the Child*. Translated by Margaret Cook. New York: Basic Books. 1954.

Piaget, Jean. *The Mechanism of Perception*. Translated by G. N. Seagrim. New York: Basic Books. 1969.

Piaget, Jean. *Understanding Causality*. Translated by Donald and Margaret Miles. New York: Norton. 1974.

Piaget, Jean, and Barbel Inhelder. *The Child's Conception of Space*. Translated by F.L. Landon & J. L. Lunger. London: Routledge and K. Paul. 1956.

Piaget, Jean, and Barbel Inhelder. *The Psychology of the Child*. Translated by Helen Weaver. New York: Basic Books. 1969.

Pirie, Gordon. *Running Wild*. London: W. H. Allen & Co., Ltd. 1961.

Pirsig, Robert. *Zen and the Art of Motorcycle Maintenance*. New York: Bantam New Age Book. 1988.

Piwonka, R.W., and S. Robinson, V. L. Gay, R. S. Manalis. "Preacclimatization of Men to Heat by Training." *Journal of Applied Physiology*. Volume 20, 1965, pages 379-384.

Podell, Richard N., and William Proctor. *The G-Index Diet*. New York: Warner Books, Inc. 1993.

Popov, Ilia. "The Pros and Cons of Altitude Training." Published by the IAAF, Volume 9, Number 2, 1994, pages 15-21.

Popov, T. "3000 meter Steeplechase Hurdle Clearance," *Track and Field Quarterly Review*. Volume 79, Number 3, 1979, page 60.

Posterino, G.S., and T.L. Dutka, G.D. Lamb. "L (+)- lactate does not affect twitch and tetanic responses in mechanically skinned mammalian muscle fibers" *Pflugers Archiv: European Journal of Physiology*. Volume 442, Number 2, May, 2001, pages 197-203.

Pruett, E.D.R. "FFA Mobilization During And After Prolonged Severe Muscular Work In Men." *Journal of Applied Physiology*. Volume 29, Number 6, 1970, pages 809-815.

Pugh, L.G.C.E. "Air Resistance in Sport." *Advances in Exercise Physiology*. E. Jokl, Editor. Basel, Switzerland: Karger. 1976.

Pugh, L.G.C.E. "The Influence Of Wind Resistance In Running And Walking And The Mechanical Efficiency of Work Against Horizontal Or Vertical Forces." *Journal of Physiology*. Volume 213, 1971, page 255.

Pugh, L.G.C.E. "Oxygen Intake in Track and Treadmill Running with Observations on the Effect of Air Resistance." *Journal of Physiology*. Volume 207, 1970, pages 823-835.

Raevuori, Antero, and Rolf Haikkola. *Lasse Viren-Olympic Champion*. Portland, Oregon: Continental Publishing House. 1978.

Reindell, Herbert, and Helmut Roskamm, Woldemar Gerschler. *Das Interval-Training*. Munich: Barth Publishers. 1962.

Rice, Stephen G. "The High School Athlete: Setting Up a High School Sportsmedicine Program." in *The Team Physician's Handbook*. M.B. Mellion, and W.M. Walsh, G.L. Shelton, Editors. Philadelphia: Hanley & Belfus. 1997.

Rice, Stephen G. "Update and Reflections on the Athletic Health Care System High School Injury Surveillance Study." *American Medical Athletic Association Quarterly*. Volume 1, Number 3, Summer, 1997.

Riley, Pat. *The Winner Within*. New York: G.P. Putnam's Sons. 1993.

Robbins, Steven E., and Gerard J. Gouw, "Athletic Footwear and Chronic Overloading." *Sports Medicine*. Volume 9, Number 2, 1990, pages 76-85.

Rogers, Bill, and Joe Concannon. *Updated Marathoning*. New York: A Fireside Book / Simon & Schuster. 1982.

Rosen, Mel, and Karen Rosen. *Sports Illustrated Track: The Running Events.* New York: Harper & Row Publishers. 1986.

Ross, Wilber L. *The Hurdler's Bible.* 2nd Edition. Arlington, Virginia: Yates Printing Company. 1969.

Sahlin, K. "Metabolic Changes Limiting Muscle Performance." *Biochemistry of Exercise VI.* Saltin, B., Editor. Champaign, Illinois: Human Kinetics. 1986.

Saltin, B., and J. Stenberg. "Circulatory Responses to Prolonged Severe Exercise." *Journal of Applied Physiology.* Volume 19, 1964, pages 833-838.

Saunders, Tony. "Steeplechase Technique and Training." *Track Technique.* Number 35, March 1969, pages 1102-1103.

Schmidt, R.A. *Motor Control and Learning: A Behavioral Emphasis.* 2nd Edition. Champaign, Illinois: Human Kinetics. 1988.

Schmidt, R.A. "Motor Learning Principles for Physical Therapy." *II Step Contemporary Management of Motor Control Problems.* M.J. Lister, Editor. Alexandria, Virginia: Foundation for Physical Therapy, Inc. 1991, pages 49-63.

Schmolinsky, Gerhardt. Editor. *Track and Field.* Berlin: Sportverlag. 1978.

Schneider, Howard. "Steve Ovett." *Runner's World.* August, 1979.

Seiler, Stephen. "Tighter Control on EPO Use by Skiers." *Sportsmedicine News.* January-February, 1997. http://www.sportsci.org/news/news9701/EPOfeat.html.

Sell, Jr., et al. U.S. Patent D347,106. *Bladder Element for a Shoe Sole.* 1994.

Sell, Jr., et al. U.S. Patent D347,315. *Bladder for a Shoe Sole.* 1994.

Sevene, Bob. *Conversation On Distance Running.* Eugene, Oregon. 1985.

Seydel, R., and S. Luthi, R. Fumi, K. Beard, O. Kaiser, U.S. Patent 6,266,897, *Ground Contacting Systems Having 3-D Deformation Elements for Use in Footwear.* 2001.

Shakespeare, William. *Richard III: The Bantam Shakespeare.* David Bevington et. al., Editors. Forward by Joseph Papp. New York: Bantam. 1988.

Shanebrook, J.R., and R.D. Jaszczak. "Aerodynamic Drag Analysis of Runners." *Medicine and Science in Sports.* Volume 8, Number 1, 1976, pages, 43-45.

Shapiro, Y., and A. Magazanik, R. Vdassin, G.M. Ben-Baruch, E. Shvartz, Y. Shoenfeld. "Heat Intolerance in Former Heatstroke Patients." *Annals of Internal Medicine.* Volume 90, Number 6, 1979, pages 913-96.

Shim, Sang Kyu. *The Making of a Martial Artist.* 1st Edition. Published Privately in the United States. 1980.

Shorten, Martyn. "The Energetics of Running and Running Shoes." *Journal of Biomechanics.* Volume 26, Supplement 1, 1993, pages 41-51.

Shorten, Martyn. U.S. Patent 5,197,206, *Shoe, Especially a Sport or Rehabilitation Shoe.* 1993.

Shorten, Martyn. U.S. Patent 5,197,207, *Shoe, Especially a Sport or Rehabilitation Shoe.* 1993.

Shorten, Martyn. U.S. Patent 5,201,125, *Shoe, Especially a Sport or Rehabilitation Shoe.* 1993.

Shorten, Martyn, and G.A. Valiant, L.B. Cooper. "Frequency Analysis of the Effects of Shoe Cushioning on Dynamic Shock in Running." *Medicine and Science in Sports and Exercise.* Volume 18, Supplement. 1986, pages 80-81.

Shorten, Martyn, and Darcy S. Winslow. "Spectral Analysis of Impact Shock During Running." *International Journal of Sport Biomechanics.* Volume 8, Number 4, November, 1992, pages 288-304.

Shorten, Martyn, and S.A. Wootton, C. Williams. "Mechanical Energy Changes and the Oxygen Cost of Running." *Engineering in Medicine*. Volume 10, Number 4, 1981, pages 213-217.

Shorter, Frank. *Conversation on Athletic Training*. Boulder, Colorado. 1999.

Sim-Fook, Lam, and A. Hodgson. "A Comparison of Foot Forms Among the Non-Shoe and Shoe-Wearing Chinese Population." *The Journal of Bone and Joint Surgery*. Volume 40-A, Number 1, January 1958, pages 1058-1062.

Sims, Graem, *Why Die? The Extraordinary Percy Cerutty, Maker of Champions*. Melbourne, Australia: Lothian Books. 2003.

Sleamaker, R.H. *Serious Training For Serious Athletes: Comprehensive Training Plans For Endurance Sports*. Champaign, Illinois: Human Kinetics. 1989.

Snell, Peter, and Garth Gilmour. *No Bugles, No Drums*. Auckland, New Zealand: Minerva, Ltd. 1965.

Sparks, Ken, and Garry Bjorklund. *Long Distance Runner's Guide to Training and Racing*. New Jersey: Prentice/Hall, Inc. 1984.

Spear, Michael. "Emil Zatopek gives Modern Day Runners the Truth Behind the Myth." *Runners World Annual*. 1982.

Spence, Gerry. *How to Argue and Win Every Time*. New York, St. Martin's Press. 1995.

Squires, Bill with Raymond Krise. *Improving Your Running*. Lexington, Massachusetts: Stephen Greene Press. 1982.

Stacoff, A., and J. Denoth, X. Kaelin, E. Stuessi. "Running Injuries and Shoe Construction: Some Possible Relationships." *International Journal of Sport Biomechanics*. Volume 4, 1988, pages 342-357.

Stacoff, A., and X. Kaelin. "Pronation and Sportshoe Design." *Biomechanical Aspect of Sport Shoes and Playing Surfaces*. B. M. Nigg and B.A. Kerr, Editors. Calgary, Alberta: University of Calgary, 1983, pages 143-151.

Staheli, Lynn. "Shoes for Children: A Review." *Pediatrics*. Volume 88, Number 2, August, 1991.

Stampfl, Franz. *Franz Stampfl on Running*. London: Herbert Jenkins Ltd. 1955.

Suslov, Felix. "Basic Principles of Training at High Altitude." Published by the IAAF. Volume 9, Number 2, 1994, pages 45-50.

Suzuki, Daisetz. *Zen and Japanese Culture*. Princeton, New Jersey: Bollingen Foundation, Inc., Princeton University Press. 1973.

Suzuki, Shunryu. *Zen Mind, Beginner's Mind*. New York / Tokyo: Weatherhill. 1970.

Swami Vishnu-devananda. *The Complete Illustrated Book of Yoga*. New York: Crown Trade Paperbacks. 1988.

Takuan Soho. *The Unfettered Mind*. Translated by William Scott Wilson. New York: Kodasha International USA Ltd. / Harper & Row. 1986.

Tames, Roger. Steve Cram: *The Making of An Athlete*. London: W. H. Allen. 1984.

Tanaka, H., and J. Cleroux, J. de Champlain, J.R. Ducharme, R. Collu. "Persistent Effects of a Marathon Run on the Pituitary-Testicular Axis." *Journal of Endocrinological Investigation*. Volume 9, Number 2, April, 1986, pages 97-101.

Thucydides. *The Peloponnesian War: The Landmark Thucydides*. Robert B. Strassler, Editor. Introduction by Victor Hanson. New York: Free Press. 1996.

Tohei, Koichi. *Ki In Everyday Life*. Tokyo, Japan: KI NO Kenkyakai, H.Q. 1981.

Torrence, E. P., and R. E. Myers, *Creative Learning and Teaching*. New York: Dodd, Mead. 1972.

Tschiene, Peter. "The Further Development of Training Theory." *Science Periodical on Research and Technology in Sport*. Volume 8, Number 4, 1988.

Tzu, Lao. *Tao Te Ching*. Translated by D.L. Lau. Middlesex, England: Penguin Books Ltd. 1963

Ueshiba, Kisshomaru. *The Spirit of Aikido*. Tokyo: Kodansha International. 1987.

Unold, E. "Erschuetterungsmessungen beim Gehen und Laufen auf verschiedenen Unterlagen mit verschiedenem Schuhwerk." *Jugend und Sport*. Volume 8, 1974, pages 280-292.

Urhausen, A., and H. Gabriel, W. Kindermann. "Blood Hormones as Markers of Training Stress and Overtraining." *Sports Medicine*. Volume 20, Number 4, October, 1995, pages 251-276.

Voss, Dorothy, and M.K. Ionta, B. Myers. *Proprioceptive Neuromuscular Facilitation*. 3rd Edition. Philadelphia, Pennsylvania: Harper & Row. 1985.

Waitz, Grete, and Gloria Averbuch. *World Class*. New York: Warner Books, Inc. 1986.

Walnum, Paul K., A.T.C. "Heat Illness and the Runner." *Track and Field Quarterly Review*. Volume 89, Number 2, 1989, pages 37-39.

Walsh, Chris. *The Bowerman System*. Los Altos, California: Tafnews Press 1983.

Ward-Smith, A.J. "Air Resistance And Its Influence On The Biomechanics And Energies Of Sprinting At Sea Level And At Altitude." *Biomechanics*. Volume 17, 1984, pages 339-347.

Warhurst, Ron. "Training for Distance Running and the Steeplechase." *Track and Field Quarterly Review*. Volume 85, Number 3, 1985, pages 13-14.

Watman, Mel. Editor. *The Coe and Ovett File*. Kent, England: Athletics Weekly. 1982.

Watts, Denis. "Hints on Steeplechasing." *Track Technique*. Number 41, September. 1970, pages 1306-1307.

Weiner, Melvin. *The Cognitive Unconscious: A Piagetian Approach to Psychotherapy*. Forward by Jean Piaget. Davis, California: International Psychology Press. 1975.

Weissbluth, Marc. *Healthy Sleep Habits, Happy Child*. New York: Fawcett Columbine / Ballantine Books. 1987.

Weissbluth, Marc. "Naps in Children: 6 Months-7 Years." *Sleep*. Volume 18, Number 2, 1995, pages 82-87.

Werner, Chick. "The Steeplechase." *Track in Theory and Technique*. Richmond, California: Worldwide Publishing Co. 1962.

Westmoreland, Barbara, et al. *Medical Neurosciences*. Third Edition. New York: Little, Brown and Company. 1994

Wiger, Chick. "The 3000 meter Steeplechase." *Track and Field Quarterly Review*. Volume 79, Number 3, 1979, pages 53-56.

Will, George. *Statecraft as Soulcraft*. New York: Touchstone Book/Simon & Schuster, Inc. 1983.

Williams, Melvin H., and Sid Wesseldine, Thomas Somma, Rudolf Schuster. "The Effect of Induced Erythrocythemia Upon 5-Mile Treadmill Run Time." *Medicine And Science In Sports And Exercise*. Volume 13, Number 3, 1981, pages 169-175.

Willman, Howard. "Steve Ovett." *Track & Field News*. Los Altos, California: Tafnews Press. November, 1985.

Will-Weber, Mark, Editor, *The Quotable Runner*, Halcottsville, New York: Breakaway Books, 2001.

Wilson, Harry. *Running Dialogue*. London: Stanley Paul. 1982.

Wilt, Fred. *Run, Run, Run*. Los Altos, California: Tafnews Press. 1964.

Wyndham, C.H., and N.B. Strydom. "The Danger of Inadequate Water Intake During Marathon Running." *South African Medical Journal*. Volume 43, 1969, pages 893-896.

Yakovlev, N.N. *Sports Biochemistry*. Leipzig, DHFK. 1967.

Yasuo, Yuasa. *The Body*. Thomas Kasulis, Editor. Translated by Nagatomo Shigenori and Thomas Kasulis. New York: State University of New York Press. 1987.

Yoshikawa, Eiji. *Musashi*. Translated by Charles S. Terry. New York: Harper & Row Publishers. 1981.

AFTERWORD

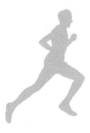

Athletics at the highest level is both a science and an art. The road to mastery is not a simple or easy one. Paradoxically, athletes must first master theory, method and technique so that they can ultimately be liberated from it. Musicians study and practice for many years so that, when inspired, they can put it all aside and play jazz. But in mastering any art, there is also need for emotional and experiential maturation from within—or what the blues musicians refer to as mileage. The challenge is no different for the aspiring coach or athlete. I wish you success and enlightenment along the way.

—Robert M. Lyden
Portland, Oregon 2003

PHOTO INDEX

Robert M. Lyden earned two M.A. degrees from the University of Minnesota, one in Modern European History, and another in Public Administration at the Hubert H. Humphrey Institute. He still writes on the subject of U.S. foreign policy. Lyden also received K-12 Teaching and Coaching Certification through St. Thomas College, St. Paul, Minnesota.

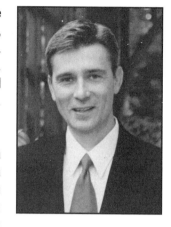

He has advised elite athletes, including Steve Plasencia (1988 and 1992 U.S. Olympic Teams), and Karl Keska (2000 British Olympic Team). Lyden served as an assistant collegiate coach, and was also associated with several high school state champions and title teams in the state of Minnesota. He has consulted to owners and trainers of Arabian and Thoroughbred racehorses, and written a training plan entitled "On Winning the Triple Crown."

Lyden was employed and later served as a consultant to Nike, Inc. An inventor and entrepreneur associated with over two-dozen patents, he creates innovative products for the sporting goods industry. He has also written several screenplays, including one based on the story of 1960 Olympic Champion Herb Elliott and his late coach Percy Cerutty. Lyden continues to write and lecture on both distance running and sports psychology.